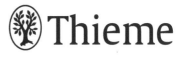

The Coordination of Clinical Research

A Handbook for Research Coordinators

Mohit Bhandari, MD, PhD, FRCSC
Professor
Department of Surgery
Canada Research Chair
Evidence-Based Orthopaedic Surgery
McMaster University
Hamilton, Canada

Esther M. M. Van Lieshout, MSc, PhD
Associate Professor
Research Coordinator
Trauma Research Unit
Department of Surgery
Erasmus MC
University Medical Center Rotterdam
Rotterdam, The Netherlands

35 illustrations

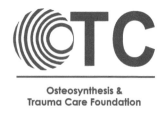

Osteosynthesis &
Trauma Care Foundation

Thieme
Stuttgart • New York • Delhi • Rio de Janeiro

Library of Congress Cataloging-in-Publication Data is available from the publisher

© 2020. Thieme. All rights reserved.

Georg Thieme Verlag
Rüdigerstrasse 14, 70469 Stuttgart, Germany
+49 [0]711 8931 421, customerservice@thieme.de

Thieme Publishers New York
333 Seventh Avenue, New York, NY 10001 USA
+1 800 782 3488, customerservice@thieme.com

Thieme Publishers Delhi
A-12, Second Floor, Sector-2, Noida-201301
Uttar Pradesh, India
+91 120 45 566 00, customerservice@thieme.in

Thieme Publishers Rio, Thieme Publicações Ltda.
Edifício Rodolpho de Paoli, 25º andar
Av. Nilo Peçanha, 50 - Sala 2508
Rio de Janeiro 20020-906 Brasil
+55 21 3172 2297 / +55 21 3172 1896

Cover design: Thieme Publishing Group
Typesetting by DiTech Process Solutions, India

Printed in Germany by CPI Books   5 4 3 2 1

ISBN 978-3-13-242229-2

Also available as an e-book:
eISBN 978-3-13-242230-8

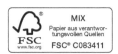

Contents

Preface   xv

Acknowledgments   xvi

Contributors   xvii

Part I   Getting Started   1
Esther M. M. Van Lieshout, Parag Sancheti

1   Leadership and Management: The Principal Investigator and Research Coordinator   2
Heather Dwyer

1.1	**Introduction**	2	**1.5**	**Communicating with Staff**	6
1.2	**Leadership Styles**	2	1.5.1	Communication Strategies	6
1.2.1	Autocratic Leaders	2	1.5.2	Communicating with	
1.2.2	Democratic Leaders	3		External Staff.	7
1.2.3	Laissez-Faire Leadership	3	1.5.3	Relationship/Team Building	7
1.3	**Building a Motivational Workplace**	3	**1.6**	**Organization**	8
			1.6.1	Documentation	8
1.3.1	Emotional Intelligence	3	1.6.2	Time Management.	8
1.3.2	Physical Environment.	4	**1.7**	**Management Competence**.	10
1.3.3	Mandates and Vision	4	1.7.1	Managing Up and Managing	
1.4	**Mentoring New Staff**.	4		Down	10
1.4.1	Orientation	4	1.7.2	Professional Development.	10
1.4.2	Mentoring.	5	**1.8**	**Conclusion**	11
1.4.3	Performance Reviews.	6			

2   Roles: Why a Research Coordinator Is Critical   12
Kelly Trask

2.1	**Introduction**	12	2.2.2	Data Management	17
2.1.1	Why a Research Coordinator is Necessary	12	2.2.3	Study Planning, Coordination, and Administration	18
2.1.2	Education and Certification	13	2.2.4	Further Tasks.	20
2.1.3	Delegation of Duties	14	**2.3**	**Practical Application**.	20
2.2	**Duties**	15	**2.4**	**Conclusion**	22
2.2.1	Study Participant Care	16			

3   Hiring: Characteristics of a Highly Qualified Research Coordinator   24
Milena R. Vicente

3.1	**Introduction**.	24	**3.2**	**Desirable Characteristics**	29
3.1.1	The Research Coordinator Role	24	3.2.1	Communication Skills	29
3.1.2	The Decision to Hire.	24	3.2.2	Team Building Skills	30
3.1.3	Hiring Process.	25	3.2.3	Interpersonal Skills.	30
3.1.4	The Interview	28	3.2.4	Positive Attitude.	31
3.1.5	Making a Decision	29	3.2.5	Professional Skills	31

v

Contents

3.2.6   Regulatory and Ethics Guidelines   32

3.2.7   Computer Skills and Project Management   33

3.2.8   Clinical Experience   34

3.2.9   Writing Skills   34

3.2.10   Financial or Grant Management   34

3.3   **The Newly Hired Research Coordinator**   35

3.4   **Conclusion**   35

4   Growth: From 0 to 100, Real Quick!   37
Nicole M. Harris, Darren M. Roffey

4.1   **Introduction**   37

4.2   **Protocol Development**   37

4.3   **Informed Consent Form**   39

4.4   **Communication**   39

4.5   **Enthusiasm**   40

4.6   **Training**   41

4.7   **Recruitment**   42

4.7.1   Identifying Eligible Patients   43

4.7.2   Who will approach the patient?   44

4.7.3   When will the patient be contacted?   44

4.7.4   Where will the patient be contacted? . . .   44

4.7.5   How will patient contact occur?   45

4.8   **Practical Application**   45

4.8.1   Designing a Recruitment Plan   45

4.9   **Conclusion**   46

Part II   What Every Research Coordinator Needs To Know   49
Ernesto Guerra Farfán, Dinesh Kumbhare, Anthony Adili

5   What Is Evidence-Based Medicine?   50
Ellie B. M. Landman

5.1   **Introduction**   50

5.2   **The History of Evidence-Based Medicine**   50

5.3   **Principles of Evidence-Based Medicine**   51

5.3.1   Best Available Evidence   51

5.3.2   Evaluate Available Evidence   52

5.3.3   Application of Evidence in the Care for Individual Patients   53

5.4   **Where Do We Stand in Evidence-Based Medicine Today?**   54

5.4.1   Criticism of Evidence-Based Medicine   54

5.4.2   Clinical Research   55

5.5   **Practical Application**   55

5.5.1   Clinical Example   55

5.6   **Conclusion**   56

6   Randomized Controlled Trials   58
Miriam Garrido Clua

6.1   **Introduction**   58

6.2   **What Is a Randomized Controlled Trial?**   58

6.2.1   Study Population   59

6.2.2   Randomized Controlled Trial Study Design   59

6.2.3   Random Assignment (Randomization)   60

6.2.4   Blinding   61

6.3   **Outcome Measurement**   62

6.3.1   Reliability and Validity of Outcomes Measures   62

6.4   **Quality Control and Data Collection**   62

6.5   **Recruitment of Study Participants**   63

6.5.1   Tips for Coordinators   63

6.6   **Participant Adherence**   64

6.7   **Assessing and Reporting Adverse Events (AEs)**   64

6.7.1   Monitoring a Randomized Controlled Trial   65

6.8   **Ethical Considerations**   65

6.9   **Practical Application**   66

6.10   **Conclusion**   66

7   Observational Studies.. 68
Pieta Krijnen

7.1   **Introduction**.................. 68
7.2   **Types of Observational Studies** .. 68
7.2.1   Cohort Studies 68
7.2.2   Case–Control Studies.............. 68
7.2.3   Case Series 69
7.3   **Pros and Cons of Observational Studies** 69
7.4   **Types of Bias Associated with Observational Studies**.......... 69
7.5   **Designing Observational Studies** .. 70
7.5.1   General Information................ 70
7.5.2   Define Research Questions Based on a Literature Review 70
7.5.3   Choose the Study Design........... 71
7.5.4   Define the Study Population 72
7.5.5   Describe the Treatment and Procedures.................... 72
7.5.6   Describe the Study Parameters....... 73
7.5.7   Outcomes and Other Study Parameters 73
7.5.8   Study Procedure.................. 74
7.5.9   Statistical Analysis Plan 74
7.5.10   Ethical Considerations/Data Handling 74

7.6   **Performing the Study** 75
7.6.1   Initiation Phase.................... 75
7.6.2   Data Collection.................... 75
7.6.3   Patient Inclusion in Prospective Studies........................ 76
7.6.4   Keep the Staff Informed and Committed during the Study 76
7.7   **Data Analysis** 76
7.7.1   Dealing with Confounding.......... 76
7.7.2   Handling Missing Outcome Data 77
7.8   **Reporting** 77
7.9   **Practical Application** 78
7.9.1   Background....................... 79
7.9.2   Study Objective 79
7.9.3   Study Design..................... 79
7.9.4   Patients 79
7.9.5   Treatment 79
7.9.6   Study Outcomes and Other Parameters 79
7.9.7   Sample Size...................... 79
7.9.8   Statistical Analysis 80
7.9.9   Ethical Considerations 80
7.10   **Conclusion** 80

8   Surveys 81
Miriam Garrido Clua

8.1   **Introduction**.................. 81
8.1.1   What Is a Survey Study?............. 81
8.2   **Research Methods** 82
8.2.1   Questionnaires 82
8.2.2   Face-to-Face Interviews 83
8.2.3   Telephone Interviews.............. 83
8.3   **Selecting the Survey Method**.... 84
8.3.1   Population....................... 84
8.3.2   Research Question 84
8.3.3   Content of the Study 85
8.3.4   Bias Issues 85
8.3.5   Resources 85
8.4   **Sample and Sampling** 85
8.4.1   Random Sampling 86
8.4.2   Nonrandom Sampling 86

8.5   **Research Tool Design** 86
8.5.1   Types of Questions................. 86
8.5.2   Questionnaire Layout.............. 87
8.5.3   Question Wording 88
8.5.4   Question Order.................... 88
8.6   **Training the Interviewers** 88
8.7   **Pilot Testing** 89
8.8   **Translation** 89
8.9   **Reliability and Validity** 90
8.10   **Analysis of Survey Data** 90
8.11   **Ethics of Survey Research**....... 90
8.12   **Practical Application** 91
8.13   **Conclusion** 92

Contents

9   **Qualitative Studies** 94
Patricia Schneider

9.1   **Objectives** 94

9.2   **Introduction** 94

9.2.1   Why Qualitative Research? 94

9.2.2   What is Qualitative Research? 94

9.2.3   Qualitative versus Quantitative Research 94

9.2.4   Advantages of Qualitative Research 94

9.3   **Designing and Conducting the Study** 95

9.3.1   General Study Details 95

9.3.2   Research Question 95

9.3.3   Research Objectives 95

9.4   **Study Methods** 95

9.4.1   Ethnography 95

9.4.2   Grounded Theory 95

9.4.3   Phenomenology 95

9.5   **Sampling** 95

9.5.1   Purposive Sampling 96

9.5.2   Quota Sampling 96

9.5.3   Chain-Referral (Snowball) Sampling 96

9.6   **Sample Size** 96

9.7   **Qualitative Data Collection** 97

9.7.1   Observation 97

9.7.2   Interview 97

9.7.3   Focus Group 97

9.7.4   Discussion Guide/Interview Script Development 98

9.7.5   Interview/Focus Group Question Development 99

9.7.6   Collecting Initial Demographic Details 99

9.7.7   Obtaining Adequate Responses 99

9.7.8   Transcription of Interviews and Focus Groups 100

9.8   **Data Analysis and Interpretation** 100

9.8.1   Qualitative Data Analysis Approaches 100

9.8.2   Qualitative Data Coding 100

9.8.3   Data Management Software 101

9.9   **Reporting and Disseminating the Study** 101

9.9.1   Where to Publish? 102

9.9.2   Authorship 102

9.10   **Ethical Implications** 102

9.10.1   Informed Consent 102

9.10.2   Protecting Confidentiality 102

9.11   **Other Considerations** 102

9.11.1   Generalizability 102

9.11.2   Ambiguities 102

9.11.3   Frequency 103

9.12   **Types of Bias Associated with Qualitative Studies** 103

9.12.1   Strategies for Managing Bias 103

9.13   **Practical Application** 103

9.13.1   Background 103

9.13.2   Study Objective 104

9.13.3   Study Design 104

9.13.4   Participants 104

9.13.5   Discussion Guide 104

9.13.6   Sample Size 104

9.13.7   Ethical Considerations 104

9.13.8   Analysis 105

9.13.9   Reporting 105

9.14   **Conclusion** 105

9.15   **Appendix A: Collaborative Research Focus Group Discussion Guide** 107

9.15.1   Welcome, Introductions, and Informed Consent 107

9.15.2   Discussion Topics 107

10   **Principles of Good Clinical Practice and Research Conduct** 109
Naveen Khan

10.1   **Introduction** 109

10.2   **History of Good Clinical Practice** . 109

10.2.1   Revisiting a Drastically Different Era of Clinical Studies 109

10.3   **The History of GCP Guidelines** 110

10.4   **The ICH-GCP Guidelines** 111

10.4.1   Introduction and Major Principles 111

10.4.2   Roles and Responsibilities of Involved Parties 111

10.4.3   Essential Documents 113

10.4.4	Advantages of the ICH-GCP Guidelines............................	115
10.5	**Future Directions and Challenges**......................	115
10.5.1	Globalization and the Universal Adoption of GCP...................	115

10.5.2	Technological Advancements........	116
10.6	**Practical Application**.............	116
10.6.1	Good Clinical Practice Checklist for Clinical Research Coordinators.......	117
10.7	**Conclusion**......................	117

Part III From Idea to Study Start-Up....................................... 119
Rebecca Ivers, Jack Chun-Yiu Cheng

11   Principles of Grant Writing: Tips for a Successful Experience.................. 120
Milena R. Vicente, Sarah Desjardins

11.1	**Introduction**....................	120
11.2	**Getting Started**..................	120
11.2.1	Start early........................	120

11.3	**Conclusion**......................	128
11.4	**Practical Application**.............	128
11.4.1	Common issues That Result in Grant Rejection....................	129

12   Dollars and "Sense": A Guide to Research Finances......................... 130
Johanna Dobransky, Darren M. Roffey

12.1	**Introduction**....................	130
12.2	**Planning and Creating a Research Budget**................	130
12.2.1	Preplanning Phase.................	130
12.2.2	Funding Source....................	130
12.2.3	Centralized versus Decentralized Budgetary Management............	131
12.2.4	Financial Lifecycle.................	131
12.2.5	Planning the Budget...............	131
12.2.6	Key Expenses.....................	131
12.2.7	Direct and Indirect Costs...........	132
12.2.8	Negotiating the Study Budget........	132

12.2.9	Need for a Contingency Budget......	134
12.2.10	Pitfalls Associated with Budgetary Planning.........................	135
12.3	**Ongoing Monitoring of a Research Budget**................	135
12.3.1	Invoicing and Payments.............	135
12.3.2	Amending the Study Budget.........	136
12.4	**Study Termination**...............	136
12.4.1	Premature Study Termination........	136
12.5	**Practical Application**.............	136
12.6	**Conclusion**......................	138

13   Maintaining Records and the Trial Master File.............................. 143
Alisha Garibaldi

13.1	**Introduction**....................	143
13.1.1	What Is a Trial Master File?..........	143
13.1.2	Why All of the Documentation?......	149
13.1.3	Setting up a Trial Master File at a Participating Clinical Site...........	149
13.1.4	Setting up a Trial Master File at a Methods Center..................	151
13.1.5	Document Control and the Trial Master File.......................	152

13.1.6	When the Methods Center Is also a Participating Clinical Site...........	152
13.1.7	Do I Really Need a Binder?..........	152
13.1.8	Spotlight: The Clinical Site Manual....	152
13.1.9	Internal audits....................	153
13.1.10	Practical Application...............	153
13.2	**Conclusion**......................	154

14   Ethics Submissions.. 155
Bregje J. W. Thomassen, Michel Sourour, Kesh Reddy

14.1	**Introduction**....................	155
14.1.1	Research Ethics Committee..........	155
14.1.2	Research Ethics Committee Submission......................	157

14.1.3	Review Process....................	157
14.1.4	Multicenter Human Studies and International Studies...............	159
14.2	**Conclusion**......................	160

Contents

15   **The Basics of Research Contracts** 161
Caroline Woods

15.1   **Introduction** 161

15.2   **Different Types of the Agreements** 161

15.2.1   Grant Funding 161

15.2.2   Collaboration 161

15.2.3   Sites 162

15.2.4   Industry Involved in Investigator Initiated Study 162

15.2.5   Industry-Initiated Study Agreement 162

15.3   **The Parts of an Agreement** 162

15.3.1   The Parties 162

15.3.2   The Preamble 163

15.3.3   The Clauses 163

15.3.4   Signatories 165

15.4   **Practical Application** 165

15.4.1   Examples of Clauses 165

15.5   **Study Budget** 165

15.5.1   Overview 165

15.5.2   The Terms 166

15.6   **Intellectual Property** 166

15.6.1   Overview 166

15.6.2   The Terms 166

15.7   **Publication Clause** 167

15.7.1   Overview 167

15.7.2   The Terms 167

15.8   **Conclusion** 167

16   **How to Start-Up a Study** 169
Ellie B. M. Landman

16.1   **Introduction** 169

16.2   **Study Start-Up Phase** 169

16.2.1   Identify and Contact Sites 170

16.2.2   Feasibility 171

16.2.3   Clinical Trial Agreement Negotiation 171

16.2.4   Regulatory and Ethics Approval 172

16.2.5   Site Initiation Visit 172

16.2.6   Site Activation 173

16.3   **Challenges Encountered During Start-Up** 173

16.3.1   Protocol Adherence 173

16.3.2   Meeting Recruitment Goals 173

16.3.3   Delaying Factors 174

16.3.4   Guidelines for Good Clinical Practice 174

16.3.5   Drug, Device, or Procedure 174

16.4   **Practical Application** 174

16.5   **Keys to Success** 174

16.6   **Conclusion** 175

Part IV Study Execution and Close-Out 177
Aaron Nauth, Kim Madden, Paul Tornetta

17   **Screening and Recruiting Participants** 178
Nienke Wolterbeek

17.1   **Introduction** 178

17.2   **Recruitment, prescreening, and study screening** 178

17.3   **Barriers for Inclusion** 179

17.4   **Ethical Considerations** 179

17.5   **How to Improve Recruitment and Screening** 180

17.5.1   Target Population 180

17.5.2   Recruitment Plan and Contact Methods 180

17.5.3   Screening Mechanism 182

17.5.4   Study Design 182

17.6   **Practical Application** 182

17.6.1   Recruitment 184

17.6.2   Prescreening Phase 184

17.6.3   Screening Phase 185

17.7   **Conclusion** 185

18 Obtaining Informed Consent 187
Chandni Patel, Nazanin Barkhordari

18.1	Introduction: What Is Informed Consent? 187	18.7	Consent Is an Ongoing Process ... 190
18.2	The Informed Consent Process ... 187	18.8	Decision-Making Capacity 190
18.3	Voluntary Consent............... 188	18.9	Language Understandable to the Participant and the Legally Authorized Representative....... 190
18.4	Consent Should Be Informed..... 188		
18.5	Basic Elements of Informed Consent...................... 188	18.10	Practical Application............. 191
18.6	Participants Must Be Free to Withdraw 189	18.11	Conclusion 192

19 Collecting Data: Paper and Electronic Data Capture Systems 193
Esther M. M. Van Lieshout, Stephanie M. Zielinski

19.1	Introduction 193	19.7	Datasheets on Paper versus eCRF........................... 195
19.2	The Aim of Data Collection in a Clinical Study................... 193	19.8	Examples of Available EDCs 195
19.3	What Data Should Be Collected .. 193	19.9	Case Report Form Design Guidelines...................... 197
19.4	Source Data................... 194		
19.5	Multidisciplinary Approach 194	19.9.1	Response Types and Coding 199
19.6	Case Report Forms, Remote Data Entry, and Electronic Data Capture................... 194	19.10	Conclusion 199

20 Follow-Up: Why It Is Important and How to Minimize Loss to Follow-Up 203
Stephanie L. Tanner

20.1	Introduction 203	20.4.1	Study Design Strategies............ 205
20.2	Why Is Follow-Up Important? 203	20.4.2	Methods Center/Sponsor Study Management 207
20.3	Why Are Participants Lost to Follow-Up (Why Do Patients Leave a Study)?................. 204	20.4.3	Local Site Study Management to Maintain Follow-Up 207
		20.4.4	Retention Strategies............... 211
20.4	Strategies to Minimize Loss to Follow-Up..................... 205	20.5	Practical Application............. 212
		20.6	Conclusion 212

21 How to Close Out a Study 214
Kelly Trask

21.1	Introduction 214	21.5.1	Closing the Study with the Ethics Committee 217
21.2	Reasons for Study Closure 214		
21.3	The Process of Study Closure..... 215	21.6	Record Retention 217
21.3.1	Preparing for the Closeout Visit 215	21.7	After the Study Closure 218
21.4	The Closeout Visit 216	21.8	Practical Application............. 219
21.4.1	What if There Isn't a Closeout Visit?... 217	21.9	Conclusion 219
21.5	After the Closeout Visit 217		

Contents

22   Knowledge Dissemination: Getting the Word Out! 222
Cheryl Kreviazuk, Darren M. Roffey

22.1   Introduction 222
22.1.1   Knowledge Dissemination 222
22.1.2   Maximizing Uptake of Knowledge Dissemination 223
22.1.3   Developing an Effective Dissemination Plan 224
22.1.4   Traditional Knowledge Dissemination 225

22.1.5   Nontraditional Knowledge Dissemination 227
22.1.6   Traditional versus Nontraditional Knowledge Dissemination: Which Is Better? 229
22.1.7   Barriers to Implementation 229
22.2   Practical Application 230
22.3   Conclusion 231

Part V   Advanced Principles of Research Coordination 235
Ydo V. Kleinlugtenbelt, Rudolf W. Poolman

23   Regulatory Trials: Key Differences from Standard Trials 236
Deborah J. Carr

23.1   Introduction 236
23.1.1   What Are Clinical and Regulatory Trials? 236
23.2   History of Regulation and International Harmonization 236
23.2.1   Role of the Regulatory Agency 237
23.2.2   Structure of Regulatory Trials 238
23.2.3   Key Differences between Standard Clinical Trials and Regulatory Trials 238
23.2.4   Good Clinical Practice Relevant in Regulatory Trials 239
23.2.5   Follow a Detailed Protocol 240
23.2.6   Trial Registration 240
23.2.7   Prompt Reporting and Public Disclosure of Interventional Clinical Trial Results 241
23.2.8   Safety Reporting 242

23.3   The Research Coordinator's Responsibilities 242
23.4   Standard Definitions 242
23.5   Expedited Reporting: When, What, Why, and How? 243
23.5.1   What and Why? 243
23.5.2   When? 243
23.5.3   Event Time Frame 243
23.5.4   How? 243
23.5.5   Documentation 243
23.5.6   Audits 243
23.5.7   Investigator Qualifications and Agreements 244
23.5.8   Clinical Study Report 244
23.5.9   Practical Application 244
23.6   Conclusion 249

24   How to Survive a Site Audit 251
Annemieke I. J. M. Schellevis-Mintiens, Esther M. M. Van Lieshout

24.1   Introduction 251
24.2   The Difference between Monitoring and Auditing 251
24.2.1   First Line of Defense: Procedures 251
24.2.2   Second Line of Defense: Monitoring 252
24.2.3   Third Line of Defense: Auditing 252
24.3   What to Do When You Find Out You Will Be Audited 253
24.4   Content of the Study: The Big Picture 253

24.5   Documentation 253
24.6   Meetings and Interviews with Auditors 254
24.6.1   Introduction or Start–Up Meeting 254
24.6.2   Audit Interviews 254
24.6.3   Daily Briefings 255
24.6.4   Informal Conversations in between Audit Events 255
24.6.5   Final Audit Meeting 255

24.7 Role of the PI, Research Coordinator, and Team 255

24.8 Practical Aspects: Travel, Space, Food and Drinks 256

24.9 Report and Corrective Action/ Preventive Action Plan (CAPA Plan) 256

24.9.1 Audit Report 256

24.9.2 Corrective Action/Preventive Action Plan (CAPA Plan) 256

24.9.3 Life after the Audit 257

24.10 Practical Application 257

25 Monitoring in a Clinical Study: Why and How? 258
David Pogorzelski

25.1 Introduction 258

25.2 Purpose of Monitoring 258

25.3 Responsibilities, Extent, and Nature of Monitoring 258

25.4 Monitor Qualifications 258

25.5 Monitoring Visits 259

25.6 Site Selection Visit 259

25.7 Site Initiation Visit 260

25.8 Routine Monitoring Visits 260

25.9 Closeout Visit 261

25.10 Monitoring Reports 262

25.11 Centralized Monitoring 262

25.12 Risk-Based Monitoring 264

25.13 Data and Safety Monitoring Committee 265

25.14 Practical Application: Ensuring an AWESOME Site Visit 265

25.15 Scheduling 265

25.16 Preparation 265

25.17 Previous Monitoring Reports 265

25.18 During the Visit 266

25.19 After the Visit 266

25.20 Managing Expectations 266

26 Managing Large Studies: Organization and Committees 267
Stephanie L. Tanner

26.1 Introduction 267

26.2 Study Management Committee .. 267

26.2.1 Study Principal Investigator 267

26.2.2 Coinvestigators 268

26.2.3 Study Manager 269

26.2.4 Database Managers 269

26.2.5 Financial Analysts/Business Analysts 269

26.2.6 Research Assistants 270

26.2.7 Study Statistician 270

26.2.8 Study Monitors 270

26.2.9 Additional Team Members 270

26.3 Additional Study Oversight Committees 270

26.3.1 Steering Committee 271

26.3.2 Data Safety Monitoring Committee/Data Safety Monitoring Boards 271

26.3.3 Adjudication Committee 273

26.4 Other Study Committees 274

26.4.1 Writing Committee/Data Dissemination Committee 274

26.4.2 Audit/Monitoring Committee 274

26.5 Practical Application 274

26.6 Conclusion 275

27 International Research: Challenges and Successes 276
Chuan Silvia Li, Mandeep S. Dhillon

27.1 Introduction 276

27.2 Study Planning Phase 276

27.3 Ethics Approval 277

27.4 Consent Process 277

27.5 Motivating Coinvestigators 277

27.6 Language Challenges 278

27.7 Time Zone Difference 278

27.8 Shortage of Research Staff 278

27.9 Data Collection Process 278

27.10 Lower Data Quality 278

27.11   Timeline Delay 278

27.12   Financial Challenges 278

27.13   Legal Considerations............. 279

27.14   Practical Application............. 279

27.14.1   Laying the Groundwork—The
           INORMUS Pilot Study 279

27.15   Conclusion 282

Part VI   A Coordinator's Toolbox 285
           Vinicius Y. de Moraes, Ashok K. Shyam

           Toolbox A.. 286

           Toolbox B.. 288

           Toolbox C.. 290

           Toolbox D.. 292

           Toolbox E 293

           Toolbox F1 299

           Toolbox F2 300

           Toolbox F3 301

           Toolbox F4 302

           Toolbox F5 303

           Toolbox F6 304

           Toolbox F7 305

           Toolbox F8 306

           Toolbox F9 308

           Toolbox F10 309

           Toolbox F11 310

           Toolbox G 312

Index 314

Preface

The Coordination of Clinical Research: A Handbook for Research Coordinators is the fourth book in our series on clinical research after *Clinical Research for Surgeons*, *Advanced Concepts in Surgical Research*, and *Getting Your Research Paper Published*. It was appropriate, for many reasons, to provide our initial offering as one of the principles of clinical research. For those who understood the principles, we provided advanced concepts in the conduct of studies with insights into newer methodological issues germane to any health care research. Successful researchers are those who are able to disseminate the results of their work. The primary output, or one might say deliverable, is a high-impact publication delivered to as many readers as possible. Our third book in the series details the anatomy of a research paper to guide researchers in telling the story of their results and maximizing impact in their message.

This book in the series is a manifesto for clinical research coordinators worldwide who understand deeply that the execution of research is as important as its design. True to the adage, "Saying isn't doing, doing is doing," most clinical research programs struggle not for the lack of ideas, but rather the lack of execution. Critical to any successful research program are passionate leaders, motivated investigators, and highly trained research coordinators. Arguably, the research coordinator is the pillar of a study's day-to-day execution.

We have leveraged an international group of authors and practising research coordinators with decades of collective hands-on experience to provide insights on their roles within a study, detail key aspects of the coordination of research, and give pragmatic tips based on their collective experience. To further assist readers, we have collated critical templates and checklists that should form a research coordinator's toolbox. These range from sample consent forms to sample budget templates.

This book is for you—whether you are new to clinical research or a seasoned researcher. Understanding the daily "how-to" activities in the conduct of clinical research is fundamental to the execution of high-quality studies. So, let's get started because "Saying isn't doing, doing is doing."

Mohit Bhandari, MD, PhD, FRCSC
Esther M. M. Van Lieshout, MSc, PhD

Acknowledgments

The Osteosynthesis and Trauma Care Foundation (OTCF) is greatly indebted to Dr. Mohit Bhandari and Dr. Esther M. M. Van Lieshout, the two editors of this book, who have supported and enriched the research program of OTCF in many ways since its inception. Their series of research methodology textbooks has become the basis for research grants and training courses, and guided many scientists and surgeons in their work. The OTCF Research Committee has benefitted from their participation and contributions over many years.

For the current book, a special thanks is due to Dr. Kim Madden, the managing editor, for her relentless coordination efforts to keep all participants on board and deliver their parts, and for her diligence, dedication, and persisting patience.

This book has 6 sections and 27 chapters in which the contributors have put in their individual knowledge and donated their time to amass a comprehensive and detailed coverage of all aspects pertinent to coordinating clinical research. Our sincere thanks to all of them, as well as to the 14 section editors who accompanied the shaping of this book from its planning to the final manuscript.

The OTCF is also grateful to Stryker for a research grant, without which the present book would have not been possible.

Richard Helmer
General Manager
OTC Foundation

Contributors

Editors

Mohit Bhandari, MD, PhD, FRCSC
Professor
Department of Surgery
Canada Research Chair
Evidence-Based Orthopaedic Surgery
McMaster University
Hamilton, Canada

Esther M. M. Van Lieshout, MSc, PhD
Associate Professor
Research Coordinator
Trauma Research Unit
Department of Surgery
Erasmus MC
University Medical Center Rotterdam
Rotterdam, The Netherlands

Managing Editor

Kim Madden, PhD
Assistant Professor
Research Methodologist
Department of Surgery
McMaster University
St. Joseph's Healthcare Research Institute
Hamilton, Canada

Section Editors

Anthony Adili, MD, P.Eng, FRCSC
Associate Professor
Orthopaedic Surgeon
Department of Surgery
McMaster University
Hamilton, Canada

Jack Chun-yiu Cheng, MBBS, MD(CUHK), FRCSE, FRCS(G), FRCSED (Orth), FACS, FHKCOS, FCSHK, FHKAM (Orthopaedic Surgery)
Choh-ming Li Research Professor
Department of Orthopaedics and Traumatology
The Chinese University of Hong Kong
Orthopaedic Surgeon
Department of Orthopaedics and Traumatology
Prince of Wales Hospital
Shatin, New Territories, Hong Kong

Vinicius Y. de Moraes, MD, PhD
Orthopaedic Hand Surgeon
Department of Orthopaedics and Traumatology
Universidade Federal de São Paulo
São Paulo, Brazil

Ernesto Guerra Farfán, MD
Orthopaedic Surgeon
Department of Surgery
Vall d'Hebron University Hospital
Barcelona, Spain

Rebecca Ivers, MPH, PhD
Professor
School of Public Health and Community Medicine
University of New South Wales
Sydney, Australia

Ydo V. Kleinlugtenbelt, MD, PhD
Orthopaedic Trauma Surgeon
Department of Orthopaedic and Trauma Surgery
Deventer Hospital
Deventer, The Netherlands

Dinesh Kumbhare, MD, PhD, FRCPC, FAAPMR
Associate Professor
Department of Medicine
University of Toronto
Toronto, Canada

Kim Madden, PhD
Assistant Professor
Research Methodologist
Department of Surgery
McMaster University
St. Joseph's Healthcare Research Institute
Hamilton, Canada

Aaron Nauth, MD, MSc, FRCSC
Orthopaedic Surgeon
Division of Orthopaedic Surgery
Assistant Professor
University of Toronto
Toronto, Canada

Rudolf W. Poolman, MD, PhD
Orthopaedic Surgeon
Department of Orthopaedic Surgery
Onze Lieve Vrouwe Gasthuis (OLVG)
Amsterdam, The Netherlands

Parag Sancheti, FRCS (Ed), MS (Ortho), DNB (Ortho), MCh (UK)
Professor and Chair
Sancheti Institute for Orthopaedics and Rehabilitation
Pune, India

Ashok K. Shyam, MS (Ortho)
Orthopaedic Surgeon
Chief Researcher
Sancheti Institute for Orthopaedics and Rehabilitation
Pune, India

Paul Tornetta III, MD
Chief and Chair
Professor
Residency Program Director
Department of Orthopaedic Surgery
School of Medicine
Boston University
Director
Orthopaedic Trauma
Boston Medical Center
Boston, Massachusetts

Esther M. M. Van Lieshout, MSc, PhD
Associate Professor
Research Coordinator
Trauma Research Unit
Department of Surgery
Erasmus MC
University Medical Center Rotterdam
Rotterdam, The Netherlands

Authors

Nazanin Barkhordari, MSc, PMP, CCRP
Research Coordinator
Department of Surgery
McMaster University
Hamilton, Canada

Deborah J. Carr, CHE, MSc
Epidemiologist and Biostatistician
Global Research Solutions
Burlington, Canada

Sarah Desjardins, BSc
Research Technician
Division of Orthopaedic Surgery
St. Michael's Hospital
Toronto, Canada

Mandeep S. Dhillon, MBBS, MS, FAMS, FRCS (Eng)
Head
Department of Orthopaedics
Department of Physical Medicine and Rehabilitation
Professor
Postgraduate Institute of Medical Education and Research
Chandigarh, India

Johanna Dobransky, MHK, CCRP
Clinical Research Program Manager
Division of Orthopaedic Surgery
The Ottawa Hospital
Ottawa, Canada

Heather Dwyer, BScH
Associate Manager
Trauma Research
Department of Surgery
McMaster University
Hamilton, Canada

Alisha Garibaldi, MSc
Associate Manager
Trauma Research
Department of Surgery
McMaster University
Hamilton, Canada

Miriam Garrido Clua, MSc
Research Coordinator
Neuroimaging and ALS Research
Division of Neurology
University of Alberta
Edmonton, Canada

Nicole M. Harris, BSc
Clinical Research Coordinator
Division of Orthopaedic Surgery
The Ottawa Hospital
Ottawa, Canada

Naveen Khan, MPH, CCRP
Research Associate
Global Research Solutions Inc.
Burlington, Canada

Cheryl Kreviazuk, BA
Clinical Research Coordinator
Division of Orthopaedic Surgery
The Ottawa Hospital
Ottawa, Canada

Pieta Krijnen, PhD
Research Coordinator
Trauma Center West Netherlands
Assistant Professor
Department of Trauma Surgery
Leiden University Medical Center
Leiden, The Netherlands

Ellie B. M. Landman, PhD
Research Coordinator
Department of Orthopaedic and Trauma Surgery
Deventer Hospital
Deventer, The Netherlands

Chuan Silvia Li, MSc
Research Coordinator
Department of Surgery
McMaster University
Hamilton, Canada

Chandni Patel, BSc
Research Associate
Global Research Solutions Inc.
Burlington, Canada

David Pogorzelski, MSc
Project Manager
Department of Surgery
McMaster University
Clinical Research Associate
Global Research Solutions
Hamilton, Canada

Kesh Reddy, MBBS, FRCSC, FACS, DABNS
Clinical Professor
Neurosurgeon
Department of Surgery
McMaster University
Hamilton, Canada

Darren M. Roffey, PhD
Clinical Research Associate
Division of Orthopaedic Surgery
The Ottawa Hospital
Clinical Epidemiology Program
Ottawa Hospital Research Institute
Ottawa, Canada

Annemieke I. J. M. Schellevis–Mintiens, MSc
Auditor
Department of Audit and Risk
Erasmus MC
University Medical Center Rotterdam
Rotterdam, The Netherlands

Patricia Schneider, BSc
Associate Manager
Orthopaedic Oncology Research
Department of Surgery
McMaster University
Hamilton, Canada

Michel Sourour, MD
Neurosurgery Resident
Department of Surgery
McMaster University
Hamilton, Canada

Stephanie L. Tanner, MS
Research Manager
Department of Orthopaedic Surgery
Prisma Health Upstate
Clinical Instructor
University of South Carolina School of Medicine
    Greenville
Greenville, South Carolina

Bregje J. W. Thomassen, PhD
Coordinator
Centre of Expertise in Health Innovation
The Hague University of Applied Sciences
The Hague, The Netherlands

Kelly Trask, MSc
Research Manager
Division of Orthopaedic Surgery
Nova Scotia Health Authority
Halifax, Canada

Esther M. M. Van Lieshout, MSc, PhD
Associate Professor
Research Coordinator
Trauma Research Unit
Department of Surgery
Erasmus MC
University Medical Center Rotterdam
Rotterdam, The Netherlands

Milena R. Vicente, RN, CCRP
Research Program Manager
Division of Orthopaedic Surgery
St. Michael's Hospital
Toronto, Canada

Nienke Wolterbeek, PhD
Research Coordinator
Department of Orthopaedic Surgery
St. Antonius Hospital
Nieuwegein, Utrecht, The Netherlands

Caroline Woods, MSc
Senior Agreements Officer
Health Research Services
McMaster University
Hamilton, Canada

Stephanie M. Zielinski, MD, PhD
Trauma Surgery Fellow
Department of Surgery
Maasstad Hospital
Rotterdam, The Netherlands

Part I

Getting Started

1 Leadership and Management:
The Principal Investigator
and Research Coordinator   2

2 Roles: Why a Research
Coordinator Is Critical   12

3 Hiring: Characteristics of a
Highly Qualified Research
Coordinator   24

4 Growth: From 0 to 100,
Real Quick!   37

I

1 Leadership and Management: The Principal Investigator and Research Coordinator

Heather Dwyer

Abstract

This chapter discusses leadership styles and when they are appropriate to use. It then considers what it takes to build a motivational workplace, approaches to use when mentoring and communicating with staff, and strategies to improve organization. Finally, it explores how to continue to develop management skills through professional development.

Keywords: leadership, management, team-building

1.1 Introduction

Clinical research involves a team of people, such as principal investigators, research coordinators, research assistants, pharmacists, statisticians, and so forth, working toward the goal of improving the lives of individuals. Each of these team members has a specific role to contribute to a research project and is all integral to the success of the project. One of the fundamental tasks of a research coordinator is to manage and expedite all aspects of a study to ensure that it is run according to the protocol and applicable guidelines and completed in a timely manner. To accomplish this, the research coordinator needs to serve as the central point of contact in the study to ensure that tasks are distributed to the right team members and that team members have all the information required to complete the task. Some research coordinators have personnel management duties in addition to project management duties. To succeed in any research coordinator role, it is important to have exceptional leadership and management skills. This chapter will outline leadership styles and will follow with practical approaches to build a motivational workplace with team members who are engaged and strategies to have a team that works efficiently and within the vision of your organization.

1.2 Leadership Styles

To successfully lead a team of junior research coordinators, research assistants, and support staff, it is important to understand varying leadership styles. Each leadership style can be effective in different situations; therefore, it is important to recognize the benefits and drawbacks of each style and when to implement them. Many great leaders employ strategies from each and having a strong understanding of when they are best implemented is key for a strong research team. Additionally, knowing how the principal investigator leads his/her team will help create a strong working relationship with the research coordinator, who can then delegate tasks appropriately to the staff. On a very basic level, leaders can be classified as autocratic, democratic, and laissez-faire.

1.2.1 Autocratic Leaders

Autocratic leaders traditionally control decision-making without input from group members. They make choices based on their own ideas and do not involve suggestions from others. Autocratic leadership is often seen in military settings or dangerous work environments where there is no room for error and tasks must be completed a certain way. Additionally, in times of uncertainty, people often look for autocratic leaders who are strong and direct to provide a clear path to follow.[1] This leadership style can also be beneficial for employees who are unmotivated or inexperienced. The autocratic leader takes all responsibility for team decisions, is focused on completing the task at hand and not the well-being of the team, is not involved socially with the team, and often motivates with threats and punishments instead of rewards. These types of leaders are often busy individuals who are dealing with high stress levels. A principal investigator or research coordinator leading the team in an autocratic style can lead to employees becoming workhorses as staff are not encouraged to contribute ideas and experiences that may enhance the research. An autocratic principal investigator or research coordinator will be demanding and uncompromising. Staff who are intrinsically motivated and highly skilled will feel dampened by an autocratic leader and will hinder the team's creativity and productivity. With that being said, when a crisis arises, an autocratic leader can be very successful at handling the matter at hand effectively and with confidence.

1.2.2 Democratic Leaders

Democratic leaders promote idea sharing and encourage all team members to be included and involved in the decision-making process. A democratic leader will encourage staff to complete training and continue education to ensure the completion of assigned duties, will use democratic deliberation when decisions are to be made, and will ensure that all team members are heard and a respectful environment is maintained. Democratic leadership often leads to high job satisfaction although the decision-making process can be cumbersome and time-consuming.[2] Democratic leaders find solutions to difficult problems by engaging the team, who generally feel supported and have a sense of a strong team environment. Democratic leaders can be construed as indecisive during a crisis when they are looking for the team's input and can often spend a great deal of time reaching a solution when all team members need to be consulted. If a crisis arises, it is important for democratic leaders to recognize that decisions need to be made in a timely matter and their preferred choice of leadership may not be ideal. Democratic leadership is an ideal style in theory due to the high team satisfaction; however, it is important to remember that a true democratic leader is often impeded by the slow process and practical results require a great deal of time and effort.

1.2.3 Laissez-Faire Leadership

The laissez-faire leader is often seen as an "avoidant" leader where team members make decisions and solve problems on their own.[3] These leaders have a hands-off approach and give complete freedom to their team. Laissez-faire leaders often give little support to their subordinates but provide them with the required tools and resources needed to complete a task. This leadership style works best with an experienced team where the tasks at hand become easier when the laissez-faire leader steps back and allows the experts to do their best. Additionally, laissez-faire leadership is useful in situations where there are many decisions to be made, the decision-making is not complex, and

when team members have routine duties that are dictated by established regulations.[4] Conversely, team members that are inexperienced and unmotivated will find this leadership style challenging and can thus lead to decreased job satisfaction.

1.3 Building a Motivational Workplace

A work environment that is encouraging and motivational will benefit any study that is being conducted. As a rule, people want to feel included and know that their input is valued and being considered. If the team is feeling this way, there is a greater sense of camaraderie and staff will often go above and beyond to ensure a successful study. Leaders who are mindful of people's needs, both emotionally and physically, will be seen as an inclusive, empathetic, and approachable manager.

1.3.1 Emotional Intelligence

The idea of emotional intelligence came to light in the 1990s when Goleman (1995) wrote a best-selling book titled *Emotional Intelligence: Why It Can Matter More than IQ*. There have been alternate models of emotional intelligence that have been developed since but simply stated, emotional intelligence is the ability to use both thoughts and feelings while making decisions. Recognizing your own emotions and those of others and using this emotional information to steer thinking and behavior show a high level of emotional intelligence. The Mayer–Salovey–Caruso Emotional Intelligence Test is the gold standard for testing emotional intelligence. This test is available to take online and will provide you with a debriefing guide to help you focus on the areas that need improvement. Having strong emotional intelligence has been linked to increased job satisfaction, successful interactions with colleagues, and excellent strategies for conflict management.[5] High emotional intelligence scores in managers have also been shown to correlate positively with managerial performance. Generally speaking, your team members come to work to contribute to the best of their ability and to be productive. If you are finding that this is not the case, then it is up to you to determine why. Perhaps there are issues in the team member's personal life that are monopolizing her attention. Maybe the team member has had an altercation with a colleague or feels overworked.

It is a manager's responsibility to have the strong emotional intelligence to see when the team is not functioning at its best and come up with solutions to help the team. Having grace when you notice a team member is struggling shows empathy and will allow the team members to work through the issues plaguing them and refocus their attention to the task at hand. A conversation with a team member where it is acknowledged that you have noticed that they have not been themselves for the last few weeks and asking if there is anything that you can do to help is a great way to build a strong relationship with your team. The team member may not divulge what is bothering them, but they will know that you are available if and when they feel they need to discuss the issue. Being kind and empathetic in your managerial position will encourage your team members to do the same and will help to build strong relationships.

1.3.2 Physical Environment

A work environment that is inclusive of everyone's needs will foster a strong team dynamic and ensure that all team members feel valued. Ideally, an office that provides spaces to work independently such as separated desks as well as rooms for meetings and brainstorming sessions will provide an opportunity for all staff to contribute and work efficiently. Basic necessities must be considered such as clean air, appropriate lighting, adequate temperature control, and ergonomic desks. Ideally, the office space will have natural light, desks that are able to adapt to all team members' needs, and an appropriate break room to allow staff to step away from their desks to recharge. If your workspace is not ideal, it is important to listen to your team members and hear their needs when voiced. Making workspaces more comfortable does not need to be an expensive venture and responding to your team member's needs in creative ways will show your high emotional intelligence. Additionally, encouraging staff to step away from their desks during breaks and lunch will not only improve the overall health of the staff but will also show that you appreciate your team as individuals, not just employees.

1.3.3 Mandates and Vision

As we know, a motivated team is a team that works together toward a common goal. It is essential that the vision of the organization and the specific department is introduced early in a new team member's career during orientations and reinforced often. In large groups, yearly retreats can gather all stakeholders and team members to share ideas, discuss challenges, and plan for the future. Smaller groups may find it enough to reiterate the vision at staff meetings and in daily communication. As a manager and leader, being excited and engaged in the vision yourself will help your team members feel the same way. It is important to remember that the team grows to continue engaging with your team to promote the vision of your group.

1.4 Mentoring New Staff

Hiring new staff can be a daunting task. Staffing can be one of the most expensive components in clinical research but is also the most important. It is critical to consider not only the qualifications of a potential new hire but also the disposition of the candidate and potential fit into the program. An inexperienced candidate who is personable and excited about the position can make a better team member than one that has the practical experience required who is simply looking for a job. The time and energy invested into a new hire are extensive; therefore, it is important to find a team member whose work ethic and attitude are appropriate for the program and someone who is committed to the vision of the program. An accomplished manager will understand that investing time and energy into new staff will not only help the new team member feel welcome and included but will also benefit the team long term. More information on hiring can be found in Chapter 3.

1.4.1 Orientation

A strong orientation program for new hires is of the utmost importance to help new staff understand the day-to-day operations of their new workplace as well as promote a sense of community and unity within the group. There may be many types of orientation programs that are needed depending on the size of the research institution. Large groups may need to introduce institutional policies in the form of a welcome package or online training modules as well as departmental information in the form of a tour of the facility, standard operating procedures (SOPs), and specific study documents. It is also beneficial to take advantage of predeveloped training programs such as the International Conference on Harmonization or technical requirements for registration of pharmaceuticals for human use and other regional specific guidelines (e.g., Tri-Council Policy Statement 2 in Canada and Clinical Trials Regulations in the United Kingdom). It can be helpful to have a personnel binder in place to ensure that all staff have completed the required training and orientation material before beginning to work independently. ▶ Fig. 1.1 shows an example of a "New Personnel Checklist" that can be adapted for your needs. It includes items such as SOPs, institutional orientation, contact form, and so forth.

1.4.2 Mentoring

Now that you have made the important decision of hiring a new team member and have oriented them to your clinical research team, it is time to develop a positive mentoring environment. This means having a transparent relationship with your new hire; therefore, they are aware of what your expectations are and how you will supervise them. This may mean for the first few months of a new hire's employment to start the week with a list of tasks that are required and then following up at the end of the week to see how these tasks were accomplished. Or, it may mean partnering a new hire with an experienced team member to double check work until the new team member is comfortable with the procedures and workflow within your team. Having clear expectations of the work that needs to be accomplished will allow the new hire to not only feel included in the team but also have a sense of accomplishment for completing assigned tasks. Being direct with your vocabulary is also incredibly important to ensure that there is no discrepancy in the message that is being delivered. For example, saying: "This report is very important, please make it a priority and have it back to me

Title: New personnel/learner checklist	Version No: 001
	Creation date: February 2014
	Last revised: N/A

Name   Title

Start date (dd/mm/yy)

Description	Date completed (dd/mmm/yy)	Confirmed by: (name)	Confirmed by: (signature)	Date completed (dd-mmm-yy)
Contract, consulting agreement, or offer of employment letter with McMaster University				
Signature log				
Current CV (signed and dated)				
Contact information form				
Building access card				
Access to file server				
Email address activated				
Personal computer activated				
Other, specify:				
Other, specify:				

Fig. 1.1 New personnel checklist example.

as soon as possible" may mean to a new employee that you expect the report by the end of the day. For you, this may mean you need it back by the end of the week. Instead, saying: "This report is very important, please have it back to me by Friday at 5 pm" is much more direct and does not leave any room for interpretation. With that being said, having an open dialogue with your new hire will allow them to discuss with you the feasibility of your expected timeline. Additionally, being approachable with your new hire is incredibly important. Remember, investing your time and energy in a new hire will benefit the team long term. Another way to include your new hire in the team and to encourage an excellent team dynamic is to inform them of who to approach with various questions. For example, identifying who in your team is the expert on ethics applications or database development will allow the new hire to reach out to all team members to start to develop relationships with each person and to relieve some of the burdens from you. In smaller groups, you may be the go-to person for all inquiries. In this case, informing your new hire that you are there to offer support and build competence and not simply to correct all of their errors will show that you are trusting of their decisions and will ease some insecurity that new team members often have. Additionally, involving new staff early in team meetings, teleconferences, and meetings with key stakeholders in the research group will allow them to learn from the rest of the group and to help build confidence to share their own ideas and thoughts. A new team member is joining the group with his/her own experiences and expertise and it is important to respect different opinions and allow the newest team member an opportunity to share the ideas and solutions to problems that may arise. New team members may not have much to contribute in the early days, but active listening is a great way to learn the inner workings of the group.

1.4.3 Performance Reviews

Regular performance reviews within the first year of a new hire's employment can be beneficial for many reasons. It can allow you, the manager, to remedy any performance issues that arise immediately to prevent bad habits from forming. Performance reviews can also give the new team member an opportunity to share the experience with the team and to raise any concerns that they

have. These performance reviews can be in many formats. For example, formal reviews with a written report at 3, 6, and 12 months can be reviewed by the team member and filed in the new employee's personnel file and you can offer informal reviews monthly by having one-on-one meetings to discuss work performance. It is also important to consider more experienced team member's feedback regarding the new hire. Other team members often work closely with the new team member and their input and thoughts should be considered. This will help the existing team members feel included and valued and will also help to resolve any internal conflicts that arise quickly and efficiently.

1.5 Communicating with Staff

Having exceptional communication within the research group is paramount to ensure the study runs efficiently, ethically, and without errors. Strong communication from the principal investigator is incredibly important. The principal investigator, who is ultimately responsible for the study, must be able to communicate what is needed for a specific study to the managing research coordinator who can then delegate to the rest of the team. Conversely, the research coordinator must be able to communicate to the principal investigator how the study is progressing, any action items the principal investigator needs to resolve, and any study problems or issues that arise. The research coordinator is responsible for ensuring that the rest of the team knows what is required of them to run a study and having an honest and open relationship with all team members will encourage junior staff to raise concerns, share innovative ideas, and feel as though they are part of the team.

1.5.1 Communication Strategies

A managing research coordinator that is accessible for day-to-day communication will again strengthen the sense of team and camaraderie within your research group. This can be achieved by checking in with your team members face to face if you are in the office, emailing the staff to inform them of your availability, and being accessible by phone if urgent issues arise. Additionally, weekly team meetings are an excellent way to ensure that all staff stay up-to-date with a specific study. They provide the team the opportunity to share milestones that have occurred over the last week and issues that have arisen. They also allow the team to be prepared for what is coming next and to delegate tasks appropriately. Furthermore, it is important for team members to understand processes beyond their specific role to encourage self-development and growth. A concern many have with weekly meetings is that they can often be time-consuming and it can be challenging to stay on topic. Running an efficient meeting comes with practice and a specific, detailed agenda. It is possible to run efficient meetings that are not a waste of time! Practice and consistent agendas will help promote a well-organized and efficient meeting. Another communication strategy is one-on-one meetings with each team member in turn. Although incredibly time-consuming, this method of communication does have its benefits. The research coordinator is able to ensure that each team member is meeting the deadlines and can discuss sensitive information in a private setting. Alternately, this approach can diminish the team dynamic and make individuals feel isolated and in the dark about study matters outside their direct role. Ideally, one-on-one meetings would occur quarterly or on an as-needed basis, with other communication methods taking precedence. In addition to meetings, it is important to be very clear when communication about a specific task that needs to be accomplished. For example, you may have a big picture idea to translate study material into many languages to introduce the study in various countries. Team members, specifically junior and inexperienced staff, will often need task-specific directions to accomplish this. A good leader will be able to share the big picture idea and work with the staff to facilitate it. It may be as simple as giving your staff a list of resources to get them started with a specific task. Setting your team up for success by being available and communicative about tasks with specific instructions will promote a sense of accomplishment.

1.5.2 Communicating with External Staff

Depending on the size of your research group, communication with external stakeholders can be an important aspect of the managing research coordinator role. Developing a good working relationship and a strong rapport with members from other teams is beneficial for all parties. It is important to remember when working with external sites (e.g., when collaborating with site principal investigators) that what you are asking of them is likely not their priority. Another research coordinator may be working on his/her own 10 projects and you asking him/her for an update on recruitment numbers may seem like a simple task, but the coordinator may need to speak with other people on his/her team to find this information. Being mindful of this reality and giving your external colleagues time and realistic deadlines can help strengthen the working relationship. Additionally, when external colleagues ask you for information or help, it is important to be transparent about your time and other commitments. Being open and honest about your expected timeline for completing the task will help to build a rapport with external colleagues and a trusting relationship. Keeping in mind the demands of other allied professionals' time constraints will also help you stay organized and on top of tasks that you need others to complete for you. For example, working with the contracts office, ethics committee, statisticians, and so forth is a necessary part of clinical research and can often feel very challenging. Being respectful of their time, other job responsibilities, and offering realistic deadlines will make these interactions smoother and help to build strong working relationships.

1.5.3 Relationship/Team Building

Building strong working relationships within your team is also essential. As mentioned above, strong relationships with external colleagues will make tasks that can often feel challenging more rewarding. Using similar techniques within your group will benefit all team members. Understanding that your team has daily/weekly/monthly responsibilities when asking for additional tasks to be done shows that you are being empathetic and supportive, especially during times of increased work, such as grant writing and other high-stress situations. Team building is a term that is often seen as activities outside the realm of a normal workday that the entire group performs together, such as escape rooms or corporate picnics with games. These types of activities are often approached with a groan from the team rather than excitement. Instead of promoting extracurricular team building, incorporating strategies into everyday office life can be more beneficial in building relationships. For example, during a brainstorming session, employees may be hesitant to speak up for fear of their ideas being rejected. To remedy this, start the meeting by banning words or sayings that are negative (we have tried that before, that will never work), do not allow negative disclaimers (I have not really thought this through …), and encourage positive sayings (great idea, I love that). Additionally, assigning a humorous code word to be called out when these prohibited sayings are heard can bring a sense of levity to the session. Then, write down ALL of the ideas that are shared and assign them to individual team members to investigate further. Simple tweaks to what can traditionally be an uncomfortable meeting can build trusting relationships within the group.

1.6 Organization

Being well organized in your managing role can be beneficial not only to the study you are managing but also for your staff. Think about the managers and leaders you have encountered throughout your career. Were you more confident in the abilities of the person who was scattered and all over the place? Or, the person who was well organized and on the ball? I suspect most people prefer the latter. A manager who is organized shows the team that they can handle the responsibilities of the role and deal with any crises that arise. Being organized does not come naturally to everyone but with practice and some tools, everyone can improve own organizational ability.

1.6.1 Documentation

As we know, a clinical research environment lends itself to a great deal of documentation. Ultimately, the research coordinator is the gatekeeper of all documents and is responsible for version controls and ensuring staff have access to what they need. It is critical to ensure that information is shared correctly and without errors. Patient data, regulatory requirements, ethics applications, protocols, and grant applications are just a few of the documents that need to be organized. Depending on the size of your research group, the amount and types of documents that will need to be accounted for will vary. In larger groups with many projects, a shared server on the computer is a great way to ensure staff have access to all study material and

access to specific folders (e.g., grants, personnel, and financial information) can be restricted to maintain confidentiality. Trackers that are kept on the shared server are an excellent way to organize grant and manuscript submissions (▶Table 1.1, ▶Table 1.2), personnel information, and other study-specific documents. In smaller groups, a binder system may be sufficient to stay organized. Whatever method of organization you choose, it is important to stay consistent and make organization a priority. Maintaining meeting minutes is also a great way to make sure that your staff know what tasks were discussed in the previous meeting and action items that still need to be completed.

1.6.2 Time Management

In addition to staying organized with documents, managing and organizing your time and your staff's time will improve the efficiency of the team. Inexperienced and junior team members may need mentoring to learn how to prioritize tasks and responsibilities, while experienced staff will likely have a great system that works well. A respected manager will appreciate that no two people work the same way and will respect the way the staff complete tasks. Additionally, effective delegation is critical to ensure that your team members have appropriate work, and everyone is working toward a common goal. To successfully delegate, you must give clear expectations as to what the end result should be. Delegating the steps to complete the task can be inefficient knowing that everyone works differently but being open with the amount of support you will offer through the task will allow the team members to approach you if they run into challenges. Moreover, it is important to consider what tasks should be delegated and what tasks you should do yourself. For example, asking a team member to create a presentation that you will be giving may seem like a great way to free up your time, but phrasing and word choices are personal. Delegation of tasks such as these often end up with multiple revisions that are very time-consuming for the team member that you delegated to and for yourself to review the presentation again and again. Additionally, if you require a report to be completed in 2 hours, it may be inefficient to spend half an hour explaining it to a team member to complete. It is important to be aware of the tasks you are delegating, the amount of time these tasks will take to complete, and the level of

Table 1.1 Grant tracker example

Granting Agency	Application Deadline	Study	PIs	Personnel Working on Application	Date Submitted	Budget	Grant Period	Expected Date of Decision	Status	Comments
Canadian Institutes of Health Research	30-May-18	AWESOME (Angina With Extremely Serious Operative Mortality Evaluation)	Jane Smith, Co-I: Greg Marsail	Jane, Heather	28-May-18	$250,000	3 years	?	Applied	
Department of Defence	15-Jun-18	BATMAN (Bisphosphonate and Anastrozole Trial - Bone Maintenance Algorithm Assessment)	Shirley Moffat, Fred McKay	Shirley, Fred, Sofia	01-Jun-18	$4,000,000	3 Years	01-Sep-18	Funded	

Table 1.2 Manuscript tracker

Manuscript Title	Authors	Contacting Author	Journal	Date (submitted/last status check)	Status	Manuscript #/Full Reference	Submitted by	Notes (include revisions and who is responsible)
Clinical Research in North America	Jane Smith, Andrew Jones	smith@email.com	Lancet	27-Mar-18	Under Review	LAN-18-0018	Heather	
The Role of the Research Coordinator	Mary Johnson, Fred Irwin, Shirley McNab	johnson@email.com	New England Journal of Medicine	07-Apr-18	Accepted	NEJM-18-1089	Sofia	Revisions sent 30-May-18

detail required when delegating the task to junior team members. Finally, involving your team in the delegation process can help your team discover their strengths and weaknesses, and you can help them develop skills to complete tasks they consider a personal weakness. Another aspect of time management in a research group is organizing vacation requests and time off for employees. Allowing your team members to take time off when they would like to will help to create a positive work environment. Although it is not always realistic to approve all vacation requests, having a policy as to when people can take time off (e.g., based on seniority), and communicating openly with your team will make this process less challenging. Additionally, coverage for your team members while they are on vacation is of the utmost importance. Everyone needs a chance to recharge and having redundancy in your group will make vacation times and unexpected absences easier to manage. Ideally, everyone in your group should have at least one person that can handle any urgent issues that arise when they are not in the office.

1.7 Management Competence

1.7.1 Managing Up and Managing Down

A managing research coordinator has many responsibilities. Not only does the research coordinator need to manage her/his study and team but she/he also must have the foresight to anticipate the needs of the principal investigator. The term "managing up" can have negative connotations, but the ideas are valid. Often people see managing up as a way of self-promotion, but in the clinical research world, managing up to your principal investigator is essential to protect the research being conducted. Principal investigators are generally busy individuals with many responsibilities and it is the research coordinator that will inform the principal investigator when they are needed for research meetings and other research-specific duties. Managing up to your principal investigator by reminding him/her when he/she is required to submit reports, when grant deadlines are approaching, and with other study-specific information will ensure that he/she stays informed of all relevant information. Ultimately, the principal investigator is responsible for all aspects of a clinical study,

even when delegating tasks; therefore, having a strong working relationship with your principal investigator will ensure that all information is shared appropriately. As seen throughout this chapter, the managing research coordinator needs to be able to manage down to the team. There have been many strategies that have been discussed to help build a team and increase managing competency, but ultimately, a great manager leads by example. Remember to practice what you preach and not expect your staff to complete tasks you are not willing to complete yourself. Be trustworthy. If a team member comes to you regarding personal issues or challenges within the group, treat the information confidentially and be as empathetic and helpful as you can. Be a strong mentor. Continue to develop your leadership ability by sharing your knowledge with your team and build them up into leadership roles. Having a team with strong confident leaders will create an efficient team.

1.7.2 Professional Development

Continuing to learn throughout your career will make you an exceptional manager. Often people are placed into management positions with no training and are expected to excel. Learning to manage people with various personalities can be challenging and professional development classes can be of great assistance. Taking professional development courses on dealing with difficult people, active listening, and providing feedback can help you understand how you are interacting with your team and give you strategies to make these relationships better. You often hear people being praised as natural-born leaders, but you do not hear the same about managers. Being an excellent manager requires you to hone your skills and be willing to change and adapt to your team. You are not always going to make the right decision and manage your team in the most efficient manner, and that is okay. If you are open and honest with your team and are willing to accept help from others, continue to better yourself, and encourage your staff to do the same, your team will benefit. Encouraging your staff to take part in professional development, specifically in leadership and management skills, will show that you have confidence in your team to become leaders/manager and will create a cohesive team.

1.8 Conclusion

Understanding various leadership styles and adopting strategies to develop a strong team dynamic will make you an exceptional manager. Building your emotional intelligence and being empathetic to your team's needs will increase the efficiency and success of your team. Additionally, learning how to organize your time, your staff's time, and various documents will allow each team member to be productive and work at the best. Finally, continuing education and professional development will allow you to continue improving your managing ability and will ultimately benefit the field of clinical research.

References

[1] Rast DE, Hogg MA, Giessner SR. Self-uncertainty and Support for Autocratic Leadership. Self Ident 2013;12(6): 635–649

[2] Ojokuku RM, Odetayo TA, Sajuyigbe AS. American Journal of Business and Management AJBM. 2012;1(4):202–207. http://www.worldscholars.org/index.php/ajbm/article/view/212/122. Accessed July 17, 2018

[3] Koech PM, Namusonge G. The Effect of Leadership Styles on Organizational Performance at State Corporations in Kenya. Int J Bus Commer 2012;2(1):1–12. www.ijbcnet.com. Accessed July 17, 2018

[4] Zareen M, Razzaq K, Mujtaba BG. Impact of Transactional, Transformational and Laissez-Faire Leadership Styles on Motivation: A Quantitative Study of Banking Employees in Pakistan. Public Organ Rev 2015;15(4): 531–549

[5] Brackett MA, Rivers SE, Salovey P. Emotional Intelligence: Implications for Personal, Social, Academic, and Workplace Success. Soc Personal Psychol Compass 2011;5(1):88–103

2 Roles: Why a Research Coordinator Is Critical

Kelly Trask

Abstract

A research coordinator is a research professional who works closely with and under the direction of the investigator. There are a wide range of educational backgrounds among research coordinators and individual job descriptions vary based on the type of institution, size of the research team, and the requirements of the study. The research coordinator typically manages the daily activities of a clinical study and takes on many of the duties of the investigator. Specifically, the role of a research coordinator is to ensure that the study is compliant with all regulations, the data are credible, and the safety and well-being of participants are protected. In the most simplistic terms, the research coordinator is responsible for recruiting participants, collecting the study data, and maintaining study documents. After reading this chapter, you will have an appreciation for the tremendous number of tasks those simple statements encompass.

Keywords: research ethics, good clinical practice (GCP), delegation, training, documentation, reporting, source data, participant advocate

2.1 Introduction

The research coordinator plays a critical role in the study team. Working directly with and under the supervision of the investigator, the research coordinator is the key element that makes a study successful. Defining the role of a research coordinator is difficult as responsibilities can vary based on the requirements of the study protocol, the composition of the research team, and the experience and educational background of each coordinator. In addition, research position titles differ across sites: research coordinator, research manager, research assistant, research aide, research nurse, research associate, study coordinator, study nurse, and so forth can all refer to the same job description. For the purposes of this chapter, "research coordinator" will be used to encompass all of these titles with the understanding that the duties described could be delegated entirely to a single person or there may be a hierarchical division of responsibilities within a site.

Generally, the research coordinator manages the administrative duties of the study. This includes preparing the ethics submission, acquiring necessary supplies and service agreements, creating source documents and standard operating procedures (SOPs), and training other staff on the study protocol. Throughout the study, the research coordinator remains the primary contact for both the ethics committee and the study sponsor and is responsible for responding to any queries from the sponsor.

The research coordinator is often responsible for recruiting participants and conducting the informed consent discussion, as well as collecting the study data and outcomes. This can involve reviewing medical charts and interviewing participants, administering questionnaires, arranging tests and procedures, and collecting samples. Once collected, the coordinator enters the source data into the study case report forms (CRFs), which can be paper-based, electronic, or web-based. The coordinator also documents any adverse events (AEs) experienced by participants and reports them, as required, to the sponsor and the ethics committee. He or she maintains all essential documents and approvals required for the duration of the research study.

Most importantly, the research coordinator is an advocate for the participant. The coordinator's knowledge of research ethics, good clinical practice (GCP), and relevant regulations is an assurance that the safety, rights, and well-being of participants are protected. The research coordinator is the primary contact person for participants to answer any questions and address any concerns.

2.1.1 Why a Research Coordinator is Necessary

Investigators often underestimate the amount of effort involved in data collection. Attempting to do it alone or relying on other clinical staff can negatively affect the quality of the data collected as clinical care will always take precedence. A dedicated research coordinator is necessary to ensure that the collection of reliable research data is a priority. The duties of the research coordinator are numerous. Research ethics, national regulations, and GCP guidelines have evolved over time and the size and complexity of clinical studies have been increasing. The onus to be in compliance with all

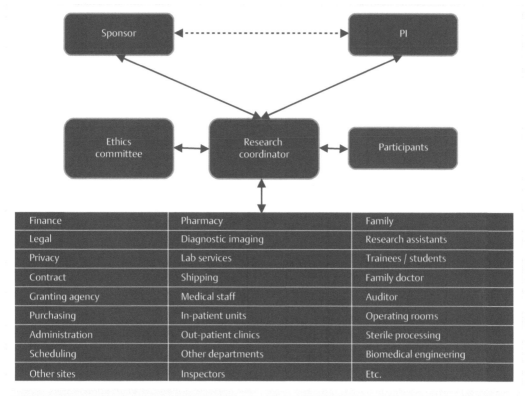

Fig. 2.1 Lines of communication in a clinical study.

applicable standards is on the investigator and having a research coordinator is recognized as an essential means to achieving this.[1,2,3,4,5]

The research coordinator is the key contact person for all parties involved in the study. Although the investigator is responsible for all aspects of the study, the research coordinator is the liaison for most study communication (▶Fig. 2.1).

2.1.2 Education and Certification

There is no single qualifying educational background for a research coordinator, although individual institutions may have their own requirements for this position. Historically, the title of research coordinator was synonymous with "research nurse" but today research coordinators come from a variety of backgrounds, both clinical and nonclinical. In reality, the qualifications are most likely related to the field and type of research being performed. A survey of intensive care research coordinators in Australia and New Zealand revealed that 94% were nurses.[6] A 2008 survey of over 1,500 clinical research coordinators working at the National Institute of Health's Clinical and Translational Science Awards program centers found that only one-third of coordinators were registered nurses.[2] A survey of research coordinators for the Spanish Lung Cancer Group found that 16.2% had a nursing degree, 21.6% had a medical degree, biology and pharmacy degrees made up 13.5% each, and the remainder had another university degree or no degree.[7]

Having a background in medicine is certainly useful in the role of a research coordinator. Many studies take place within hospital or clinic settings; therefore, being comfortable working within that environment is an asset. Those within medicine are familiar with the terminology when communicating with other health care providers; and of course, the clinical skill set and core competencies a nurse or other medical professional brings with them are valuable assets for the study. Ultimately, the needs of the research program at a given institution will dictate the skills and experience required for the role.

Clinical research degree and certificate programs are now available at colleges and universities, nevertheless many research coordinators get their training on the job. Peer-to-peer mentoring is one of the best ways for a new coordinator to learn the ins and outs of the research coordinator role. Finding ways to connect with other research coordinators at your institution, at investigator meetings, at conferences, or even online is helpful in sharing best practices. Many research coordinators work alone; thus, having a peer group to call on for advice is invaluable.

Institutions with a large research program will offer educational sessions for research staff in areas of ethics, GCP, and regulatory topics. Opportunities are also available online, for example, the Collaborative Institutional Training Initiative (CITI Program, www.citiprogram.org), and at conferences of the research associations Society of Clinical Research Associates (SoCRA) and the Association of Clinical Research Professionals (ACRP). Documented self-study of research topics can also be acceptable training. There are often training opportunities available from study sponsors that may be specific to the protocol or general enough to apply to all research (e.g., GCP).

Research coordinators (and everyone else on the study team) must be qualified to perform the duties they have been assigned. You must keep track of any training you receive or the courses you complete. Your study sponsor will require you to keep training documentation in the investigator site file (ISF). Keep a personal file with copies of training documentation to build your educational portfolio. When sponsors select sites for future clinical studies, it is beneficial to show the experience of the coordinator. It also helps in tracking continuing education credits if you decide to become certified.

Although not required, many experienced research coordinators will have certification. The two most commonly recognized organizations that provide certification are SoCRA (www.socra.org), which provides the Certified Clinical Research Professional designation, and ACRP (www.acrpnet.org), which provides the Certified Clinical Research Coordinator designation. Both organizations have minimum work experience requirements to qualify and require passing a standardized certification exam. Both also require maintenance of certification and proof of continuing education.

Certification provides assurance of a standard of knowledge, education, and experience that is recognized internationally.

2.1.3 Delegation of Duties

The investigator is responsible for the overall conduct of the study at his or her site; however, he or she can delegate some or even most of the study tasks to others who are qualified. The delegation of these tasks must be documented. Most sponsors will provide a delegation of authority log for this purpose, but you can create your own (▶ Fig. 2.2). It is often combined with the site signature log. Each person on the delegation log must be able to demonstrate that they are qualified to perform the task assigned to them: this includes documentation of training on the protocol and study manual, SOPs, GCP, and any relevant policies and regulations.

The investigator will sign the delegation log as the evidence of oversight of the study. He or she should sign off on the start and end date of each person assigned study tasks and should initial and date any changes made to the log. The start date for anyone listed on the delegation log must be after they have been trained in their study-specific tasks and after the study has been approved by the ethics committee.

There are some responsibilities that cannot be delegated. The lead, or "principal," investigator cannot delegate overall responsibility of the study to someone else. In addition, medical decisions may only be delegated to a physician (or dentist if applicable). That includes determining participant eligibility for a regulated clinical trial and determining causality of AEs.

Any tasks delegated to a research coordinator must be within their scope of practice and scope of employment. Scope of practice refers to the procedures and responsibilities permitted within the limits of a professional license. Scope of practice is well understood by licensed healthcare practitioners, such as nurses, but for research coordinators without a medical background, the scope of employment will dictate their limits of practice. For example, measuring blood pressure is typically a core competency for a health professional and within their scope of practice; whereas a coordinator without any medical background can be trained to measure blood pressure, but an institution may not allow that task to be performed by nonmedical staff regardless of training. Although

Delegation of authority and signature log

Study:_____ PI:_____ Site #_____

Please print	Study tasks (See below)	Start date	PI initial/ date	Stop date	PI initial/ date
Name:					
Role:	Signature: Initials:				
Name:					
Role:	Signature: Initials:				
Name:					
Role:	Signature: Initials:				
Name:					
Role:	Signature: Initials:				

Study Tasks, *modify as needed to suit study requirements*

1. Obtain informed consent
2. Source document completion
3. CRF completion
4. Determine eligibility
5. Physical exam

6. Medical history
7. Concomitant medications
8. Collect vital signs
9. Specimen / lab collection
10. Query completion

11. Essential documents management
12. Investigational product accountability
13. AE inquiry and reporting
14. AE interpretation (causality, severity)
15. Other:_____

I attest that the above designated study personnel were appropriately trained on the protocol, delegated duties, and pertinent sections of relevant regulations and Good Clinical Practice guidelines, and were authorized to conduct the various study-related procedures under my supervision as specified in the study protocol.

Signature of PI: _____ Date: _____

Page ___ of ___

Fig. 2.2 Sample delegation of authority and signature log.

the responsibility of appropriate delegation lies with the investigator, performing duties outside your scope of practice/employment can put participants at risk of harm and put you personally at risk of malpractice or negligence.

2.2 Duties

The role of the research coordinator varies between institutions, disciplines, and types of studies. Large academic institutions may have research teams where study tasks are distributed among a number of research employees. Other sites may have a single coordinator for multiple studies and even multiple investigators. The type of study will also influence the tasks required. If the study is sponsored by an external party, you may be provided with an ISF, CRFs, study binders or folders, and a study monitor to train you and your team members. If the study is investigator-initiated at your site, you may need to create these documents and ensure the training needs of the rest of your team are met. Duties are also based on whether the study is a single site or multisite, a randomized controlled study, an observational study, or a regulated trial (investigational devices or drugs). Despite the variability in specific tasks assigned, there are many duties and tasks commonly delegated to the research coordinator.[6,7,8,9,10]

2.2.1 Study Participant Care

Protection of Human Participants

The most important role of the research coordinator is ensuring the safety and well-being of study participants. This requires the research coordinator to be familiar with the applicable regulations, such as Health Canada Division 5 or the US Code of Federal Regulations Title 21; local policies and SOPs; and the documents that form the foundation for ethical research in humans.* These documents include:
- The Declaration of Helsinki.
- The Belmont Report.
- The Nuremberg Code.

Local policies or funding bodies may also require adherence to additional standards. For example, to be eligible to receive and administer research funds from Canada's three federal research agencies institutions must comply with the Tri-Council Policy Statement: Ethical Conduct for Research Involving Humans.* In the United States, a number of federal agencies are governed by the Common Rule.*

Research coordinators (and all study staff) must conduct the study in accordance with GCP standards. Internationally accepted standards include the International Conference on Harmonization of Technical Requirements for Registration of Pharmaceuticals for Human Use (ICH) E6, Good Clinical Practice: Consolidated Guideline* for drug trials and the International Organization for Standardization (ISO) Standard 14155: Clinical Investigation of Medical Devices for Human Participants—Good Clinical Practice* for medical device trials.

Last but certainly not least, the research coordinator must be fully trained on the study protocol. The protocol is a detailed description of the rationale and objectives of the study, the study design, the methodology, and the proposed analysis. It will describe the eligibility criteria for participants and what information is to be collected or tests are to be completed at all stages of the study.

Participant Advocate

The research coordinator is involved in a participant's journey throughout the study. As the initial point of contact for participants, the research coordinator is expected to answer questions or address problems or concerns and follow-up as appropriate. The role of participant advocate cannot be understated. Being available to listen to and address concerns can go a long way in keeping participants in your study. Losing study participants to drop out can have devastating effects on study data and outcomes. You are the cheerleader that will keep the participant motivated to be compliant with the protocol and return for all study visits.

The trust developed between a participant and the coordinator can be the difference between a positive research experience and a negative one. Research participation often involves time and effort above and beyond standard medical care. Part of the research coordinator role is to help the participants understand the importance of the research and how their cooperation is meaningful, even if they may not benefit personally.

Informed Consent

In some countries, research coordinators are delegated the task of obtaining informed consent. This is typically the initial introduction of the research coordinator to the potential participant and sets the tone of the relationship for the duration of the study. Informed consent is more than just a signature. Truly informed consent involves a discussion about the study, a review of all pertinent information, and answering any questions that arise. It is a process that is often not completed in one visit. Potential study participants require time to read the information presented to them and often will want to discuss it with family members or their own physician. If not involved directly in the informed consent discussion, the investigator must be available to answer questions or concerns if they arise. The entire process must be documented to prove that the participant was given ample time and information to make a decision, that he or she gave consent voluntarily, and that all questions and concerns had been addressed. Informed consent does not end with the signing of the consent form. Participants must be notified of new information as the study progresses; therefore, they may decide whether to continue participating in the study. Further information on obtaining informed consent can be found in Chapter 18.

---

*Websites for these documents can be found in the "Further Reading" section at the end of this chapter.

Conducting Study Visits

The research coordinator assists the investigator by collecting information at study visits, beginning with the screening visit. The screening visit is the first visit after informed consent has been signed when information is collected to determine eligibility for the study. This may include obtaining medical and family history from the participant or their medical records, administering questionnaires, and performing assessments as required (and within your scope of practice/employment). There may be laboratory tests or other examinations to arrange (e.g., X-rays). Although the investigator will ultimately determine eligibility (for a regulated study), the research coordinator will arrange for all necessary screening procedures so that the required information is available to the investigator.

The research coordinator is usually responsible for training the participants on the aspects of the study that are relevant to their involvement. This may include how to take study medication or how to operate a device. It also includes explaining how to complete questionnaires or participant diaries. Most importantly, it includes teaching the participant how to recognize and report side effects or other problems and how to reach the study team if there are questions or concerns related to the study.

The research coordinator will schedule follow-up appointments in accordance with the timelines defined in the protocol. Again, the research coordinator will ensure that all required information is collected at each visit and that it is complete. If any AEs are reported by the participant (or discovered in test results or medical records), the research coordinator is usually tasked with reporting them to the sponsor (and ethics committee as required). If the AE is serious, there are timelines for reporting, which may be dictated by the protocol, ethics committee, or regulatory authority. The investigator must determine the causality of the AE—whether or not, it was related (or possibly related) to the study, but gathering the necessary information to make that determination is often the responsibility of the coordinator.

2.2.2 Data Management

Study data are collected on a CRF provided by the sponsor. CRFs may be paper-based or electronic. All data collected on the CRF must be supported by a source document. A source document is any document where the data are first recorded. Source documentation permits the reconstruction of the study as it happened. It should enable an independent observer to reconfirm the data. Documentation should be such that it is able to provide an audit trail to permit investigation if and when required.

Examples of source documents include the medical record, electrocardiograms, X-rays, and laboratory reports. There should be no discrepancies between source documents and CRFs and if there are, they must be explained. In some cases, the CRF will be the source document (e.g., a self-administered questionnaire). In other cases, you may need to create source documents to capture information that would not be recorded elsewhere (e.g., a worksheet that captures a study-specific measurement, like grip strength, that would not normally be measured or recorded). Information that you record on CRFs, worksheets, or other source documents should be consistent with GCP guidelines. Further information on data collection can be found in Chapter 19.

The key elements of good documentation practice are often termed "ALCOAC":

- *Attributable*: It should be obvious who wrote it. If a record is changed, it should be obvious who changed it, when, and why the change was made.
- *Legible*: The documentation must be readable. When a mistake is made or something is not legible, it should be corrected by striking it through with a single line, re-writing it, and then noting the correction with initial and date. Never obliterate information with whiteout or scribbles.
- *Contemporaneous*: Events should be documented as they are observed. Data should be existing, occurring, or originating during the same time.
- *Original*: Documents should be original, not photocopies.
- *Accurate*: Study records should be thorough and correct.
- *Complete*: Records are only complete when all fields are entered properly. If data entry is complete and there are blank fields, they should be marked to indicate that the empty field was deliberate (e.g., "not applicable" or "N/A"). Multiple empty fields or pages can be marked with a diagonal line through the fields, writing "N/A" above the line, initial, and date. An explanation for blank fields may also be required.

Once data are collected, the research coordinator is responsible for submitting it to the sponsor. This may entail entering it into an electronic data capture system, faxing, emailing, or sending by courier. If the investigator is also the sponsor, the research coordinator may be responsible for creating spreadsheets or databases or otherwise summarizing data.

The research coordinator usually responds to any queries from the sponsor on the study data. Queries may be automatically generated in an electronic system (e.g., a date or laboratory value outside an expected range) or may be entered manually by the sponsor representative after reviewing the data and source documents (e.g., a discrepancy between source and CRF that must be explained).

The research coordinator must keep the participant files organized and secure for the duration of the study. Maintaining participant confidentiality is imperative. Access to study documents must be limited only to appropriate study staff.

2.2.3 Study Planning, Coordination, and Administration

The first step in preparing for a study is the ethics submission. The research coordinator will gather all documents required for submission and prepare the initial submission to the ethics committee. The coordinator also prepares the informed consent documents, which are comprised of a study information form and informed consent signature form. They are often combined into a single document. The sponsor will provide a sample consent and the ethics committee will likely have its own template that must be used. The research coordinator will combine these into the informed consent form in consultation with the investigator, sponsor, ethics committee, and in accordance with regulations and guidelines. Further information on ethics applications can be found in Chapter 14.

In preparing for the study to start, the research coordinator is typically involved with contract negotiations within the institution (and possibly with the sponsor). As the liaison between collaborating departments, the coordinator will work to negotiate internal service agreements for study procedures as necessary. For example, the local laboratory may process and ship blood samples to the sponsor, the pharmacy may be needed for drug storage and dispensing, or the study protocol may require participants to have specialized imaging, such as an MRI, which involves subcontracting those services. Further information on study contracts can be found in Chapter 15.

The research coordinator will procure all the supplies required for the study. This includes not only the investigational product but also all other materials required: office supplies, CRFs, study binders or folders, participant diaries, sample containers, blood collection tubes, and equipment as necessary.

Training

Sponsors provide training for their study, typically at an investigator meeting. It is common for the research coordinator to also attend investigator meetings; however, there can be many staff involved at a site that are not able to attend. The investigator and research coordinator must bring back the knowledge from the investigator meeting to other staff and ensure that each person involved in the study is trained appropriately for their part in the study and that the training is documented. The research coordinator is generally tasked with scheduling and arranging training sessions for support staff, and may even be tasked with providing the training if appropriate.

Training is an ongoing process. Any amendments to the protocol or changes to any study procedures have to be communicated to all parties involved. This may be as simple as reading a protocol amendment and documenting the self-study, or it may require scheduling further training sessions.

Standard Operating Procedures

Prior to the start of the study, the research team should ensure that all research-related activities are described in written SOPs. SOPs are a quality measure providing documentation that everyone is performing tasks in the same way. They assist in ensuring compliance with the protocol, GCPs, and regulatory requirements.

Even in established sites with existing SOPs, the research coordinator will need to create written procedures for any new tasks that are specific to the study protocol. They may also need to modify existing SOPs if there have been changes in procedures. Creating SOPs is a simple task—but not an easy one. Some tips for creating SOPs include:

- Use a consistent format for all your SOPs.
- Adopt an approval process (reviewed, accepted, signed, and dated by the appropriate authority).
- Have a unique number/version control (archive previous versions).
- Keep the SOP organized and simple.
- Determine an official repository for SOPs (where the approved SOPs will be accessible to all staff).
- Dictate periodic review to ensure they still comply with local policies and regulations.
- Update the SOP whenever processes change.
- Ensure all necessary personnel are trained on the SOP.

Communication with the Ethics Committee

Once the study is approved by the ethics committee and has started, the research coordinator must maintain ongoing communications with the ethics committee throughout the study. This includes:

- Reporting protocol deviations (instances where the requirements of the protocol were not followed, whether intentional or not).
- Safety reporting (e.g., serious adverse reactions and safety summary reports from the sponsor).
- Maintaining ongoing approval for the study (at least annually, the ethics committee must be updated on the status of the study and give favorable approval for it to continue).
- Obtaining approval of any changes to study documents such as protocol amendments or changes to the informed consent.

Communication with the Sponsor

The research coordinator is the liaison to the sponsor and sponsor representatives, such as the study monitor. The coordinator must facilitate monitor visits, audits, and inspections by the sponsor or regulatory authorities, if applicable. This includes arranging a secure space for the monitor or inspector to work, making sure necessary study and medical charts are available and accessible, providing proof of qualifications of study staff, and gathering other documentation as required. After each monitoring visit, the research coordinator

must ensure all issues identified are corrected and develop a preventative action plan, if necessary, to prevent the same issue from reoccurring.

Essential Documents Management

Throughout the study, the research coordinator will manage the essential documents for the study, keeping them filed in the ISF. A comprehensive overview of maintaining records is provided in Chapter 13, but briefly the documents in the ISF include:

- Current, and previously approved, versions of the study protocol, informed consent, CRFs, and investigator brochure (or product monograph or surgical technique guide).
- Regulatory authority documents and correspondence (e.g., No Objection Letter, Qualified Investigator Undertaking, Food and Drug Adminstration Form 1572, Statement of Investigator, etc.).
- Ethics correspondence: initial and ongoing approvals, reports of protocol deviations, list of ethics committee members, letter of attestation, and so forth.
- Staff curricula vitae and medical licenses, training, and delegation of authority log.
- Safety reports from the sponsor, AEs, and data safety monitoring board (DSMB) reports.
- Investigational product accountability.
- Pharmacy and/or laboratory documents.
- Screening and enrollment log.
- Site visit log and monitoring visit reports and sponsor correspondence.
- Agreements and contracts (e.g., confidentiality, data transfer, material transfer, and service agreements).

In addition to managing documents, the research coordinator often manages the investigational product (e.g., drug or device). This means maintaining records of shipping, receipt, dispensing, return, and final disposition. As the liaison to other departments, the research coordinator should also ensure the storage conditions for the product are adequate, even if someone else has been delegated the storage of the product, for example, a drug that is stored and dispensed from the pharmacy.

At the end of the study, the research coordinator is often delegated the process of closing the study with the assistance of the study monitor, if applicable. The coordinator ensures all study activities are complete and all financial obligations are met.

The research coordinator prepares the final report for the ethics committee to close the study and arranges for the retention of study records for the required length of time. Further information on study closeout can be found in Chapter 21.

2.2.4 Further Tasks

Research coordinators come with a variety of experience and skill sets. Some coordinators assist with protocol development and applying for funding in the form of research grants. Still, others remain involved after the study ends by assisting with data analysis, manuscript preparation, and dissemination of study results.

A research coordinator may be asked to evaluate a research protocol for feasibility. The research coordinator is probably the one best suited to determine if the workload of the study is feasible given other studies that are ongoing at the site. This will include reviewing the participant eligibility requirements to determine if the practice will be able to recruit the required number of participants, which may entail submitting data requests to estimate the sample population (e.g., the number of hip fractures admitted to the hospital per year if that is your target population) or surveying physicians to see how many patients they treated with a specific condition in a given timeframe. The protocol also needs to be reviewed to determine if the site has all the resources required to do the study (equipment, personnel, space, materials, etc.). Moreover, finally, the research coordinator may be responsible for determining if the study is financially feasible by reviewing (or possibly developing) the study budget.

Some sites have research teams where tasks are divided among various roles. It is not uncommon for the research coordinator to be the supervisor of other team members such as research assistants, research administrative personnel, or students.

Research coordinators are often involved with study finances, managing payments to participants (if applicable), submitting receipts for research-related expenses, and invoicing the sponsor for study payments or ensuring internal services are paid.

Although not part of a study protocol, research coordinators are often asked to prepare internal reports or give updates on study progress. For example, recruitment challenges are a common issue in studies. Regular reports of screening numbers and the reasons for screen failures or exclusions may identify areas where local recruitment can be improved (e.g., extending recruitment hours or adding additional investigators).

For investigator-initiated studies, a research coordinator may be asked to summarize data in charts or tables. Experienced research coordinators may also prepare presentation slides or posters and even write abstracts.

2.3 Practical Application

The following anecdote is an example of how the role of a research coordinator can differ, even within the same study.

Several years ago, I attended an investigator meeting and spent the lunch break speaking to a research coordinator from another site. Although we were both coordinating the same study, our sites were completely different and so were our duties.

I work at an academic hospital with a large, established research program and a local ethics committee. At the time, I was coordinating about 25 studies ranging from chart reviews to regulated trials. I worked with more than a dozen investigators, and I do not have a medical background.

This research coordinator was a nurse at a small community hospital and had many years of experience in research. She had one investigator and this was her only study.

The study was a drug trial looking at the effects of a specific dose of the drug in specific patients and at the levels in the blood at defined time points. There were local laboratory tests required to determine eligibility, dispensing of the study medication at the study dose, vital signs, and blood draws during the screening visit and at follow-up visits. The blood had to be processed according to the protocol, frozen and shipped to a central laboratory for analysis.

Her site did not have a local ethics committee; therefore, she was able to use the central ethics committee for her local approval. She could also use the informed consent provided by the sponsor as it was already approved by the central ethics. She arranged for receipt of the study drug and ensured it was appropriately stored and locked in the research office. As the study team consisted of two people (investigator and coordinator), there was very little training required of other staff. She had to arrange to pay the cost of screening blood work but was trained in the transportation of dangerous goods and had all the equipment and expertise necessary to process and store the blood before shipment.

She obtained informed consent and scheduled the screening visit where she was able to draw the blood herself and take the participant's vitals. She sent the blood for analysis at her local laboratory and her investigator confirmed eligibility once the results were back. She stored the study drug in the research office, under the appropriate conditions. Once a participant was enrolled, her investigator (a physician) was able to dispense the study medication from the office. She was able to schedule all follow-up visits with herself and her investigator where she took the vitals and drew the blood. She had access to a centrifuge where she processed the blood herself. She froze the samples and shipped them to the central laboratory herself.

My job involved more up-front coordination. As I was required to use my local ethics committee, I had to prepare a full application, including creating informed consent that met the requirements of both the sponsor and my ethics committee. I also had to begin the process of organizing internal agreements. I required agreements with pharmacy, the clinical laboratory (for analyzing blood work), phlebotomy (to draw all the required blood samples), the research laboratory (for processing and storing samples), and local shipping service for packaging and sending the samples to the central laboratory.

As I was contracting out so many services, I spent a lot of time prior to study start-up, doing study training with each service. I also needed to gather documentation of qualifications as these personnel would be on the delegation of authority log. In the case of large departments, like phlebotomy, the manager would be listed on the delegation log and would also sign a note to file stating that he or she was responsible for ensuring that all personnel were trained in the required elements of the protocol and licensed or certified to perform the task.

I obtained informed consent and scheduled the screening visit during a standard-of-care clinic appointment. I ordered blood work through the clinical pathway, paid by the research study, so that the screening results that I needed would be in the medical records. Once the investigator determined eligibility, I was able to train the participant on the study procedures and how to take the study medication and record it in the diary. With more than a dozen investigators, there was always someone available to answer questions if I did not know the answer.

I scheduled all study visits in the hospital clinic during standard-of-care visits for the participant's condition. Fortunately, the visit windows in the study matched our standard-of-care for this study. However, this meant I also had to train all the clinic staff in the study protocol as I would be using their source notes for my study, that is, the clinic nurses would be recording the participant's vital signs as required by the protocol.

I do not have a location in my office that is temperature controlled nor do I have SOPs regarding storing and dispensing study medications. I also had no way to ensure that the study medication was securely stored and yet still accessible to all my investigators; therefore, I used pharmacy to store and dispense the medication. My institution has a research subsection within its pharmacy; therefore, this is common practice and it makes far more sense to put it in their hands. We used standardized prescription orders created by the pharmacy for the study to order the study drug for study participants.

I arranged for phlebotomy to draw the blood during each study visit and had the research laboratory process and freeze it until it was shipped. I do not have a suitable location to process the blood myself nor do I have the SOPs in place regarding safety and spills.

While I appreciate the simplicity of doing everything yourself and knowing it was done correctly, I recognize the best quality comes from having each task performed by an expert in that task. At her site, she had the training and experience to perform all the tasks herself, but at mine, I used the many services available to me. That is not to say it all happened in the background, as I coordinated every step. I attended every visit to ensure the vitals were not missed; I paged phlebotomy and watched to make sure the blood was drawn; I phoned the laboratory to make sure it received the blood and processed it within the protocol timelines; and I oversaw all the shipping to make sure all the correct samples were in the inventory.

Of course, the other big difference between our sites was the management of the study budget. Most of her budget went directly to her salary as she did all the work. My budget was divided up among all my services and salary. That may explain why she coordinated only one study and I coordinated 25.

In the beginning, she was surprised to find out I was not a nurse and could not understand how I could coordinate a drug trial without a medical background. In the end, we both ran successful sites in different ways.

2.4 Conclusion

The definition of "coordinate" is: "to make many different things work effectively as a whole."[11] The research coordinator undertakes the many varied tasks described in this chapter to effectively manage the day-to-day activities of the study. From participant care to data collection and document management, the research coordinator is the key player in the research team.

Definitions

- **Adverse event:** Any untoward medical occurrence in a study participant; whether or not there is a causal relationship with the study treatment.
- **Case report form:** A document (written or electronic) designed to capture all protocol-required information on each study participant.
- **Data safety monitoring board:** An independent group of experts that oversees the study and reviews results to ensure they are acceptable. The DSMB can decide to modify or close a study to protect participants.
- **Essential documents:** Study documents that permit evaluation of the conduct of a study and the quality of the data produced.
- **Ethics committee:** An independent committee, board, or group that reviews research involving human participants. The ethics committee approves the initiation of studies and provides periodic review for the purpose of protecting the rights, safety, and well-being of human participants in research. The ethics committee may be known locally as an independent ethics committee, institutional review board, medical research ethics committee, or research ethics board.
- **Good clinical practice:** Regulations and guidelines that describe the responsibilities of sponsors, investigators, and ethics committees involved in clinical studies. Their purpose is to protect the safety, rights, and welfare of participants and ensure the accuracy of data collected during the study.
- **Informed consent:** The process by which a participant confirms his or her willingness to participate in a study. It also refers to the written documents that accompany this process, namely the participant information and informed consent signature form.
- **Investigator:** A person responsible for conducting the study at a study site. The lead investigator who holds the overall responsibility is referred to as the principal investigator or qualified investigator and the others may be referred to as subinvestigators.
- **Investigator site file:** The collection of essential documents for a study, which are held by the investigator. It is sometimes referred to as the site "regulatory binder" or the site master file.
- **Monitor:** A person who is appointed by the sponsor to monitor the study by overseeing its progress and ensuring it is being conducted in accordance with the protocol, good clinical practice, written procedures, and regulatory requirements. The monitor is sometimes called the clinical research associate.
- **Participant:** A human subject participating in a study.
- **Protocol:** A document that describes the rationale, objective(s), design, methodology, statistical plan, and conduct of a study. It is sometimes called a clinical investigation plan.
- **Protocol deviation:** A planned or unplanned change from, or noncompliance with, the approved research protocol.
- **Query:** A request for clarification on a data item collected for a study to resolve an error or inconsistency discovered during data review.
- **Source documents:** Original documents, data, and records, that is, a document where the data are first recorded.
- **Sponsor:** The person, company, or institution that is responsible for the initiation of a study.
- **Standard operating procedure:** A set of step-by-step instructions that describe the activities required to complete a task.
- **Trial master file (TMF):** The collection of essential documents for a study. The TMF is normally composed of a sponsor master file,

held by the sponsor organization, and an investigator site master file, held by the investigator (often called ISF). These files together comprise the TMF for the study.

References

[1] Woodin KE. The CRC's Guide to Coordinating Clinical Research. Boston, MA: Thomson CenterWatch; 2004

[2] Speicher LA, Fromell G, Avery S, et al. The Critical Need for Academic Health Centers to Assess the Training, Support, and Career Development Requirements of Clinical Research Coordinators: Recommendations from the Clinical and Translational Science Award Research Coordinator Taskforce. Clin Transl Sci 2012;5(6):470–475

[3] Kee AN. Investigator Responsibilities for Clinical Research Studies: Proper Staffing Can Ensure an Investigator is Compliant. J Med Pract Manage 2011;26(4):245–247

[4] Leighton RK, Trask K. The Canadian Orthopaedic Trauma Society: A Model for Success in Orthopaedic Research. Injury 2009;40(11):1131–1136

[5] Fedor CA, Cola PA, Pierre C. Responsible Research: A Guide for Coordinators. London, UK: Remedica; 2005

[6] Rickard CM, Roberts BL, Foote J, McGrail MR. Intensive Care Research Coordinators: Who are They and What Do They Do? Results of a Binational Survey. Dimens Crit Care Nurs 2006;25(5):234–242

[7] Rico-Villademoros F, Hernando T, Sanz JL, et al. The Role of the Clinical Research Coordinator—Data manager—in Oncology Clinical Trials. BMC Med Res Methodol 2004;4:6

[8] Larkin ME, Lorenzi GM, Bayless M, et al. Evolution of the Study Coordinator Role: The 28-year Experience in Diabetes Control and Complications Trial/Epidemiology of Diabetes Interventions and Complications (DCCT/EDIC). Clin Trials 2012;9(4):418–425

[9] Honari S, Caceres M, Romo M, Gibran NS, Gamelli RL. The Role of a Burn Research Coordinator: A Guide for Novice Coordinators. J Burn Care Res 2016;37(2):127–134

[10] Kang HS, Son HM, Lim NY, et al. Job Analysis of Clinical Research Coordinators Using the DACUM Process. J Korean Acad Nurs 2012;42(7):1027–1038

[11] Cambridge Dictionary. https://dictionary.cambridge.org/dictionary/english/coordinate. Published 2018. Accessed June 6, 2018

Further Reading

Declaration of Helsinki. https://www.wma.net/policies-post/wma-declaration-of-helsinki-ethical-principles-for-medical-research-involving-human-subjects/. Published March 19, 2018. Accessed May 28, 2018

Health Canada. Part C, Division 5 of the Food and Drug Regulations (Drugs for Clinical Trials Involving Human Subjects). https://www.canada.ca/en/health-canada/services/drugs-health-products/drug-products/applications-submissions/guidance-documents/clinical-trials/links.html. Accessed June 4, 2018

ICH E6(R2) Good Clinical Practice (GCP) Guideline. http://www.ich.org/products/guidelines/efficacy/article/efficacy-guidelines.html. Accessed May 30, 2018

International Organization for Standardization. Clinical investigation of medical devices for human subjects–Good clinical practice (ISO Standard No. 14155). 2011. https://www.iso.org/standard/45557.html. Accessed May 30, 2018

The Belmont Report. https://www.hhs.gov/ohrp/regulations-and-policy/belmont-report/read-the-belmont-report/index.html. Published April 18, 1979. Accessed June 11, 2018

The Common Rule Subpart A. Part 46: Protection of Human Subjects, of Title 45: Public Welfare, in the Code of Federal Regulations (46 CFR 45). https://www.hhs.gov/ohrp/regulations-and-policy/regulations/45-cfr-46/index.html. Published January 15, 2010. Accessed May 28, 2018

The Nuremberg Code (1947). BMJ 1996; 313:1448. https://doi.org/10.1136/bmj.313.7070.1448. Published 7 December 1996. Accessed May 14, 2019

Tri-Council Policy Statement. TCPS2 (2014). http://www.pre.ethics.gc.ca/eng/policy-politique/initiatives/tcps2-eptc2/Default/. Published October 12, 2017. Accessed May 28, 2018

3 Hiring: Characteristics of a Highly Qualified Research Coordinator

Milena R. Vicente

Abstract

A qualified and experienced research coordinator (RC) is vital to ensure the success of a clinical study. Selecting the ideal candidate for this multifaceted, complex role is challenging in part due to the lack of standardization and a clear definition of the RC role. This chapter reviews the process for selecting and hiring a qualified research professional and includes information from the authors' own experience. Emphasis is placed on desirable interpersonal qualities and key personality traits as well as professional skills. Sample interview questions and a job posting example as well as tips on how to ensure continued job satisfaction are provided.

Keywords: research coordinator, leadership, communication, networking, interpersonal skills

3.1 Introduction

Research coordinators (RCs) are an integral part of the research team, overseeing all aspects of clinical study conduct. The RC profession is currently unregulated and lacks a clear definition and a standardized education trajectory, making selecting the ideal candidate challenging. Superior interpersonal or "soft skills" are highly desirable traits in a research professional. In addition, given the many responsibilities assigned to the RC, those who are proactive with a strong work ethic and are able to manage their time and workload will be most effective in the research realm.

3.1.1 The Research Coordinator Role

RCs can be critical to the success of the clinical study. Although they have less authority in study conduct than the principal investigator (PI), they often have a greater number of daily duties and study-related tasks that frequently go unnoticed.[1] The role of the RC has received limited attention in the literature. Historically, the field of study coordination has lacked clear and consistent definition and standardization. Because of the lack of formal career structure, roles and responsibilities of the RC are often department or study-specific. On-the-job learning is common, and the occupation has numerous job titles worldwide.[2] Examples include study coordinator, clinical coordinator, site coordinator, clinical RC, research assistant, and research associate. These designations, among others, are often used interchangeably when referring to someone who manages or conducts clinical studies. Regardless of job title or educational background, the RC plays an important role in clinical study management, making a diligent selection of the appropriate candidate crucial to the success of the research program.

It is important to understand that the PI and the RC have a close interdependent working relationship. While PIs have complete oversight of the research, are typically lead authors on study publications, and are ultimately responsible for the proper conduct of the trial, RCs are rarely highlighted and tend to be the invisible players in much of the general scientific literature.[3] However, they typically work closely with the PI, keeping the study on track and monitoring progress, ensuring clinical trial compliance, preserving data quality and study integrity, and maintaining effective communication.[4] A collaborative rapport, mutual trust, and respect between these two individuals are essential.

3.1.2 The Decision to Hire

The first step in hiring an RC is to determine the needs of the research program and the role that the new employee is expected to play. All stakeholders (coinvestigators, collaborators, program managers, etc.) with whom the new RC will interact on a regular basis must be identified to determine the degree of their involvement in the hiring process.

Clearly define the position being filled, including the actual job title. While the RC title differs across multiple institutions, research employment categories may already exist within the organization or department. It is recommended that you follow the existing job title structure within the your own institution to avoid confusion and ensure uniformity.

Decide what level of experience is required. While this chapter focuses on hiring a highly qualified, experienced professional, consider the needs of your specific clinical study. Will the RC oversee an entire research portfolio, multiple projects, or a single study? Do you require someone with sufficient knowledge and experience to perform the job with limited supervision? Are there resources within your department to train someone with limited experience? Will the RC report directly to a single investigator, multiple investigators, or a research manager? Will they be required to supervise other staff or students within the department?

Ensure that your department has the means to financially support the new RC, and consider opportunities to share resources if funding is limited. Review available staffing within your research program and evaluate if current personnel resources are being utilized to their full potential. For example, part-time experienced RCs in other departments may consider increasing their work hours or taking on new tasks. Perhaps there are opportunities to promote current staff to new roles and responsibilities. Assessing the current staffing landscape and exploring resource-sharing opportunities are an excellent way to fully utilize your personnel assets and make the most of scarce research dollars. Be mindful that a permanent position offers a degree of job security and is more attractive to prospective applicants. Although not always possible, it is always preferable to hire someone on a permanent basis rather than on a temporary/contract assignment. Employment security promotes commitment and increased job satisfaction, which in turn has the potential to decrease staff turnover.

3.1.3 Hiring Process

Once you decide that you must hire a new RC, the next step is to create a job description (job posting) that outlines duties and responsibilities. A typical job posting describes expected tasks and responsibilities as well as education, training, and knowledge requirements (▶ Fig. 3.1). Decide which requirements are of critical importance for the role based on the needs of the program and ensure it is reflected in the job description. Design the posting with absolute "must-haves," adding nonessential skills as assets. Be clear on what constitutes "must-have" (requirement) and "nice to have" (asset). If you absolutely must have a coordinator with prior experience in your specific area of research (e.g., diabetes, oncology, etc.), ensure that is listed as a requirement. However, research-specific knowledge may be attained with on-the-job

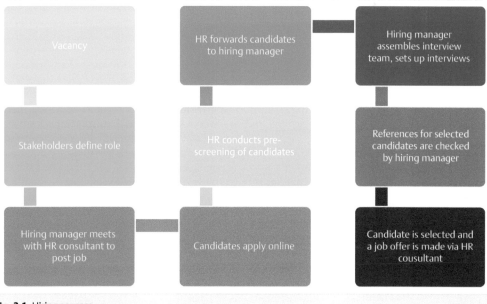

Fig. 3.1 Hiring process.

training. Listing this element as a requirement in the job posting instead of a "nice to have" might discourage otherwise excellent candidates from applying for the position.

Be aware of the financial commitment required when hiring a new RC. Calculate total employer costs by adding salary and any payable benefits, vacation, and pension, as applicable. Verify salary ranges and benefit rates with your human resources department. Employer paid benefits can range from 22 to 26% or even higher, depending on your institution. Be realistic when deciding on a salary range for the position. Match required qualifications with the available role and corresponding salary. Candidates with higher education, significant clinical expertise, and years of research experience will not likely apply for (or be content with) an entry-level position and base salary.

Work with your human resources department when drafting the job posting (▶ Box 3.1). Human resources professionals can provide advice and guidance on the hiring process and have a vast knowledge of applicable regulations, employer relations, and obligations. Appoint one individual as the main contact for all communications with the human resources department and other stakeholders.

Most career opportunities are advertised online with a web link directing candidates to an online application. Decide where the RC position will be advertised (posted):

- Internally, in the career/job opportunities page of the institution's intranet, available only to current employees, usually free.
- Externally, in the career/job opportunities page on the institution's own website, viewable to the general public, usually free.
- Externally, on publically available job websites typically for a set fee.

Decide on the number of weeks to keep the job opportunity advertised and include the cutoff date in the posting.

It is not uncommon for a large academic research institution to receive over 100 applicants for externally advertised positions. In some institutions, human resources department personnel can do a basic prescreening of candidates, making the selection process more efficient. The prescreening may include verifying (by way of online screening questions) that candidates are legally able to work in the country and that they have the education and the number of years of experience required. Provide specific yes/no questions for "screening out" candidates, relevant to your requirements. Candidates who answer in the negative will be screened out. For example:

- "Do you have at least 3 years of clinical research experience?"
- "Do you have a bachelor's or master's degree in a health-related field?"
- This initial process may vary among each organization, depending on local and national employment regulations. The goal of this prescreening is to narrow down the number of candidates to only those who meet the minimum requirements set out in the job posting. Only candidates who meet these requirements should make it through the next phase of the selection process.

Once human resources have prescreened the most suitable candidates, ensure that all stakeholders carefully review the applicant resumes and cover letters. This can be a burdensome task; therefore, it might be a good idea to divide the applications among stakeholders. Review cover letters and resumes, selecting candidates that have the required qualifications and that also seem most proactive and knowledgeable. Look for action words such as "create," "influence," "accomplish," and "lead." Evaluate their education, career accomplishments, and extracurricular activities to determine if they would be able to fulfill the requirements of the positions and be a good fit within the team. Arrange a meeting with all stakeholders to review and discuss these applications in greater detail to determine which to select for an interview. There is no secret formula to determine the number of candidates selected for an interview, but 6 to 10 would be reasonable. If the quantity and quality of applicants are overwhelming, you may wish to conduct a structured telephone or web-based interview as an additional screening procedure. During this interview, confirm items on applicants' resume and inquire about salary expectations. This might help narrow the selection to the most suitable contenders for the position. Selected candidates for in-person interview are contacted by the human resources department or by the hiring manager. Typically, only those selected for an interview are contacted.

Box 3.1 Sample RC job posting

Job Title: Research Coordinator

The Research Coordinator (RC) performs research activities involving project design, and collecting, summarizing or analyzing data. They may assist in study administration. This position requires the ability to adhere to research protocol and work with the study coordinator/REB/investigator to carry out various aspects of conducting a clinical trial. The RC reports to higher level coordinators, research associate and principal investigators. All positions must be flexible to work beyond the job description at times as work demands.

Duties and Responsibilities

The research coordinator will:
- Oversee the collection and transcription of study-related data and/or review data previously transcribed by other research staff.
- Assist investigators in the initiation of new research including grant application preparation and submission.
- Assist investigator in the development and implementation of study protocols.
- Maintain ongoing communication with representatives at sponsoring agencies/firms.
- Prepare REB submissions relative to the initiation and conduct of individual studies.
- Design and revise consent forms.
- Assist in the design, development and management of a clinical database.
- Edit and submit abstracts and manuscripts.
- Administer the Letter of Information and Consent Form to study participants.
- Conduct informed consent discussions and interviews with research participants, administer standardized questionnaires, and conduct education of participants regarding treatment schedule and/or the use of data collection tools.
- Conduct chart audits and liaise with interdisciplinary teams to support ongoing quality improvement projects.
- Oversee the ongoing collection, tabulation and analysis of study related data and ongoing review and development of study databases.
- Supervise research students, medical elective students and research volunteers.
- Ensure payments are forthcoming during conduct of study.
- Ensure appropriate regulations are adhered to in the conduct of research.
- Present research related information including written study reports where necessary.

Qualifications, Knowledge, and Skills

- Bachelor's degree in science or related field, Master's preferred
- Minimum of 1–3 years of experience in research and coordination of clinical trials
- Knowledge of applicable regulatory guidelines (e.g. GCP, TCPS2, FDA)
- Advanced computer skills
- Clinical experience (in specific area) preferred
- Prior knowledge of database design and management
- CCRP or ACRP designation is an asset
- Experience with statistical data analysis (SAS, SPSS, R) is an asset
- Superior writing skills: academic writing and experience in critical appraisal of literature is preferred
- Experience with grant, budget and financial management in a clinical research environment
- Excellent communication skills
- Proven ability to successfully work in a team environment and demonstrate a positive team culture
- Exceptional Interpersonal Skills and ability to create successful collaborations
- Positive attitude and self-motivated professional
- Strong analytical skills and an aptitude for accuracy, detail and problem-solving
- Proven ability to learn new skills
- Superior organizational skills; must be able to manage multiple projects in a timely manner and have the flexibility to adapt to changing workload.

3.1.4 The Interview

Determine who should be present during the interviews and schedule a time that is convenient, ensuring that all involved stakeholders are able to fully dedicate their attention to the interview process. Within clinical research, it is not uncommon to conduct interviews in the early morning or late evening to accommodate clinicians' schedules. A human resources representative may be present during the interview, depending on institutional policy, although this is not required in most instances.

A typical interview for an RC position should last between 30 and 60 minutes. This will allow sufficient time for introductions, icebreaker questions, review of the resume and previous experience, specific questions for the position as well as questions relating to compatibility, salary expectations, and next steps. It will also allow time for the hiring manager to share more detailed information about the company and role. Interviews should follow the 80–20 rule in which the candidate speaks for 80% of the time during the meeting and the interviewer speaks for 20% of the time at the end.[5]

When conducting the interview, avoid questions that do not provide useful information as to the candidates' suitability for the position. Instead, ask for examples of the biggest professional or educational achievement or successes. Inquire as to what professional skill the candidate is most passionate about and what makes them stand out among their peers. Asking open-ended questions allows the candidates to express themselves freely and elaborate on their accomplishments (▶Table 3.1).[5] When hiring a more experienced RC who may be tasked with writing publications or presenting data, you may consider "testing" their professional skills during the interview. For example, provide the candidate with a clinical trial publication prior to the interview and ask them to prepare a critical appraisal of the paper and present it to stakeholders during the interview, or request that they prepare a brief presentation of the trial results. This allows stakeholders an opportunity to appraise the candidates' critical thinking and presentation skills.

Table 3.1 Sample interview questions

- What would your current supervisors say make you the most valuable to them?
- How many hours a day do you find it necessary to work to get your job done?
- How sensitive are you to accepting constructive criticism?
- Describe the pace that you typically work in the office—moderate, fast, or hair-on-fire?
- How much structure, direction, and feedback do you generally prefer on a day-to-day basis?
- Do you generally ask for permission or forgiveness when making decisions?
- Why would you want to work here, and what do you know about our organization?
- What makes us stand out in your mind from other institutions?
- How would this role with our institution provide a link to your future career progression?
- What was the most difficult ethical decision you have ever had to make in your career or during your education, and what was the outcome?
- How do you approach your work from the standpoint of balancing your career with your personal life?

Sample questions to ask a referee

- How structured an environment would you say this individual needs to reach his/her maximum potential?
- Can you comment on this persons' ability to accept constructive criticism?
- How would you grade this individual's capacity for analytical thinking and problem-solving?
- In terms of this individual's energy level, how would you grade the capacity to hustle?
- How would you describe this individual's disposition in terms of optimism and general outlook?

Adapted from Falcone 2018.[5]

3.1.5 Making a Decision

Once you have conducted interviews, contact prior supervisors, managers, or coworkers to obtain references of qualification, skills, and qualities for each candidate. Ask for an overview of duties and responsibilities; investigate work ethic, analytical thinking and problem-solving skills, ability to accept constructive criticism, and any concerns during previous employments. Inquiring about known reasons for leaving may also provide some insight into the candidates' motivation and interest in the new position. Following the reference check, arrange a meeting with all stakeholders to decide which candidate to hire. Review skills and key personality traits observed during the interview and reported during reference checks (▶Table 3.2). Ensure that everyone, especially investigators who will work closely with the RC, is able to provide input and to speak freely about what they liked and disliked about each candidate. Stakeholders with apprehensions with regards to a particular candidate should be heard and their concerns should be considered in an objective and unbiased manner. Ideally, all stakeholders should be able to agree on the candidate selected with minimal or no reservations.

3.2 Desirable Characteristics

A few studies have been conducted on the RC role, although much of the information consists of single-center descriptions of study-specific duties or anecdotal material.[2,6,7] The top skills necessary for success as reported by RCs include clinical research knowledge, creative problem-solving, the ability to identify ethical questions, objectivity, organizational and management skills, communication, and attention to detail.[6,8,9] Higher rates of success in the role of RC are identified in those who also possess "soft skills" such as excellent communication, team building, interpersonal skills, and positive attitude.[10] Furthermore given that RCs are often the driving force behind study progress and help to keep the PI on track, they should demonstrate initiative and self-motivation, integrity, and honesty. The next sections will provide an overview of some characteristics to look for when hiring an RC.

3.2.1 Communication Skills

Often confused with the ability to produce eloquent speech, communication skills encompass an important set of subskills: listening, nonverbal

Table 3.2 Key personality traits of a successful research coordinator (RC)

1. Proactive, hands-on attitude

With mountains of other responsibilities, including clinics, surgery, and call schedules, investigators often let their research projects sit in the back burner. The RC must be confident, practical, and have a positive hands-on approach to getting the job done. This will ensure that staff is kept on task and that the clinical trial progresses as planned

2. Effective task management

The RC must be able to manage multiple tasks and ensure that they all get proper follow-up and resolution. This requires someone with a good memory, organization skills, and the ability to juggle without dropping the balls

3. Excellent coordination skills

A clinical trial will run smoothly if the RC can coordinate workload, staff, departments, and contracts while meeting all GCP guidelines and adhering project timelines

4. Aware of limitations

Successful RCs have confidence in their ability to do the job while recognizing their strengths and weaknesses. Recognizing potential obstacles and limitations and working to resolve them within set timelines are critical

5. Flexible and open to change

The RC must be able to work beyond the job description at times and exercise flexibility in working hours. They must also be willing to adapt to an ever-changing environment

Abbreviation: GCP, Good clinical practice.

communication (body language, eye contact, hand gestures, and tone), clarity and concision of the message, friendliness, confidence, empathy, open-mindedness, and respect. Whether these skills are applied during contract negotiations, communication with ethics boards, speaking to patients about the study, contacting funding agencies or study sponsors, or team consultations on a new study proposal, a successful RC must be an active, respectful, empathetic, and effective communicator. Evaluate these skills during the in-person interview. Does the candidate appear credible? Do they instill trust; demonstrate knowledge and passion for the position? Are they engaging? Do they hold attention and speak in a clear, organized manner? Do they reply to interview questions in a genuine, articulate fashion? Pay attention to body language, facial expressions, eye contact, stance, and posture and ensure that the candidate displays the appropriate communication skills for the role. Keep in mind that although candidates may be nervous during the interview process, a highly qualified RC should have the confidence and ability to successfully navigate unfamiliar, stressful situations with aplomb. Even novice coordinators with limited research experience should demonstrate above average communication skills during the interview.

3.2.2 Team Building Skills

Team building begins with working toward a common goal. There are key elements to building a collaborative and effective team, which are not dependent on the number of people within the team. Furthermore, "the team" as it refers to clinical research is not limited to the people working on the project, but rather on all individuals or departments, which contribute in some form to the clinical trial.[11] Successful RCs do not need to be employed in a management position to apply team building skills; they build trust, establish open communication and transparency, foster passion and commitment to the project, demonstrate a positive team culture, value and show appreciation of contributions of all members, are self-aware, and apply the principles of emotional intelligence to build relationships within the team as well as with external parties.[12] This capacity for team building is a key determinant of success in many professional careers. In applying the principles of team building, RCs establish positive relationships

and collaborations with their peers, investigators, coinvestigators, research ethics board members, contracts officers, granting agencies, coordinators from participating sites, and departments within the institution (e.g., medical imaging, laboratory, fracture clinics, etc.) The best leaders surround themselves with people who have skills and strengths in different areas.[10] The ability to work as a team throughout the study allows for individuals with complementing skills to come together and strive to reach a common goal, such as study success. During the interview process, ask for specific, real-life examples of leadership skills and abilities. For example:

- "Tell us about a time when something went wrong at work and you took control of the situation."
- "How have your professional or personal experiences helped you to become a good leader?"
- "Did you ever take charge of a project and what was the outcome?"
- "What do you like about managing people?"

Look for individuals who are willing to put in the effort to lead the team out of a bad situation rather than take a back seat when situations are tough to deal with. Negative comments toward previous team members, signs of arrogance, and blaming others for past challenges are red flags and could indicate someone who does not function well in a team environment. A good team builder engages members of the team, listens to suggestions and ideas, and allows all members to feel part of and take ownership of the whole project, even if their direct contributions are limited to one task. Working collaboratively enables team members to reach their full potential and promotes a good culture within the research group.[11]

3.2.3 Interpersonal Skills

The ability to "get along" with other people while getting the job done is another characteristic of a highly qualified RC. This is not meant to indicate being overly agreeable. Rather, interpersonal skills refer to one's ability to create good relationships with others. It includes traits such as likeability, to be perceived by others as being pleasant, honest, approachable, receptive, and insightful, indicating the ability to connect with others by relating to them on a personal basis.[10] It is one of the most critical leadership skills in the professional world and a desirable trait for an RC. Insightfulness and awareness of the needs and wants of other individuals are noteworthy skills in situations involving disputes or divergent opinions. This is particularly evident during project initiation and trial setup with various new individuals, departments, and institutions, each with their own set of guidelines, rules, and conflicting ideas on the best course of action. An RC who is capable of viewing the situation from the perspective of the other party will be able to better overcome these challenges and collaborate on a mutually agreeable solution. RCs often report that a significant challenge of the role is the process of ethics committee approval. Ask a group of RCs about their personal dealing with ethics committees and you will undoubtedly hear one frustrating story after another. From the screening process and consent design to study analysis plan, getting a study approved by ethics committees takes considerable time and patience. It also requires the ability to see the issue from the committee's perspective: protection of human subjects. The RC with highly developed interpersonal skills is able to establish a good rapport with members of the ethics committee, is receptive to proposed changes, has insight as to the concerns raised by the committee members, and is able to arrive at a (perhaps creative) solution to ensure participant rights are protected while still maintaining study feasibility.

Creating and maintaining positive collaborations in clinical research can increase efficiency, minimize duplication of services, increase accountability, improve the capacity to plan and evaluate the project, and strengthen the teams' ability to complete the tasks. Qualified RCs exhibit empathy and insightfulness, allowing them to understand the other side of a situation and to navigate tough conditions, strengthening relationships with others in the process. To evaluate interpersonal skills during an interview, ask candidates to provide an example of working with someone who was difficult to get along with. How did they handle interactions with that person? Did they seek feedback from others to understand the problem, for example? How was the problem resolved? Ask candidates to provide examples of prior errors and how they dealt with them. Again, look for warning signs such as blaming others for bad outcomes or refusing to admit they have ever made a mistake. A capable RC is able to show honesty and humility by admitting past errors, reflecting on them, and demonstrating changes made to avoid repeating that mistake.

3.2.4 Positive Attitude

The successful RC continually seeks out the "win/win" or mutually beneficial solutions or agreements in every situation. Through further discussion and review of difficult situations, a positive attitude can help find solutions that are mutually agreeable and satisfying for all parties involved. Along with interpersonal skills, the ability to exude positivity and optimism leads to motivation, inspiration, and development of trusting relationships and is an important characteristic of any successful professional. Focusing on the positive side to everyday situations does not mean ignoring conflicts or negatives, but rather seeking the "silver lining" in the most challenging circumstances and pursuing ways to improve the situation. Optimistic people are generally able to achieve goals by envisioning success right from the start. They do not let mistakes stand in their way, using every setback as an opportunity to learn and grown. As people are naturally drawn to those who are positive and have cheerful dispositions, relationships and collaborations are easier to develop. Furthermore, a positive attitude can have a beneficial effect on one's ability to deal with challenges and stress, conditions often encountered during the conduct of clinical research.

Include "positive attitude" in the job posting when hiring an RC. Seek references from previous employers or supervisors and ask referees to describe the candidates' disposition to evaluate whether they possess this characteristic. Make note of terms such as "cheerful," "good-natured," and "good sense of humor," which could indicate a generally positive person. Positivity is also found in those individuals who have confidence in their own person. A self-confident person is able to inspire others, is not afraid to ask questions, and is willing to admit mistakes, recognizing their own strengths and weaknesses. They have the utmost confidence in their ability to do the job without the need to show off, and this is often manifested in their positive attitude and outlook on life.

3.2.5 Professional Skills

Instruction on the conduct of clinical research is not typically taught in postsecondary health science educational programs. Although some postsecondary institutions offer certification courses in Clinical Trial Management, for example, the RC role is not regulated by a professional body.[11] Professional certification is offered through some research organizations such as the Society of Clinical Research Associates (SOCRA) or Association of Clinical Research Professionals (ACRP).[13,14] SOCRA provides education and certification to all persons involved in clinical research activities. ACRP provides certification for clinical research associate, clinical RC, PI, and ACRP-certified professional. Certification in these and other research societies is voluntary. It typically requires that candidates meet specific requirements such as demonstrated experience in managing clinical trials and minimum number of full-time hours employed in a clinical research role. Certification may provide evidence of prior experience in the field of clinical research and would certainly be considered an asset. However, RCs need not have certified clinical research professional, certified clinical RC, or other designations to be qualified to conduct clinical studies. Given the multifaceted and complex nature of the role and the diversity of clinical research subspecialties, certification in clinical research does not ensure that the candidate possesses the professional skills or experience required to perform the duties required of the position. Some of the professional skills required by a qualified RC include:

- Knowledge of national regulatory guidelines.
- Computer and project management skills.
- Clinical expertise in the specific area of research.
- Grant, budget, and financial management.
- Writing skills and experience in critical appraisal of literature (as required).

It should be highlighted that historically, on-the-job experience has been the most common educational model available to the RC. Many professional and clinical skills acquired by coordinators currently working in clinical research were acquired through self-learning methods. Others were taught by highly qualified mentors who dedicated time to impart their knowledge and experiences to teach novice professionals the role over the course of many years. In today's competitive employment landscape, there is a tendency to rank formal education above years of experience or to dismiss a candidate that does

not have postgraduate education (master's or PhD). When hiring an RC, it is advisable to always take into consideration the hands-on experience and on-the-job training knowledge for a good overall impression of the candidates' professional qualifications.

3.2.6 Regulatory and Ethics Guidelines

Research ethics and regulations have evolved over time: The Nuremberg Code, established after World War II, focused on voluntary informed consent; the Declaration of Helsinki in 1964, stresses that the well-being of the research participant should take precedence over the interests of science and society; the Belmont Report: Ethical Principles and Guidelines for the Protection of Human Subjects of Research resulted from awareness of the Tuskegee study in which 400 men with latent syphilis were followed for the natural course of the disease rather than receiving treatment.[15] Current advanced knowledge of accepted ethical principles in human research helps to ensure that all research studies are conducted according to the highest ethical, scientific, and safety standards. Guiding ethical principles include:
- Respect for human dignity.
- Respect for free and informed consent.
- Respect for vulnerable persons.
- Respect for privacy and confidentiality.
- Respect for justice and inclusiveness.
- Balancing harms and benefits.
- Minimizing harm.
- Maximizing benefits.[16]

Staff involved in the conduct of clinical research must be able to perform their duties in an ethically sound manner. Regulatory guidelines may vary worldwide and knowledge of the relevant local and national ethical and regulatory guidelines is essential. In fact, specific ethics certification and training are required by many institutions before staff can begin conducting research with human subjects. Potential candidates should be able to provide proof of certification and training during the hiring process. RCs with prior clinical research experience will be aware of these regulatory requirements and will most likely have completed the training modules.[19,20] Novice coordinators should obtain information on requirements and complete training prior to starting their careers in clinical research. Depending on where the study is being conducted, RCs should know the following:

- Good Clinical Practice (GCP): GCP is an international ethical and scientific quality standard for designing, conducting, recording, and reporting trials that involve the participation of human subjects.[17] It was developed by the International Council for Harmonization[18] and adopted by many countries, including Health Canada's Therapeutic Products Directorate and the Food and Drug Administration. It is an essential standard that should be part of the RC's knowledge base.
- Tri-Council Policy Statement 2 (TCPS2): The TCPS2 is a Canadian guideline to establish principles to guide the design, ethical conduct, and ethics review process of research involving humans and/or human biological materials.[16] Familiarity with TPCS is required for any RC involved in research involving humans and/or human biological materials in Canada.
- Health Canada Division 5—Drugs for Clinical Trials Involving Human Subjects: Training in Part C, Division 5 of the Food and Drug Regulations is a Health Canada-required expectation for anyone involved in conducting research activities for Health Canada-regulated clinical drug trials.[21]
- The Code of Federal Regulations (CFR): The CFR is the codification of the general and permanent rules published by the departments and agencies of the US Federal Government. It is divided into 50 titles that represent broad areas subject to Federal regulation. The US Food and Drug Administration Regulations: Good Clinical Practice and Clinical Trials govern the conduct of clinical trials for studies with both human and nonhuman animal subjects.[22]
- Clinical trials—Regulation EU No 536/2014: The Clinical Trials Regulation is set to replace the current Clinical Trials Directive, which governs clinical trial conduct in the European Union (EU). It is expected that the regulation will ensure a greater level of harmonization of the rules for conducting clinical trials throughout the EU.[23]

There are many other regulatory bodies that govern the conduct of research. A list of regulatory agencies across the world can be found online.[24] RCs seeking a position in the field should familiarize themselves with the national and local regulations governing clinical trial conduct in their specific part of the world.

3.2.7 Computer Skills and Project Management

The use of computers in clinical research has been evolving rapidly. The data collection and management process have moved progressively from paper to digital form, ethics submissions are often web-based, and electronic signatures are becoming more commonly accepted in legal contracts. Instances of electronic consent form and questionnaire administration are emerging, although still not legally acceptable in every country. In today's digital world, computer skills are essential in almost all work environments and are a must-have in clinical research. RCs must be able to effectively use advanced search engine tools, have a good understanding of electronic data entry systems and data validation, and have the ability to learn and adapt to different systems. Highly qualified RCs have knowledge of software applications (e.g., Excel spreadsheets, Word processing), presentation software (e.g., PowerPoint), and database management programs (e.g., REDCap, Medidata, etc.). More experienced RCs may have advanced knowledge of these programs using advanced formulas and transforming grids of data into charts and graphs for presentations and analysis. These skills can be attained by online course work or through employer learning programs. Experience with statistical analysis programs is not always a requirement for the coordinator occupation, although it is a worthy skill to have.

It is important that RCs consider the implications of using electronic media in clinical research, given the continuously expanding virtual environment. Special attention must be given to the protection of privacy when making use of electronic systems and processes that may employ multiple electronic media to conduct research, including obtaining informed consent, collecting questionnaires, or obtaining signatures electronically. Online security is a significant challenge and keeping current on evolving technologies and practices is crucial to the research profession. The successful RC works collaboratively with the information technology (IT) department within their institution to develop security procedures for the transmission of data electronically. They are acutely aware of online threats such as malware, virus threats, and email "phishing" scams in their many forms and are able to take measures to ensure security and privacy when transmitting sensitive data in the course of clinical trial conduct.

3.2.8 Clinical Experience

RCs have diverse backgrounds (e.g., nursing, physiotherapy, etc.) and work in a multitude of research settings (e.g., cardiology, oncology, trauma, critical care, etc.). Clinical expertise in specific areas can be important to this role, especially in complex care trials. In previous studies, coordinators working in intensive care research units reported spending 47% of their time on managing clinical care while 97% of critical care RCs indicated that clinical research knowledge is one of the top skills to have in that role.[2,6] In some research areas, coordinators with nursing background have significantly more involvement in the clinical care of research participants than non-nurse coordinators.[25] While the responsibility of medical oversight of clinical trials falls with the PI, an RC with clinical knowledge of the condition being studied, especially in high-risk complex trials, may be better equipped to perform screening activities, communicate with patients and families about their condition and complications, describe study treatments in greater detail, and may be more apt to differentiate between study related, unrelated, and critical complications needing immediate assessment. In-depth clinical knowledge of the disease or condition being investigated is also extremely valuable when discussing the study or conducting research consent discussions with patients and their families. Prior specialized background knowledge may be an asset in most clinical trials but it is not always essential. Regardless of clinical background, a highly qualified RC has highly developed critical thinking skills and is able to identify and analyze problems deliberately in a systematic fashion. Novice coordinators can hone these skills by practicing active listening and carefully considering the problem by systematically reviewing each issue while setting aside their own biases and opinions, to arrive at a solution.

3.2.9 Writing Skills

Proficiency in writing takes time and practice. Academic writing involves a clear focus and logical structure, evidence-based and well-informed discussion, and objectivity. While a potential RC candidate may not be proficient at writing for academia, they should be able to demonstrate superior writing aptitude and ability to convey a message in a clear and succinct manner. RCs often compose sections of the protocol, prepare ethics submissions forms, write grant applications, and contribute to abstract and manuscript preparation and publication. They are the communication link between the investigator and various other stakeholders such as the ethics board, the study sponsor, participating centers, and so forth, producing high-quality reports, study memos, emails, and other written communications. RCs should have an excellent command of language, spelling, grammar, punctuation, and should be able to effectively deliver information that is easily and quickly understood. Candidates applying for an RC position should present a clear and error-free resume and cover letter for review. The formatting of the resume is not nearly as important as demonstrating proper grammar and punctuation, attention to detail (e.g., correctly spelling the hiring managers' name), and a good command of language. Writing with clarity, conviction, and passion is vital to research.

3.2.10 Financial or Grant Management

The PI generally oversees the study budget and makes final budgetary decisions as to financial spending. Frontline research staff is usually involved in smaller financial tasks such as ordering supplies and monitoring grant funds. A more senior and experienced RC, however, is often tasked with larger financial aspects of study conduct, including the development of a study budget, negotiation of budgets with internal and external parties, managing invoices, and making payments. Some of the more common duties given to RCs include:

- Negotiating with external parties to secure appropriate funding.
- Assisting the legal department with a study contract review to assess the appropriateness of the proposed compensation schedule.
- Receiving external funding and managing the PI's research accounts.
- Ensuring proper allocation of expenses and monitoring all research spending.
- Preparing expense reports for the PI or the department.
- Keeping track of grant cycle end dates to ensure appropriate reports are submitted to funding agencies in a timely manner.

- Keeping track of monies due from sponsors and issue appropriate invoices.
- Submit study-specific payments to participating sites.

While the position does not require a business degree, someone with a solid understanding of money management is better equipped to perform financial tasks required in the research environment.

3.3 The Newly Hired Research Coordinator

Any RC needs guidance when starting a new position. Be sure to provide your new employees with the resources and tools they need to perform the duties expected of them. Because of the lack of standardization of the RC role, individual institutions often set their own standards and define the position, depending on the research specialty and needs of the program. Confirm that your new employees clearly understand their role and responsibilities, and provide them with the training and education necessary to succeed. Allocate time for teaching and job shadowing, and set realistic expectations for task completion. A mentor is a great resource for a new employee; ensure that the mentor has the experience, knowledge, and availability to train and guide the newly hired RC. Make certain that there is appropriate physical space and equipment (e.g., desk, computer station, etc.) to accommodate the new coordinator on their first day and that they have access to clinical or research-specific software applications they may require. This ensures that the coordinator feels welcome and valued in the organization and within the research department. Explain the organizational or departmental structure and hierarchy, ensuring they know who they report to and who to contact if they need help or have questions. While RCs have an extensive list of common responsibilities and your new hire may have prior research work experience, be aware that other organizations may have different expectations of their coordinators. During the initial employment period, plan frequent in-person meetings with the new employee to ensure that expectations are being met. Understand that it will take time for them to become proficient in their new role.

Once your new hire is settled, it is essential to take steps to promote continued job satisfaction. This is important for the entire research team particularly when introducing a new member, as changes in the hierarchy may cause friction. Maintaining a high degree of job satisfaction and engagement avoids staff turnaround and enables the uninterrupted success of the research program. Because the RC role has been given little attention in the scientific literature, not much is known about job satisfaction.[2,6,7] The RC position offers patient contact, continued professional development, and the challenge of conducting research, all of which appear to contribute to self-reported satisfaction with the job.[2] It also provides an opportunity to work independently or with minimal direct supervision. Some of the reasons for dissatisfaction in the RC role include increased workload, lack of time to maintain high standards, lack of recognition, feelings of isolation, lack of support, and limited funding.[6] This is not surprising given that many RCs are involved in concurrent multiple studies, including investigator-initiated and complex pharmaceutical-sponsored trials, their duties and responsibilities expanding well beyond the recruitment of participants and data collection. Staff must be valued and respected within the department and this esteem conveyed regularly. RCs should take advantage of opportunities for further education and training and request access to resources and tools required for professional success. RCs should embrace opportunities to be involved in relevant decision-making and to provide feedback on new ideas or changes. Given their unique perspective on frontline workload, they can provide valuable input on study feasibility and their experience allows them to anticipate potential challenges. Engaging the entire research team is a significant accomplishment in a research program and professional development is an important contributor to job satisfaction.

3.4 Conclusion

A highly qualified RC is a vital member of the clinical research team and can be a key element for the successful conduct of clinical research. Hiring a qualified RC involves selecting candidates with research-specific professional qualifications as well as superior interpersonal skills. Important "soft skills" include the ability to create successful collaborations, positive attitude, and flexibility to adapt to changing workload. Because the role itself lacks standardization, it is important to ensure that the RCs clearly understand their role and responsibilities and that they are provided with training and resources necessary to succeed.

Definitions

- **Soft skills:** The Collins English Dictionary defines the term "soft skills" as "desirable qualities for certain forms of employment that do not depend on acquired knowledge: they include common sense, the ability to deal with people, and a positive flexible attitude."
- **Phishing scams:** "Phishing" stems from a malicious email disguised as a trustworthy entity in an electronic email, in an attempt to obtain sensitive information such as usernames, passwords, and credit card.

References

[1] Fisher JA, Kalbaugh CA. Altruism in Clinical Research: Coordinators' Orientation to Their Professional Roles. Nurs Outlook 2012;60(3):143–148, 148.e1

[2] Rickard CM, Roberts BL, Foote J, McGrail MR. Intensive Care Research Coordinators: Who are They and What Do They Do? Results of a binational survey. Dimens Crit Care Nurs 2006;25(5):234–242

[3] Davis AM, Hull SC, Grady C, Wilfond BS, Henderson GE. The Invisible Hand in Clinical Research: The Study Coordinator's Critical Role in Human Subjects Protection. J Law Med Ethics 2002;30(3):411–419

[4] Bhandari MA, ed. Clinical Research for Surgeons. 1st ed. New York: Thieme Publishing Group; 2009:315

[5] Falcone P, ed. 96 Great Interview Questions to Ask Before You Hire. 3rd ed. New York: HarperCollins Leadership; 2018:356

[6] Eastwood GM, Roberts B, Williams G, Rickard CM. A Worldwide Investigation of Critical Care Research Coordinators' Self-Reported Role and Professional Development Priorities: The Winner Survey. J Clin Nurs 2013;22(5)(–)(6):838–847

[7] Larkin ME, McGuigan P, Richards D, et al. Collaborative Staffing Model for Multiple Sites: Reducing the Challenges of Study Coordination in Complex, Multi-Site Clinical Trials. Appl Clin Trials 2011;20(1):30–35

[8] Honari S, Caceres M, Romo M, Gibran NS, Gamelli RL. The Role of a Burn Research Coordinator: A Guide for Novice Coordinators. J Burn Care Res 2016;37(2):127–134

[9] Pelke S, Easa D. The Role of the Clinical Research Coordinator in Multicenter Clinical Trials. J Obstet Gynecol Neonatal Nurs 1997;26(3):279–285

[10] Campo MA. Leadership and Research Administration. Res Manag Rev 2014;20(1):1–6

[11] Baer AR, Zon R, Devine S, Lyss AP. The Clinical Research Team. J Oncol Pract 2011;7(3):188–192

[12] Goleman D. The Emotionally Competent Leader. Healthc Forum J 1998;41(2):36, 38, 76

[13] SOCRA. The Society of Clinical Research Associates. Chalfont, PA. https://www.socra.org. Accessed July 2, 2019

[14] ACRP. Association of Clinical Research Professionals. Alexandria, VA: ACRP. https://www.acrpnet.org. Accessed July 2, 2019

[15] Fowler SB, Stack K. Research and the Clinical Trials Coordinator. J Neurosci Nurs 2007;39(2):120–123

[16] Canada Go. Tri-Council Policy Statement: Ethical Conduct for Research Involving Humans. 2014. http://www.pre.ethics.gc.ca/eng/policy-politique/initiatives/tcps2-eptc2/Default. Accessed July 2, 2019

[17] Vijayananthan A, Nawawi O. The Importance of Good Clinical Practice Guidelines and its Role in Clinical Trials. Biomed Imaging Interv J 2008;4(1):e5

[18] ICH. The International Council for Harmonisation of Technical Requirements for Pharmaceuticals for Human Use. 2018. http://www.ich.org/about/history.html. Accessed July 2, 2019

[19] CITI. Research Ethics and Compliance Training. Miami, FL: CITI Program; 2018. https://about.citiprogram.org/en/homepage. Accessed July 2, 2019

[20] Canada Go. Tri-Council Policy Statement: Ethical Conduct for Research Involving Humans—Tutorial: Government of Canada. 2014. https://tcps2core.ca/welcome. Accessed July 2, 2019

[21] Canada Go. Part C, Division 5 of the Regulations: Drugs for Clinical Trials Involving Human Subjects. 2018. https://www.canada.ca/en/health-canada/services/drugs-health-products/drug-products/applications-submissions/guidance-documents/clinical-trials/links.html. Accessed July 2, 2019

[22] Regulations FDA US. Good Clinical Practice and Clinical Trials: United States Food and Drug Administration. 2018. https://www.fda.gov/scienceresearch/specialtopics/runningclinicaltrials/ucm155713.htm#FDARegulations. Accessed July 2, 2019

[23] Commission E. Clinical trials—Regulation EU No 536/2014. 2018. https://ec.europa.eu/health/human-use/clinical-trials/regulation_en. Accessed July 2, 2019

[24] IAoCR. Regulatory Authorities Around the World. 2018. http://iaocr.com/clinical-research-regulations/regulatory-authority-links. Accessed July 2, 2019

[25] Rico-Villademoros F, Hernando T, Sanz JL, et al. The Role of the Clinical Research Coordinator—Data Manager—in Oncology Clinical Trials. BMC Med Res Methodol 2004;4:6

Further Reading

Goleman D. Emotional Intelligence: 10th Anniversary Edition; Why It Can Matter More Than IQ. Bantam. 0th ed. 2005:384. ISBN-13: 978-0553383713

https://www.fda.gov/science-research/clinical-trials-and-human-subject-protection/websites-information-about-clinical-trials. Accessed July 2, 2019

4 Growth: From 0 to 100, Real Quick!

Nicole M. Harris, Darren M. Roffey

Abstract

Conducting a clinical research study can be challenging and overwhelming. Preliminary protocol assessment for practicability, in addition to early communication and staff training, is necessary to expedite the start-up process. Thorough preparation and development of a recruitment plan is required to accelerate patient screening, determine eligibility, and permit patient enrollment. In this chapter, we will discuss the various stages of planning that will allow for study progress to take off rapidly and patient recruitment to ramp up quickly. Our aim is to showcase the critical tasks that a research coordinator should complete in order to increase the likelihood of success in their role and to ensure the overall efficient execution of the study.

Keywords: planning, protocol, recruitment, informed consent, training, communication, engagement

4.1 Introduction

Once ethical approval for a study has been secured, screening and enrollment conducted by a research coordinator can begin in earnest. It is important that patient recruitment is considered during protocol development and then again throughout the start-up phase to ensure an efficient ramp-up in study numbers. Starting patient enrollment within a scheduled time frame is a recognized challenge: up to 86% of clinical trials fail to enroll patients on time and 52% are delayed by 1 to 6 months.[1] Bachenheimer and Brescia[2] indicate that the formula for successful enrollment is 80% planning and 20% execution plus implementation.

Patient recruitment should be a key consideration in the development stages of a study. The protocol should facilitate ease of enrollment. There are many ways this can be accomplished, including broadening the inclusion and exclusion criterion, minimizing the burden on study participants in terms of visits, questionnaires, and tests, and ensuring that the research site has adequate resources for all study procedures. The research coordinator must be involved in the early stages to highlight any potential barriers to recruitment and study flow, and then work with the principal investigator to diminish these issues. Determining

a realistic timeline for recruitment should be based on the study sample size and the likelihood of patients within the desired population agreeing to be involved.

In this chapter, we aim to provide a guideline on how to grow a study from "0 to 100" with an emphasis on start-up and patient recruitment. Discussions will center around the research question in relation to the target population and how patients should be considered in the protocol design to devise a tailored recruitment plan. Feasibility and planning from the early stages and how this can expedite personnel training and facilitate departmental communication to enhance patient recruitment will also be highlighted. By way of a practical application, we will outline and discuss tips for a research coordinator in relation to ramping up recruitment for a randomized controlled trial comparing two types of anesthesia in elderly patients with hip fractures.

4.2 Protocol Development

Careful planning of the study design and protocol prior to the first patient being enrolled is essential for a study to run smoothly.[3] It is the responsibility of the principal investigator to ensure that the protocol is ethically sound and scientifically and clinically significant.[4,5] The research coordinator should be involved in the early stages of protocol development as it is within their scope to investigate feasibility, recruitability, logistics, and resource availability at their site.[4,5,6]

With this in mind, some logistical questions to consider during protocol development include:

Are the number of study procedures (e.g., laboratory tests, questionnaires, and medical imaging) necessary and reasonable?

Patient recruitment should be incorporated into the study design from the outset.[2] A known barrier to recruitment in clinical trials is requiring additional time from the patient.[7] Usually, if the research is directly benefiting the patient, it is reasonable to assume that they might be willing to complete more study-related procedures. To assess the burden on the participant, start with a clear understanding of their usual standard-of-care. How often and at what time points do patients follow-up in the clinic? How often do they get diagnostic imaging? How often do they get blood work? Do they routinely fill out questionnaires? Only then is it possible to assess how much extra is being asked of any research participant. The goal is to then limit any additional burden by aligning research visits with standard-of-care visits and eliminating unnecessary procedures. Each extra procedure must add value to the study and help address the study question.

Will there be a sufficient number of eligible patients?

It is useful to examine historical data to determine whether there will be enough research participants in the local population to finish recruitment in a reasonable time. Start by looking for the number of patients who fit the basic eligibility requirements (e.g., age, gender, diagnosis, and injury). Depending on how strict the inclusion criteria are, it might be possible to estimate that a certain number of patients will qualify, and a percentage of those will agree to the research study. If the prediction estimates that there will not be enough eligible patients, it may be necessary to re-examine the exclusion criteria. Are one or two criteria eliminating a large number of people? What is the importance of any such strict exclusion criteria? If possible, it is beneficial to include as much of any one patient population as possible to ensure the generalizability of the results.[8] Another option is to branch out into a multicenter study so as to increase the total patient population. Start-up procedures at other sites are often very time-consuming; therefore, involving them early on in the process will speed up their recruitment planning.[9] Alternatively, the principal investigator could make an agreement with the colleagues to refer suitable patients that might meet the eligibility criteria.[10]

Are there conflicting studies?

Multiple studies targeting the same patient population can cause a burden on the patient population and have negative effects on overall recruitment for all of the studies effected. The research coordinator may be aware of studies in the respective division (e.g., Division of Orthopaedic Surgery), but if the patient population will be seen by multiple departments (e.g., Division of Urology and Division of Endocrinology and Metabolism), communication with the affiliated research coordinators must occur to ensure that there are no conflicting studies. Learning that several studies are vying for the same patient population just before starting recruitment can be detrimental to the recruitment phase; therefore, this should not be overlooked.

Are there enough research staff available to conduct the study?

Research staff are necessary to conduct quality clinical research.[11,12] It is imperative to ensure that the site has sufficient capacity to start a new study. Determining what responsibilities will be delegated to research staff and how time-consuming these tasks will be is equally important. Research staff should forecast their day-to-day availability to ensure that they are available when needed. For example, if a research coordinator is delegated to recruit patients, they should determine whether they will have the time available to begin recruitment when asked, and how much time this will take away from any previous research engagements.

What are the potential barriers to enrollment?

It is important to consider potential obstacles to recruitment early on so that the research team can start assessing the barriers and preparing resolutions. If the time window for informed consent is short, as it is with many critical care research studies, ensure that research staff can be available quickly and with limited notice.[13] If this is not realistic, a clinical member of staff involved in the circle of care for the patient population should be trained and delegated the responsibility of obtaining informed consent. This should be resolved at the start of study development so that the impact on the department can be assessed and approved and proper training can be completed prior to the start of enrollment. In studies where the target population is unlikely to be competent to provide informed consent (e.g., patients with Alzheimer's or patients with traumatic brain injuries), a system for proxy consent should be arranged. In some situations, proxy consent will need to be completed in a matter of minutes or hours; therefore, ethical approval for proxy consent via phone should be obtained.[13] Language barriers can also be a common barrier to enrollment in clinical research.[13,14] If a language barrier will exist between the research coordinator and the target population more often than not, arrangements should be made for a translator to be on hand and/or the research team should have the study documents translated into the most predominant foreign language. Translation can be both timely and costly; therefore, accounting for this early on will limit its effects on recruitment.

It is essential to design the study with patient recruitment in mind. This will save time and money, and it will preserve and protect the patient experience.[2] It is far more efficient to address any concerns with the study design early to avoid unnecessary amendments that can later hinder patient recruitment and retention.[3] The research coordinator should be involved in the early stages of protocol development so that they can inform and establish relationships with other departments that will be involved with the study such as medical imaging or pharmacy.[3,5] Representatives from each department will be able to make informed recommendations on ways to improve the protocol to enhance recruitment and retention of study patients.[5]

4.3 Informed Consent Form

The informed consent form is an essential document in any investigational clinical research study. The ideal informed consent form will strike a difficult balance between providing sufficient information to elicit an informed decision and being easy enough to read and comprehend at a reasonable education level.[8] Clinical research studies often involve complex diseases, injuries, pharmacology, or surgeries, and their terminologies can be long and difficult to read and interpret. Typically, the research ethics board will have a set level of understanding required for the informed consent form, and it is the role of the principal investigator and research coordinator to produce a clear, concise, and easy-to-understand informed consent form accordingly. Throughout this process, keep the target patient population in mind. In general, an informed consent form should be written at an eighth-grade reading level.[4] A more simplified consent form may be required for a study that is enrolling patients from the general population compared to a study that is recruiting from a group of learned individuals (e.g., university

students and physicians). In a multicenter study, the informed consent form will vary between sites because many research ethics boards have specific guidelines and wording that must be incorporated.

It is essential to clearly indicate the risks associated with study involvement. However, do not overamplify these risk factors as it may lead to discouragement from participation.[3] For example, if the study is investigating surgical patients, the patient will have to sign a separate consent form for the surgical procedure. This surgical consent form will list all of the risks associated with the surgery. Therefore, it is not necessary to restate these surgical risks in a research study informed consent form unless the intervention directly impacts upon these previously stated surgical procedure risks.

Any appointments or procedures that are not considered standard-of-care for the patient population should be clearly indicated in the informed consent form, for example, additional blood draws, questionnaires, or study visits that the patient would not undergo if they did not consent to the research study. Risks associated with any additional procedures should be present in the informed consent form too (e.g., localized bruising from blood draws).

The informed consent form is a vital part of the recruitment process. Preparing the informed consent form should involve careful planning and discussion between research staff. Developing the informed consent form is a process that will require many revisions and drafts before a final version is produced. Even with careful planning and attention to the informed consent form, there may be information that is confusing, misleading, or missing that comes to light once enrollment begins and patients begin to pore over the study details from a different perspective. At this point, do not hesitate to amend the informed consent form accordingly and submit it to the ethics board for approval so that it is clear and concise for future patients.

4.4 Communication

It is the responsibility of the research coordinator to ensure that all relevant parties are introduced and kept up-to-date on important aspects of the study. Communication should extend to the principal and coinvestigators, research team members, applicable departmental members within the hospital, and across participating sites. The research coordinator should be the first point of contact for any questions or concerns; therefore, their contact information, including office phone, email, pager, fax, and cell phone, should be readily available.

Communication within the hospital

If an upcoming study will have an impact on a certain department or clinic within the hospital, it may be beneficial to meet with their representative to discuss how the study can best be integrated into the workflow of that environment. For example, if the plan is to recruit patients in the emergency department, arrange in advance for a meeting with a clerk, nurse, or physician who works in the department. It may be most beneficial to meet with someone who is actively working in that area but approval is most likely also required from the chief, head, or manager of the department.[5] At this meeting, introduce the study and the patient population to be recruited. The representative will be able to describe how these patients typically flow through the department. From there, jointly discuss the best time and place for the research coordinator to approach the patient. Ideally, there will be a mutually agreeable time and place for recruitment that will have minimal to no impact on the flow of the department. This approach can also be taken if a patient is being recruited from a ward or a clinic within the hospital. Clinic staff may prefer that recruitment takes place outside of an exam room as the recruitment and consent process can be time-consuming, and occupying an exam room can hinder the flow of the clinic. This information is valuable prior to the start of the recruitment so that the appropriate connections can be made and suitable measures put in place.

Communication between sites

When a study is enrolling patients at multiple centers, whether they are in the same city or across the country, continent, or around the world, it is essential for the research coordinator at the primary study site to maintain regular communication with the other sites. Additionally, it may be beneficial for subsite coordinators to communicate with one another. In many multicenter studies, start-up and recruitment is staggered between sites. There may be sites that have already been recruiting for a period of time when your site is in the prerecruitment phase. If this is not the case, it is likely that other sites have done similar studies in the past and will have valuable information to share. If there is uncertainty about a specific step in the recruitment plan, inquiring with other sites as to how they manage this issue could result in local solutions while also opening up additional opportunities for improvement in the conduct of the study at each respective site.

4.5 Enthusiasm

There is a lot of work that goes into the start-up, recruitment, and maintenance of clinical research studies. It is important throughout this process to keep all parties informed, aware, and enthusiastic about recruitment. Often, enthusiasm about a study will stem from the principal investigator and any coinvestigators involved. While physician interest is a necessary component in any successful research project, it is important to recognize that physicians have competing interests for their time. Research coordinators play a key role in maintaining enthusiasm levels as it is vital both at the start of patient recruitment and throughout the course of the study.

Research staff should have their contact information available to all parties involved in the study, especially in a situation where others are identifying eligible patients. If these individuals know who the research staff are, they are more likely to approach them with questions and suggestions or to identify eligible patients. Therefore, the research coordinator should take the time and initiative to meet with individuals and representatives from each department in person whenever and wherever possible. This approach will minimize the risk of missing patients that are eligible for the study.

It is also the role of the research coordinator to send study-related updates to the research team in the form of monthly or quarterly reports/newsletters. This applies to both the research coordinator at the lead site of a multicenter study as well as subsite research coordinators with respect to their local research teams. These updates should include recruitment-related data, including the number of patients screened, the number of patients eligible out of all that were screened, and the number of patients recruited. If eligible patients have been missed, provide details as to why they were missed (e.g., language barrier, consent form not available in the patient's language). If possible, include local and site-wide recruitment and a comparison between sites. It is also useful to compare your local site over time. While this communication is useful to inform and update research staff, it can also be used to draw attention to potential weaknesses. This way, everyone is informed as to why eligible patients are being missed, which can make it easier to spot trends and discuss solutions (e.g., translate the consent form).

4.6 Training

It is the responsibility of the research coordinator and principal investigator to ensure that all departments and individuals have the necessary training required to conduct their role in the study properly and effectively.[4] The training should be specific to the department or individual trainee, and the extent of the training should correspond with the involvement in the study. The approach, timing, and content of the training should be planned out carefully and well in advance. A research coordinator must understand the protocol, facilities, and departments involved in all aspects of the study. It may be useful to develop a comprehensive list of tasks and responsibilities and then delegate these responsibilities to the most reasonable party or individual. The task delegation log is a good starting place when developing this list, but the list itself should go into much more depth. For example, the task delegation log may state that pharmacy technicians are responsible for storing and dispensing a study drug. Without more information, it is unclear who is responsible for ensuring that the drug has not expired, disposal of expired drugs, and maintaining stock of the drug. ▶Table 4.1 provides an example of a detailed list of study-related procedures. The training schedule should be developed based on these responsibilities to ensure that each department and its individuals are aware of their roles. This is essential in the start-up phase of a study as miscommunications can delay the start of recruitment.

In most cases, training can occur prior to screening and recruitment. However, it is best to have a realistic understanding of when recruitment will begin. While delaying recruitment to conduct training is not ideal, conducting training too early is also unbeneficial as study-related protocol and responsibility retention might wane. It is best if the information is fresh and current; therefore, training sessions held 1 to 2 weeks prior to the start of the screening phase is ideal. This allows for the

Table 4.1 Example of a comprehensive list of study-related responsibilities

Task	Delegate to
• Identify potential patient	Physician; consultation appointment
• Assess eligibility criteria	Physician and research coordinator
• Obtain informed consent	Research coordinator
• Randomize	Research coordinator; online
• Inform relevant parties of randomization	Research coordinator; email
Study drug	
• Dispense drug	Pharmacy technician
• Maintain stock	Pharmacy technician
• Disposal of drug	Pharmacy technician
• Document compliance	Research coordinator; phone call and pill count
Complete follow-up visits	
• Schedule appointment	Clerk
• Inform patient of the appointment	Research coordinator; phone call
• Complete CRFs	Physician and research coordinator
• Data entry	Research coordinator

Abbreviation: CRFs, case report forms.

clarification of any issues and to ensure staff readiness. However, for studies that necessitate extensive training for advanced techniques (e.g., specialized diagnostic tests), more time may be required.

There are many methods by which personnel training can be completed. In some situations, it may be most appropriate to distribute the study protocol and a targeted training slide presentation electronically for trainees to read, review, and respond with any questions or concerns at their own leisure. For those individuals who are more involved with the study and for those who have a larger role in the conduct of the study, it is usually preferable to hold an in-person training session.[5] This way, the research coordinator is present to thoroughly explain and highlight important aspects of the study, and any questions can be discussed and answered immediately. During in-person training sessions, individuals can sign the training log there and then, eliminating the need to collect signatures at a later date. There are many other methods in which training can be completed, including via telephone, over web conference, through instructional videos, or a combination of the above. Thorough planning of each training session by the research coordinator shows respect for the time taken by the departments and individuals to complete the training. Additionally, the research coordinator should work within the schedule of the collaborating departments and individuals, and not their own. This is important in maintaining a positive relationship from the outset, which is essential for the success of the study.[5]

The research coordinator should prepare a study reference manual and distribute copies appropriately to necessary individuals and to the required locations.[5] The study manual should include the study title, research staff, contact information, objectives, importance, and study procedures. Additionally, it should outline the roles and responsibilities of each department involved in the study.[5] The study manual should be the first reference for study staff to go to in case they need to review the study procedures at any stage. It should be concise and easy to navigate. The study manual will vary with each research protocol, but flow diagrams and checklists should always be used when appropriate.

4.7 Recruitment

Planning out every aspect of patient enrollment from screening to informed consent will expedite patient recruitment, especially in the early stages of a study.[10] A recruitment plan is an in-depth blueprint that details all aspects of the recruitment process, including identifying, contacting, and consenting eligible patients for a study. Each phase of recruitment should be considered when developing a recruitment plan. ▶ Fig. 4.1 outlines the five main components of a comprehensive patient recruitment plan.

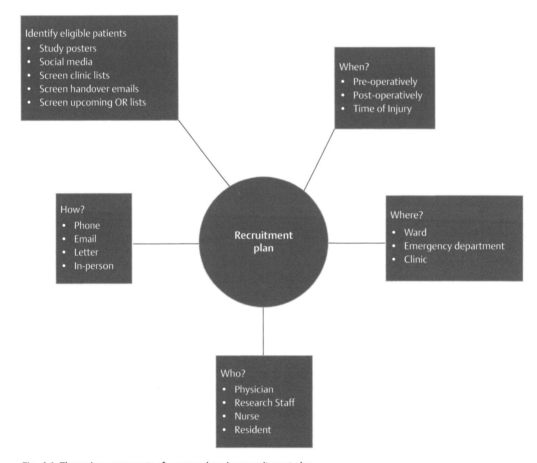

Fig. 4.1 The main components of a comprehensive recruitment plan.

It is important to consider the patient population that will be the focal point of the research question. There is no one perfect recruitment plan; rather, each recruitment plan should be individualized. For each step of the recruitment plan, consider the patient population and make informed decisions based on their demographics. There are several factors that may hinder recruitment, including a placebo arm, satisfactory existing treatments, invasive procedures, and limited prevalence of the disease.[2] Alternatively, there are several factors that may facilitate recruitment such as the lack of a satisfactory existing treatment, a large demographic population falling within the study criteria, and physician endorsement.[2]

4.7.1 Identifying Eligible Patients

The first step to a comprehensive recruitment plan is determining how eligible patients will be identified. Using a study poster or advertising on social media is an appropriate first foray for studies with minimal inclusion and exclusion criteria wherein recruitment will primarily occur from the general population. With this approach, participants will identify themselves as potential subjects and contact the research team on their own accord. Given the appropriate permissions, study posters can be placed in a hospital or clinic or even a public location such as a bus stop or shopping mall. Study posters can also be distributed electronically by email, placed on a website, or posted on social media (e.g., a Facebook page for the local hospital). ▶ Fig. 4.2 is an example of a recruitment poster for a study investigating exercise and high blood pressure. This poster includes all of the key elements, including principal investigator contact details, a brief research summary, eligibility criteria, benefits to the participants, time requirements, and additional contact information.[4]

In many studies, the inclusion and exclusion criteria are extensive, thereby narrowing the potential population pool and limiting the number of eligible patients. As such, it is far more efficient for research staff to identify eligible patients. There are many ways that this can be performed, including screening patients with clinic appointments, screening daily handover emails between residents and staff of newly consulted or admitted

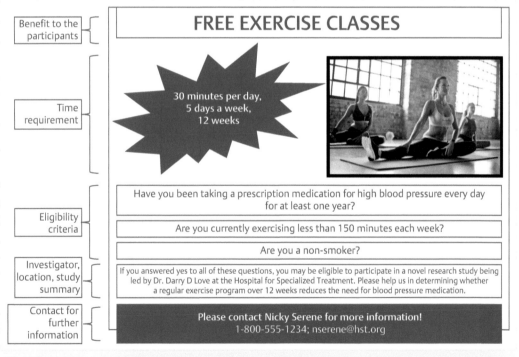

Fig. 4.2 A study recruitment poster that can be advertised around a hospital, clinic, public area, or online on a website or social media. All of the essential information that should be included in a recruitment poster are clearly indicated.

patients, or screening upcoming operating room lists. The manner in which research staff identify eligible patients will vary depending on the nature and complexity of the study. It is important to remain flexible and adapt any chosen modalities as necessary to target new or different patients.

Once eligible patients are identified, they need to be properly and ethically introduced to the study. It is important to plan out who will approach the patient, when and how the patient will be contacted, and where the initial contact will occur.

4.7.2 Who will approach the patient?

In many cases, it is advantageous for the treating physician to introduce a study to their patient. This shows the patient that the research is important to their physician and that they support participation in the study. Up to 53% of patients said they would prefer to learn about clinical research study opportunities from their physician.[1] If the physician cannot introduce the study for logistical reasons, a nurse or research coordinator should be delegated this responsibility.

Once the patient is introduced and has shown interest in participating in the study, the informed consent process must take place. Additional staff are often involved in the informed consent process. The physician may introduce the study, but the research coordinator tends to lead the informed consent discussion. Ideally, both the physician and research coordinator will be present. This way, any questions, whether they be scientific, technical, procedural, surgical, logistical, or otherwise, can be answered immediately. Preliminary research shows that having a research staff member or educator present during the consent process improves patient understanding.[15] It is up to the research coordinator in the planning phase to determine which individual will be the most knowledgeable, prepared, and available to carry out both the research introduction and the informed consent discussion.

4.7.3 When will the patient be contacted?

The protocol will dictate whether the patient is enrolled upon hospital arrival, immediately preoperatively, postoperatively while admitted, or at a consultation or follow-up clinic visit. Within the allotted time window, further consideration should be given as to when the patient should be approached. If a patient is approached preoperatively following hospital arrival, there could be minutes, hours, or days to secure informed consent. For example, if a patient presents to the emergency department with a closed midshaft tibia fracture, they may be admitted for several days before they undergo surgical fixation. In this scenario, it may be best to approach the patient the day after admission. At this point, the patient may have received a bed on the ward that provides more privacy than the emergency department. Additionally, the patient likely underwent a traumatic event leading to their fracture; therefore, if discussion about a research study can wait until the following day, it may avoid unnecessarily overwhelming the patient. Moreover, the patient may be more receptive to research once they have been given time to adjust to their environment and accept their prognosis. The specific timing of when to introduce research to patients is often overlooked, but it can have an impact on receptiveness and overall recruitment. The best time to recruit a patient will depend on the nature of the study, and it should be considered when designing the recruitment plan, prior to the starting enrollment.

4.7.4 Where will the patient be contacted?

The research coordinator has to understand how the patient flows through different departments within the hospital to decide when to introduce a research study. For example, imagine recruiting patients with wrist fractures requiring surgical fixation. It is likely that they will first present to the emergency department. However, the route the patient takes before surgery can vary greatly (▶Fig. 4.3). In this scenario, there may be more than one area to recruit patients, depending on whether they are admitted, arriving the morning of surgery or following up in the clinic. In each area, clinic or ward identify a location that is suitable for the study to be presented. The location should be private to ensure confidentiality. The patients should feel comfortable taking their time during the informed consent process. In a busy follow-up clinic environment, it may not be appropriate for recruitment and informed consent to take place in an exam room. These discussions can be time-consuming, which can negatively impact the flow of the clinic. Always have an alternative

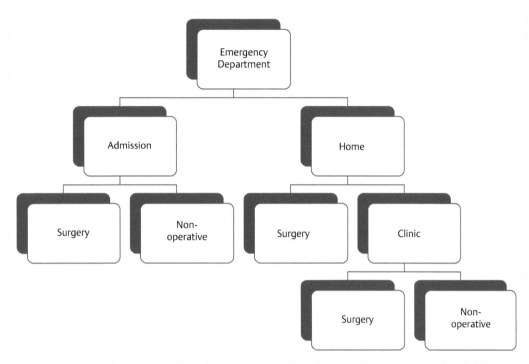

Fig. 4.3 Example of a patient flowchart from the point of the first contact to treatment.

location specified in the planning phase to facilitate multiple avenues of enrollment.

4.7.5 How will patient contact occur?

It is important to consider the method in which the study is communicated to eligible patients. In some instances, it will be most effective to introduce the study in person at an outpatient clinic visit or on the hospital ward. Other times, it may be beneficial to come at it via a different approach such as a telephone call, email, or letter. The study design and patient population may dictate one method of communication over another. For example, an in-person introduction may be advantageous versus an email when recruiting from an elderly population. However, recruiting via telephone calls may be advantageous if it allows more potentially eligible patients to be contacted in a given time frame. Research coordinators should investigate the pros and cons of each method of communication for introducing the study prior to the start of recruitment so as to reach as many patients as possible in the most efficient manner.

4.8 Practical Application

4.8.1 Designing a Recruitment Plan

In this practical application, our goal is to provide a theoretical recruitment plan for a study targeting elderly patients with hip fractures. The study aims to assess independence after hip fracture surgery between participants who are randomized to general anesthesia versus spinal anesthesia. Hip fracture patients typically present to the emergency department where their fracture is identified and the orthopaedic service is called or paged for a consultation. These patients will then be admitted and assigned a bed on the orthopaedic ward. In most cases, these patients are consented for surgical management of their fracture and have surgery within 1 to 3 days of hospital arrival. Pending circumstances and availability, these patients may also go directly from the emergency department to the operating room. The preoperative course for patients with hip fractures in this study is outlined below (▶Fig. 4.4).

The first step in this recruitment plan is determining how potentially eligible patients will be

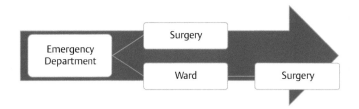

Fig. 4.4 Preoperative course for patients with hip fractures.

identified. Ideally, the on-call resident or staff will be fully versed in the research studies currently being performed within the division, and upon recognizing an elderly patient with a hip fracture, will quickly assess their eligibility against the inclusion and exclusion criteria outlined on a study poster posted in the emergency department, and then contact the research coordinator to follow-up should they deem the patient to be potentially eligible. Alas, this scenario does not always unfold seamlessly for a myriad of reasons (e.g., junior resident too busy juggling cases to prioritize research and off-service resident unaware of research study); therefore, the recruitment plan must outline numerous avenues and pathways accordingly.

As a hip fracture is a traumatic event, it is unlikely that study advertisements in the hospital or posted online via social media will be an effective method. Arguably, the best way for a research coordinator to identify patients will be through screening the daily handover emails between residents and staff. Any patient that is consulted or admitted through the orthopaedic service in the previous 8 to 12 hours will be listed and discussed on the daily handover email. Handover emails normally include a brief rundown of diagnosis, comorbidities, and a plan for surgical management. From the clinical perspective, this information allows for the efficient continuation of care between shifts. For the research coordinator, it affords the opportunity to quickly scan through emergent patients and identify potentially eligible research subjects.

Once a patient is identified, and as this is a randomized, interventional trial, it is advantageous for the physician to introduce the study to the patient. As the patient is admitted to the hospital, this can happen in person. According to the study protocol, patients must be approached preoperatively as their anesthetic provided during surgery will be randomized. Introducing the study when the patient is on the ward is beneficial as it is a quieter environment, and hopefully, the patient

has had time to settle in, consult with the family and loved ones, and come to terms with the diagnosis. However, as indicated in ▶ Fig. 4.4, not all patients will go to the ward preoperatively. Therefore, it is reasonable and necessary to handle recruitment on a case-by-case basis. If it appears as though the patient will go directly to the operating room, then it will be necessary to approach them in the emergency department; if not, then wait until the patient is on the ward.

Within this patient population, there will a percentage of eligible patients who are unable to provide their own consent due to cognitive deficits. These patients will often have a designated substitute decision maker in place (i.e., a family member, friend, or caretaker). The recruitment plan should be flexible and have contingencies in place to account for these situations. The substitute decision maker may or may not be physically present in the hospital and thus may need to be contacted via a phone call, if permissible according to the ethical regulations. If possible, it is still beneficial for the physician to be the one to introduce the study to the substitute decision maker, while the informed consent process can be led by the research coordinator. In this situation, prior to contacting the substitute decision maker, it is advisable to preliminarily check as many of the inclusion and exclusion criteria as possible so that the phone call to gain informed consent for the patient proceeds efficiently and is one of the few remaining tasks that needs to be completed for recruitment before randomization into the study.

4.9 Conclusion

In order for study progress to take off rapidly and the recruitment phase to commence as seamlessly and promptly as possible, careful thought and planning must go into the early stages of study development. The research coordinator should be involved from day 1 of the planning stages of the study. This will help to limit future pitfalls and roadblocks that may then require costly and untimely protocol amendments. The research coordinator should evaluate the study in terms of patient recruitment, logistics, and feasibility. In addition, it is advisable for the research coordinator to initiate communication early on with other departments to highlight the importance of the study and incorporate any feedback into the development of the protocol and recruitment plan. The informed consent form should be clear, concise, and informational. The target population should be kept in mind throughout the early planning stages, especially when creating a recruitment plan for the study. Consider the how, when, where, and who of patient recruitment and enrollment into the study. Communication between the principal investigator and the research coordinator to plan out each stage of the study will limit the burden on other departments and the study patients. In doing so, it will accelerate patient recruitment, expedite the overall progress of the study, and improve the perception of clinical research.

Definitions

- **Recruitment plan:** Outline of steps contrived by the principal investigator, research coordinator, and research team to ensure that the trial design and protocol development, trial feasibility and site selection, and communication are all tailored toward making patient recruitment as easy and efficient a process as possible during the conduct of the study.
- **Informed consent:** Ongoing process that starts with the principal investigator and/or research coordinator contacting a potential patient about a clinical research study and continues until the study is complete or the participant withdraws from participation. Any discussion of informed consent, the information sheet or written informed consent form, or any other written information given to participants should provide adequate information to make an informed decision about their participation in the clinical research study.
- **Eligibility:** Factors that allow a patient to participate in a clinical research study are called inclusion criteria, while factors that disqualify participation are called exclusion criteria. These criteria are based on characteristics such as age, gender, the type and stage of an injury or

disease, previous treatment history, and other medical conditions and comorbidities.
- **Substitute decision maker:** Someone whose responsibility is to make decisions for a person who is not able to make his or her own healthcare decisions. Such a person can be: a legally appointed guardian; a power of attorney for personal care; a representative appointed by the Consent and Capacity Board; a spouse, partner, child, parent, brother, sister, or any other relative by blood or marriage; a treatment decision consultant from the Office of the Public Guardian and Trustee.
- **Randomization:** Process by which subjects are assigned by chance to separate groups that compare different treatments or other interventions. Randomization gives each participant an equal chance of being assigned to any of the groups being studies in the clinical research study.

References

[1] BBK Worldwide. The Will & Why Survey: Examining America's Motivation to Participate in Clinical Studies. Needham, MA: BBK Healthcare Inc; 2003
[2] Bachenheimer JF, Brescia BA. Reinventing Patient Recruitment: Revolutionary Ideas for Clinical Trial Success. New York, NY: Gower Publishing; 2017
[3] Rosenbaum D, Dresser M, eds. Clinical Research Coordinator Handbook: GCP Tools and Techniques. Boca Raton, FL: CRC Press; 2015
[4] Liu MB, Davis K. A Clinical Trials Manual from the Duke Clinical Research Institute: Lessons from a Horse Named Jim. Chichester, West Sussex: Wiley-Blackwell; 2010
[5] Pelke S, Easa D. The Role of the Clinical Research Coordinator in Multicenter Clinical Trials. J Obstet Gynecol Neonatal Nurs 1997;26(3):279–285
[6] Rico-Villademoros F, Hernando T, Sanz JL, et al. The Role of the Clinical Research Coordinator—Data manager—in Oncology Clinical Trials. BMC Med Res Methodol 2004;4:6
[7] Friedman DB, Foster C, Bergeron CD, Tanner A, Kim SH. A Qualitative Study of Recruitment Barriers, Motivators, and Community-Based Strategies for Increasing Clinical Trials Participation Among Rural and Urban Populations. Am J Health Promot 2015;29(5):332–338
[8] Boden-Albala B, Carman H, Southwick L, et al. Examining Barriers and Practices to Recruitment and Retention in Stroke Clinical Trials. Stroke 2015;46(8):2232–2237
[9] Williams RL, Johnson SB, Greene SM, et al. Principal Investigators of Clinical Research Networks Initiative. Signposts along the NIH roadmap for reengineering clinical research: lessons from the Clinical Research Networks initiative. Arch Intern Med 2008;168(17): 1919–1925

[10] Kadam RA, Borde SU, Madas SA, Salvi SS, Limaye SS. Challenges in Recruitment and Retention of Clinical Trial Subjects. Perspect Clin Res 2016;7(3):137–143

[11] Fujiwara N, Ochiai R, Shirai Y, et al. Qualitative Analysis of Clinical Research Coordinators' Role in Phase I Cancer Clinical Trials. Contemp Clin Trials Commun 2017;8: 156–161

[12] Zielinski SM, Viveiros H, Heetveld MJ, et al. FAITH Trial Investigators. Central Coordination as an Alternative for Local Coordination in a Multicenter Randomized Controlled Trial: The FAITH Trial Experience. Trials 2012;13:5

[13] Sole ML, Middleton A, Deaton L, Bennett M, Talbert S, Penoyer D. Enrollment Challenges in Critical Care Nursing Research. Am J Crit Care 2017;26(5):395–400

[14] Haley SJ, Southwick LE, Parikh NS, Rivera J, Farrar-Edwards D, Boden-Albala B. Barriers and Strategies for Recruitment of Racial and Ethnic Minorities: Perspectives from Neurological Clinical Research Coordinators. J Racial Ethn Health Disparities 2017;4(6):1225–1236

[15] Flory J, Emanuel E. IInterventions to Improve Research Participants' Understanding in Informed Consent for Research: A Systematic Review. JAMA 2004;292(13): 1593–1601

Further Reading

Cavalieri RJ, Rupp ME. Clinical research manual: practical tools and templates for managing clinical research. Indianapolis, IN: Sigma Theta Tau International; 2013

Part II

What Every Research Coordinator Needs To Know

5 What Is Evidence-Based
  Medicine?   50

6 Randomized Controlled Trials 58

7 Observational Studies   68

8 Surveys   81

9 Qualitative Studies   94

10 Principles of Good Clinical
   Practice and Research
   Conduct   109

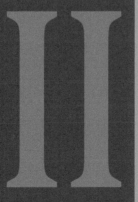

5 What Is Evidence-Based Medicine?

Ellie B.M. Landman

Abstract

A shift in medical practice from being based on clinical experience and opinion toward the use of scientific evidence as a foundation for clinical decision-making has led to the introduction of the term evidence-based medicine (EBM) in 1991. Since then, the concept of predicating decisions about the care for individual patients upon findings from medical research, in conjunction with the patients' preferences and personal circumstances, has become an accepted approach in current medicine. However, to apply EBM in daily clinical practice requires a thorough literature search, critical appraisal of the available literature, and careful consideration of a patient's opinion and circumstances. This can be a time-consuming process that requires specific skills. Although EBM is widely accepted as an important, or even necessary, aspect in medical practice, it is not always applied. The aim of this chapter is to outline the principles of EBM and the difficulties it brings along, and how to apply EBM in daily clinical practice.

Keywords: evidence-based medicine, levels of evidence, critical appraisal, shared decision-making

5.1 Introduction

To conscientiously, explicitly, judiciously, and reasonably apply the best available evidence for making decisions about the care for individual patients is what evidence-based medicine (EBM) stands for. In practice, it means that clinicians must consult appropriate literature and apply findings in discussing what is best for an individual patient. During decades before the term EBM was first introduced in 1991, the approach in clinical practice was shifting from being based on medical knowledge and experience to a more scientific foundation. However, adhering to the principles of EBM in daily practice is not as straightforward as it might seem at first. Consulting literature entails more than just finding the most recent publication. One needs to evaluate the research design, the applied analysis, and the correctness of the interpretation of data to judge literature on its true value. Next, applying research findings from a study population to an individual patient presents clinicians with completely different challenges. Each patient not only has his own personal circumstances and preferences but also characteristics such as comorbidities that should be taken into account. As EBM was accepted as an acknowledged approach in medicine, advances have been made to facilitate evidence-based clinical practice.

To apply EBM in daily clinical practice requires continuous time and effort, and conducting clinical research to support practice is inevitable. The aim of this chapter is to provide a brief history of the development of EBM, to outline the principles underlying EBM and the challenges that come along with it, and to explain what it means to apply EBM in clinical practice today.

5.2 The History of Evidence-Based Medicine

After years of work by multiple people that led to the idea of critically reviewing the literature and the concept of using scientific facts rather than personal experience or opinion as a basis for clinical practice, Gordon Guyatt first introduced the term "EBM" in 1991. The preliminary concept of EBM was already developed in the decades preceding the introduction of the term EBM. In the 1960s, new methods of medical education were developed in North America and the Canadian health system was altered to provide universal coverage of medical costs. These changes initiated a careful beginning of what would later be considered EBM. When McMaster University was founded in 1968, clinical epidemiology methods played a crucial role in the problem-based learning curriculum and it became the first university with a department of clinical epidemiology and biostatistics. From 1978, courses on "critical appraisal" were taught, focusing on the critical assessment of clinical information about diagnosis, etiology, and therapy. These courses led to several publications on the methods of critical appraisal, leading up to the introduction of EBM in 1991. Guyatt initially suggested the term "scientific medicine," but this raised objection from both clinicians and scientists. The term "EBM" seemed to appeal to everyone and quickly became a well-known term throughout the medical world.[1]

The initial publication introducing EBM led to a series of 32 articles published over the course of 11 years, comprising the latest developments in clinical epidemiology, which was termed EBM from that moment onward. The number of publications found on PubMed using the term "EBM" increased exponentially during the first decade after the term was introduced. In 2017, the term was mentioned in almost 15,000 publications, and nowadays, it is considered a generally applied approach in medical practice.[2]

5.3 Principles of Evidence-Based Medicine

The aim of EBM is to improve medical care for patients by providing a scientific basis for clinical decision-making. Finding the best available evidence, critically appraising the evidence for its trustworthiness and applicability, and weighing evidence with patients' preferences are the basic principles underlying EBM. Using a systematic approach to integrate evidence from research with clinical expertise and patients' preferences aims to result in the best care for the patient. Each step in this approach brings up challenges and requires clinicians to invest time and effort to successfully

fulfill them. Progress has been made toward providing tools and skills to optimize the necessary actions to practice EBM thoroughly and efficiently.

5.3.1 Best Available Evidence

The first principle of EBM is to apply the best available evidence as a basis for clinical decision-making. But what is the "best evidence" and how does one narrow down the required information from the massive amount of available literature? To be able to use scientific evidence as a basis for clinical practice, one needs to not only be aware of most recent medical literature but also be able to judge the reliability and applicability of available literature.

Hierarchy of Evidence

Critical appraisal, the process of systematically evaluating scientific literature to judge its reliability, validity, and relevance form the basis of practicing EBM. The hierarchical levels of evidence can provide a guide to support the decision for which piece of evidence should be considered "best" and thus used for clinical decision-making.[3] The levels of evidence classify scientific literature based on their research design and the likelihood of bias to occur (▶Fig. 5.1).[4]

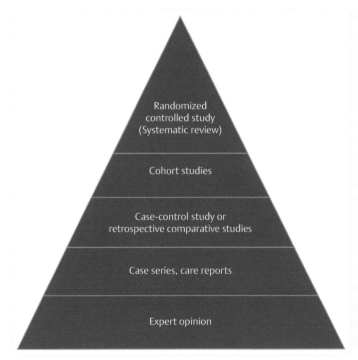

Fig. 5.1 Hierarchy of levels of evidence of different study designs.

Randomized controlled study (Systematic review)

Cohort studies

Case-control study or retrospective comparative studies

Case series, care reports

Expert opinion

Level I evidence: Randomized controlled trials (RCTs), systematic reviews, and meta-analyses

Systematic reviews of RCTs and meta-analyses, summarizing data from multiple studies, can provide reliable statements based on large sample sizes. Therefore, these are considered to provide the most reliable, level I, evidence. A good quality meta-analysis should use explicit selection criteria for relevant literature to address a specific clinical question.[5]

In RCTs, treatments are randomly allocated to patients so that potentially confounding factors are randomized as well. Therefore, RCTs are considered to provide level I evidence, as the possibility to introduce bias is minimized and conclusions can be considered more reliable.[6]

Level II evidence: Cohort studies

Ranked just below RCTs and meta-analyses are cohort studies. In this prospective study design, patients are assigned to cohorts based on the presence or absence of certain characteristics or exposures and followed for the outcome of interest. For a research question that cannot be answered by an RCT due to practical or ethical limitations, a cohort study can provide the highest level of evidence possible.[6]

Level III evidence: Case–control studies

In the retrospective design of case–control studies, patients are selected based on the presence or absence of the outcome of interest, and potentially prognostic factors are identified by comparing certain characteristics or exposure. Although no direct causative relation can be proven, case–control studies can provide useful insight into potential risk factors for the outcome of interest.

Level IV evidence: Case reports and case series

For rare conditions, case reports, describing the intervention and outcome for a single patient, or case series, describing multiple patients, can be useful. This observational study design that is not controlled provides only weak evidence.[6] It can, however, be used to describe rare cases and provide the hypothesis to set up a more elaborate study providing higher level evidence.

Level V evidence: Expert opinion

At the bottom of the pyramid are expert opinions, in which the view of an expert in the field on a specific topic is described. As expert opinions are based on the individual opinion of the author, this study design is highly susceptible to bias.

5.3.2 Evaluate Available Evidence

The second principle of EBM is to correctly value the best available evidence before applying it when making decisions about care for individual patients. As the trustworthiness of available evidence is determined by the choice of study design, proper conduct, and appropriate analysis and interpretation of data, one needs to correctly evaluate these aspects of the selected literature. Only when based on properly designed, conducted, and analyzed research, evidence should be used for the practice of EBM.

Critical Appraisal

Although the hierarchy of levels of evidence provides a comprehensive basis for the evaluation of medical literature, one cannot easily say that medical practice can only be based on the highest level of evidence. It is not correct to say that only an RCT (or a systematic review thereof) can provide the "best" evidence that is needed to support clinical decision-making. Critical appraisal of available literature plays an important role in EBM. The validity and reliability of each individual study should always be assessed, before deciding whether its results should be used for making clinical decisions. When evaluating medical literature, one should note the importance of identifying types of errors and the power of the study. An important difference in the outcome can be missed or misinterpreted when a study is underpowered. Therefore, it can be more appropriate to disregard a badly designed or conducted RCT and rely on the results of a cohort study that is properly designed and conducted.

In addition, not all research questions can be studied by performing an RCT. For certain questions, a study design ranked lower on the hierarchy of levels of evidence can be most suitable. This might be due to ethical or practical considerations. For instance, it is not possible to conduct an RCT to study the effect of a healthy versus an unhealthy diet on a certain outcome. It would be unethical to subject patients to a lifestyle that is a known cause for certain health problems. Therefore, for this situation, a cohort study would be the most suitable study design to provide the best evidence possible.

Judicious and Reasonable

To conscientiously, explicitly, judiciously, and reasonably apply evidence in making decisions about the care for patients, one needs to judge the trustworthiness of the available evidence.[7] It is important for clinicians to understand the different study designs and their advantages and drawbacks to facilitate critical appraisal of medical literature. Moreover, as medical research is continuously in progress, keeping up-to-date about the latest advances is crucial. As it is unrealistic for clinicians to be able to be up-to-date regarding all relevant scientific literature, summarizing the best available evidence in systematic reviews (and meta-analyses) has come more and more in vogue. However, caution needs to be taken when using systematic reviews for clinical decisions, as the quality of a systematic review determines its value. For a good systematic review, the question to be answered needs to be detailed and clear. The individual studies included in the systematic review (and meta-analysis) should ideally be aimed at answering the same research question in a similar population.

To facilitate finding and evaluating available evidence, preappraised sources of information can provide assistance. The Grading of Recommendation, Assessment, Development, and Evaluation framework provides a tool to rate the quality (or certainty) of evidence and the strength of recommendations. The approach is based on evaluating the inconsistency, indirectness, imprecision, risk of bias, and publication bias.[8]

Realistically, not all practical clinical questions can be answered by published findings from clinical studies providing reliable evidence. In certain circumstances, assumptions and rationale need to be used when making recommendations. Assumptions and rationale are subjective in nature and may interfere with judiciously applying EBM. However, there are cases for which it is the best one can do and it is up to the clinician to be as subjective as possible.

Furthermore, in this era of rising costs for medical care, it is important to take into account cost-effectiveness. Health insurers keep strict regulations of the treatments that they cover. Therefore, the best treatment according to literature might not always be the available treatment, when it cannot be provided in a cost-effective manner. In addition, the fact that not every hospital has the facilities to provide certain care and the need for referral might have an additional influence on the choice of treatment.

5.3.3 Application of Evidence in the Care for Individual Patients

Once the best available evidence is identified, the question of "what is best for the individual patient?" remains. One needs to take into account the personal needs and the opinion of each individual patient. The best available scientific evidence provides an indication about which treatment might be better in the study population, in terms of, for instance, survival. Although a properly designed trial with a large sample size of a heterogeneous study population provides a result that should be relevant to patients in general, results do not necessarily apply to each individual patient. Usually, the presence of comorbidities is a reason for patients to be ineligible to participate in a study, whereas many patients do suffer from multiple conditions. Therefore, study results are not directly applicable to many patients. Moreover, patients' preferences or circumstances might affect which outcome they value most. As some patients might value how long they survive after a certain treatment, others might consider the quality of their remaining life more relevant and choose a different treatment, or even no treatment at all. Thus, the best available scientific evidence might provide an indication about which treatment gives a patient, in general, the best chance of, for instance, survival, but personal circumstances and preferences might influence the decision about what is the best option for that one particular patient.

Shared Decision-Making

The process of integrating research findings with the patients' preferences and situation plays a major role in shared decision-making. To involve patients in medical decision-making requires that the clinician communicates different options and the associating benefits and harms with the patient. The clinician needs to summarize the available evidence for the patient in a comprehensible manner. This way, patients can weigh their personal preferences and what they value as important in the chances of benefits and harms.[9]

As a result of practicing EBM, guidelines for the treatment of many common health issues have been developed. The use of guidelines helps to facilitate clinicians in using the current best available evidence in clinical decision-making. However, guidelines do not take into account possible comorbidities and risks and often disregard patients' preferences. Therefore, due to the introduction of guidelines, personalized medical care based on patients' preferences might be jeopardized.[10]

5.4 Where Do We Stand in Evidence-Based Medicine Today?

Since its first introduction, EBM has become an important factor in clinical decision-making. As the concept of EBM has gained support, the necessities needed for evidence-based practicing have come in focus. The need for clinical studies, based on a clear and descriptive research question, using a solid research design, and appropriate analyses, is acknowledged. Large RCTs are generally accepted as the ideal study design to provide a reliable answer to clinical questions (providing it is the most suitable study design relevant for the particular clinical question). As a result, current clinical research is more fitted to provide reliable evidence to support evidence-based decision-making.

In addition, advances have been made in the accessibility and understanding of medical information, and the development of summarized evidence-based information. To be able to apply EBM in clinical practice, the need for clinicians to have the skills to understand and interpret clinical research has emerged. Databases, such as the Cochrane Library, enable the clinician to perform efficient searches. The Cochrane Database of Systematic Reviews provides an overview of different types of high-quality, independent evidence to support clinical decision-making.

Finally, the focus on patients' opinion and preferences in shared decision-making has increased.[11] Patients have more information available to them, and clinicians recognize the importance of patient participation in making clinical decisions. Their clinical expertise enables clinicians to deduce findings from clinical research, translate them to patients, and weigh them with patients' circumstances and preferences.

5.4.1 Criticism of Evidence-Based Medicine

With the rising popularity of EBM in medicine, so has criticism with regards to the principles of EBM increased as well. Critics claim that there is no evidence that EBM in itself has had a beneficial effect on health care. However, there are numerous examples of cases where the clinical practice was not based on thorough research, resulting in catastrophic failures, for instance, hormone replacement therapy in postmenopausal women leading to an increased risk of breast cancer and the advice to put babies to sleep on their belly resulting in an increased incidence of sudden infant death. Another argument against EBM is its strict adherence to the hierarchy of studies and the need for RCTs as the only reliable evidence is felt to be overrated. However, critical appraisal of available literature plays a key role in EBM. The quality as well as the appropriateness of the study design are reviewed before applying results. Even though RCTs, or the systematic reviews thereof, are on the top of the hierarchy, EBM does not ignore those situations for which the best available evidence is not provided by RCTs. In addition, critics consider EBM "cookbook medicine," without leaving space for clinical reasoning, or specific adjustment to a particular patient. However, the incorporation of patients' specific preferences and values is one of the key elements of EBM.[12] Clinical reasoning is inevitably applied in weighing risks and benefits with patients' preferences, to reach a joint decision about the best care for the individual patient.

Another issue that is brought up by opponents of EBM is the fact that more and more clinical research is funded by industry. The increase of industry-funded research risks concession of the objectiveness of presented data and subsequent conclusions in favor of the study sponsor. When critically assessing available literature, one needs to be aware of the sources of research funding and take into account potential underlying interests.[8]

Moreover, with the emergence of the use of electronic medical records, opportunities to use collected information in retrospective studies to assess the effectiveness of treatment and quality of care have increased. Although this information can be useful, one needs to be aware of the biases imposed by observational studies, as treatments are not randomly allocated but provided based on choice. It is important to keep in mind the hierarchy of levels of evidence and to critically evaluate the appropriateness of the study design that is used to answer a research question.[8]

5.4.2 Clinical Research

The application of EBM in clinical practice depends on clinical research and has increased the focus on potential bias and the importance of good quality research. The necessity of conducting large studies to provide adequate power to reliably answer a clinical research question is widely accepted. Understanding the drawbacks and advantages of different study designs enables researchers to properly design a study that provides solid evidence that can be used to support EBM. With the acceptance of EBM as an important aspect of modern medicine, the quality of clinical research has improved considerably.

5.5 Practical Application

To facilitate the practical application of EBM in daily clinical practice, a systematic approach is best applied. A stepwise approach enables clinicians to integrate the best evidence from the literature with clinical expertise and patients' preferences (▶Table 5.1). First, it is necessary to formulate a clear and descriptive clinical question. A patient presenting with a particular problem might comprise many details and raise multiple questions; therefore, it is important to clearly define the clinical problem at hand. A detailed question that specifies the particular patient, the intervention in question and possibly a comparative intervention, and the outcome of interest, facilitates finding the answer. Next, the specific terms used to formulate the clinical question can be used to perform a directed search. Multiple online databases of medical literature, such as the Cochrane Library and Medline, can be used. Using a combination of keywords or limiting a search to, for instance, a certain type of publication can be helpful to obtain a reasonable number of results that fit the clinical question. Subsequently, the critical appraisal of the literature is of key importance to answer the clinical question. One cannot simply choose the most recent article but should also judge the validity and relevance

Table 5.1 Application of EBM in clinical practice

	Actions
1. Formulate clinical question	Who is the patient? (Or, what is the problem?)
	What is the intervention?
	What are comparative interventions (if applicable)?
	What is the outcome of interest?
2. Search evidence	Use suitable keywords (from the clinical question)
	Use a database (e.g., Cochrane Library and Medline) to search
3. Appraise evidence	Does the study design give valid results?
	What is the result?
	Are study results applicable to the patient?
4. Apply evidence	What are patient's opinion and preference?
	Does the selected evidence fit the individual patient?

Abbreviation: EBM, evidence-based medicine.

of the literature. Finally, the theoretical "best" for the patient should be weighed with the personal preferences and opinion of the patient. The details of the evidence in terms of efficacy and risks should be discussed with the patient, in a comprehensible way, to allow the patient to make an informed decision. Conversely, the patients' preferences and personal circumstances should be taken into account when evaluating the available treatment options. Moreover, the accessibility and cost of the proposed intervention should be considered.[12]

5.5.1 Clinical Example

A 23-year-old female patient presents at the orthopaedic surgeon's office with persistent knee pain. She is an active tennis player but is impaired by the pain she experiences. After radiographic examination, she is diagnosed with osteoarthritis of the medial femoral condyle. As she is too young to undergo knee arthroplasty, the orthopaedic surgeon considers other treatment options. As the patient's legs are in a slight varus position, the surgeon considers whether an osteotomy of the proximal tibia would be an option for this patient.

Formulate a clear and descriptive clinical question

- Patient: A 23-year-old female patient with unicompartmental medial knee osteoarthritis.
- Intervention: Osteotomy of the proximal tibia.
- Comparison: There is no comparative treatment available.
- Outcome: Reducing pain and improving knee function.

Search for evidence

Searching PubMed for "tibial osteotomy" and "knee osteoarthritis" and "pain" gives 327 results, of which 20 are systematic reviews in English.

Critically appraise evidence

Regarding tibial osteotomy as the treatment for knee osteoarthritis of the medial compartment, only one systematic review[13] (and two updates thereof) and one meta-analysis[14] were considered applicable. The systematic review included 21 studies. Based on weak evidence, it concluded that tibial osteotomy reduced pain and improved function. In the meta-analysis, tibial osteotomy was compared with unicondylar medial arthroplasty, concluding that osteotomy reduced pain in younger patients with associated slightly compromised function.

Apply evidence to specific patient

In view of the age of the patient and the fact that she is impaired by pain, the orthopaedic surgeon considers tibial osteotomy a suitable treatment option. He discusses the expected improvement in pain, the recovery after surgery, and the slight impairment in function that can be expected. The patient decides she would rather play tennis at a reduced intensity without pain and decides to undergo proximal tibial osteotomy.

5.6 Conclusion

EBM has become an important aspect in current medical practice, aimed at using the best available evidence when making decisions about individual patients. The concept of EBM is based on integrating the findings from clinical research with the patients' preferences and personal circumstances to reach a joint decision about the care for the patient. To practice EBM, it is crucial for clinicians to be able to identify and evaluate available literature, communicate options with the patient, and be open to the patient's opinion and personal situation.

Definitions

- **Critical appraisal:** The process of systematically evaluating the outcome of medical research to assess its validity, reliability, and applicability to a specific situation.
- **Evidence-based medicine:** An approach to conscientiously, explicitly, judiciously, and reasonably apply the best available evidence for making decisions about the care for individual patients.
- **Hierarchy of levels of evidence:** The ranking of research designs based on the likelihood of bias.
- **Shared decision-making:** The joint process between clinician and patient, during which the clinician discusses treatments and alternatives to enable the patient to partake in making a medical decision.

References

[1] Guyatt G, Voelker R. Everything You Ever Wanted to Know About Evidence-based Medicine. JAMA 2015; 313(18):1783–1785
[2] Zimerman AL. Evidence-based Medicine: A Short History of a Modern Medical Movement. Virtual Mentor 2013;15(1):71–76
[3] Petrisor B, Bhandari M. The Hierarchy of Evidence: Levels and Grades of Recommendation. Indian J Orthop 2007;41(1):11–15
[4] Burns PB, Rohrich RJ, Chung KC. The levels of evidence and their role in evidence-based medicine. Plast Reconstr Surg 2011;128(1):305–310
[5] Montori VM, Swiontkowski MF, Cook DJ. Methodologic Issues in Systematic Reviews and Meta-analyses. Clin Orthop Relat Res 2003(413):43–54
[6] Sprague S, McKay P, Thoma A. Study Design and Hierarchy of Evidence for Surgical Decision Making. Clin Plast Surg 2008;35(2):195–205
[7] Evidence-Based Medicine Working Group. Evidence-Based Medicine. A New Approach to Teaching the Practice of Medicine. JAMA 1992;268(17):2420–2425
[8] Guyatt GH, Oxman AD, Schünemann HJ, Tugwell P, Knottnerus A. GRADE Guidelines: A New Series of Articles in the Journal of Clinical Epidemiology. J Clin Epidemiol 2011;64(4):380–382
[9] Hoffmann TC, Del Mar CB. Shared Decision Making: What Do Clinicians Need to Know and Why Should They Bother? Med J Aust 2014;201(9):513–514

[10] McCartney M, Treadwell J, Maskrey N, Lehman R. Making Evidence Based Medicine Work for Individual Patients. BMJ 2016;353:i2452

[11] Djulbegovic B, Guyatt GH. Progress in Evidence-Based Medicine: A Quarter Century on. Lancet 2017; 390(10092):415–423

[12] Akobeng AK. Principles of Evidence Based Medicine. Arch Dis Child 2005;90(8):837–840

[13] Brouwer RW, Huizinga MR, Duivenvoorden T, et al. Osteotomy for Treating Knee Osteoarthritis. Cochrane Database Syst Rev 2014(12):CD004019

[14] Spahn G, Hofmann GO, von Engelhardt LV, Li M, Neubauer H, Klinger HM. The Impact of a High Tibial Valgus Osteotomy and Unicondylar Medial Arthroplasty on the Treatment for Knee Osteoarthritis: a Meta-Analysis. Knee Surg Sports Traumatol Arthrosc 2013;21(1):96–112

Further Reading

Cochrane Library of Systematic Reviews. https://www.cochranelibrary.com/cdsr/reviews. Accessed November 20, 2019

GRADE Working Group. http://www.gradeworkinggroup.org. Accessed November 22, 2018

Guyatt G, Rennie D, Meade MO, Cook DJ; American Medical Association. Users' Guides to the Medical Literature: A Manual for Evidence-Based Clinical Practice. New York, NY: McGraw-Hill Education; 2015

6 Randomized Controlled Trials

Miriam Garrido Clua

Abstract

This chapter provides an overview of considerations for the development of a randomized controlled trial (RCT), which is the gold standard level of proof in clinical research. In this chapter, you will learn the main features of RCTs and how to design, evaluate, assess, and monitor a randomized trial. The research coordinator should be able to conduct a high-quality trial while protecting the rights and welfare of human subjects.

Keywords: randomized controlled trial, blinding, outcomes assessment, data collection, data monitoring

6.1 Introduction

The clinical trial is a relatively recent development in medical research. Its evolution dates back to the 18th century.[1] Prior to the 1950s, most research was based upon case series or uncontrolled observations. The concept of randomization was introduced by Fisher and applied in agriculture research in 1926. The randomized clinical trial or randomized controlled trial (RCT) has remained the premier source of new knowledge in medicine since then.

The RCT is regarded as one of the most valued research methodologies for examining the efficacy or effectiveness of interventions. It is considered to be the gold standard in evidence-based medicine, according to the hierarchy of evidence.[2] The majority of RCTs are drugs studies or studies of therapy.

Other study interventions can be surgical operations, physical therapy, physiological treatments, or other modalities to modify illness.

This chapter is an introduction to the major concepts and approaches involved in designing and conducting an RCT.

6.2 What Is a Randomized Controlled Trial?

An RCT is an experiment in which participants are randomly assigned to treatment conditions (i.e., they have an equal probability of being assigned to any group). Procedures are controlled to ensure that all participants in all study groups are treated the same except for the intervention that is unique to their group. RCTs incorporate methodologies that reduce the potential for bias (randomization and blinding) and that allow for comparison between intervention and control groups (▶ Fig. 6.1).

The primary goal of conducting an RCT is to test whether an intervention works by comparing it to a control condition, which is usually either no intervention (e.g., placebo) or an alternative intervention (e.g., standard-of-care). Secondary goals may include identifying factors that influence the effects of the intervention and understanding the processes through which an intervention influences change.[3]

The key to this type of study is that it is a planned experiment and can provide sound evidence of

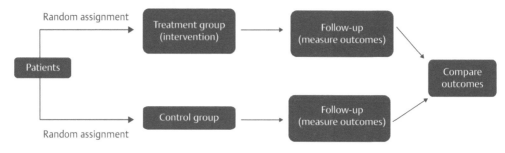

Fig. 6.1 Randomized controlled trial.

cause and effect. The effect of the intervention is measured and the events that are measured and compared are known as outcomes.

As with all study designs, RCTs have both strengths and limitations (▶ Table 6.1).

6.2.1 Study Population

One of the most important aspects when designing a study is choosing the inclusion and exclusion criteria that define the target population. The eligibility criteria are developed by the investigator before beginning the study. The eligibility criteria will define who will be included in the study and who will be excluded from the study.

The eligibility criteria should ensure a balance between generalizability and minimization of bias. Strict criteria may create challenges in recruiting suitable patients and the results will be less generalizable. On the other hand, criteria that are too broad may create challenges in identifying the true effect of the intervention and which variables make a real impact on the outcome of interest.[4] Inclusion and exclusion criteria should be directly related to the research question being answered.[3]

6.2.2 Randomized Controlled Trial Study Design

There are different types of RCT designs. The most frequently used design for randomized trials is the parallel design in which treatment and controls are allocated to two or more different groups (▶ Fig. 6.2).

There are also randomized trials with a factorial design that evaluate multiple factors simultaneously (▶ Fig. 6.3). For example, investigators could study the effects of irrigation pressure (high versus low pressure) and irrigation solution (soap versus saline) in patients with open fractures. Group 1 would receive high pressure and soap. Group 2 would receive low pressure and soap. Group 3 would receive high pressure and saline. Group 4 would receive low pressure and saline. Factorial designs permit researchers to investigate the joint effect of two or more factors on a dependent variable. The factorial design also facilitates the study of interactions, illuminating the effects of different conditions of the experiment on identifiable subgroups of subjects participating in the experiment.[5]

A randomized trial can also have a crossover design. In these types of studies, each patient receives several different treatments in a randomized order (▶ Fig. 6.4). In this study design, the patient is own control. Generally, this design requires a smaller sample size.[6]

Table 6.1 Strengths and limitations of RCTs

Strengths	Limitations
Gold standard for obtaining evidence of a treatment effect	Expensive and time-consuming
Ability to evaluate causation	Shorter duration follow-up (inefficiency of detection of delayed outcomes)
Bias minimized by allocation concealment and blinding	Ethical restrictions
Randomization avoids confounding	Strict inclusion/exclusion criteria

Abbreviation: RCTs, randomized controlled trials.

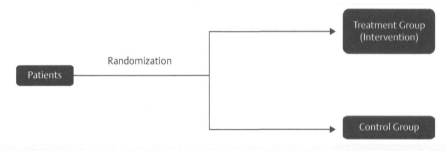

Fig. 6.2 Parallel design.

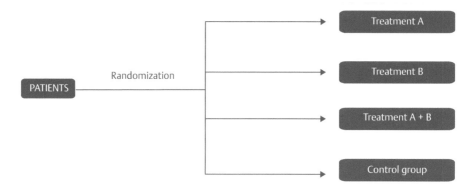

Fig. 6.3 Factorial design.

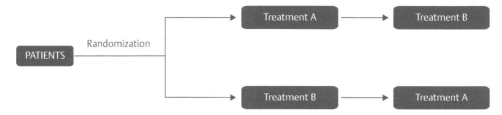

Fig. 6.4 Crossover design.

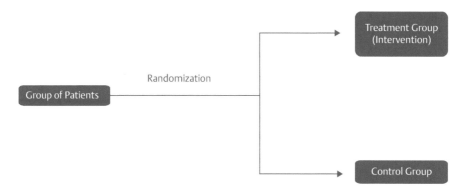

Fig 6.5 Cluster randomized trial.

A cluster RCT is an RCT in which groups of subjects are randomly assigned to one of two or more treatments, instead of individuals subjects (▶ Fig. 6.5). For example, Clinic A can be randomized to implement a program for screening patients for intimate partner violence and Clinic B can be randomized to standard care.

6.2.3 Random Assignment (Randomization)

Randomization is the procedure by which study participants or study clusters are allocated to either intervention groups. Randomization is what makes RCTs the gold standard design for performing clinical trials because, if done correctly, each group should be balanced on all prognostic factors except for the intervention that is being studied. This minimizes bias.

There are several randomization strategies. The most common ones are simple, block, and stratified randomization. There are other less common methods used for clinical trials such as biased coin, urn randomization, and minimization method.

Simple randomization is based on a single sequence of random assignments. The concept is to assign subjects to each group randomly for every subject. The analogy is flipping a coin; participants will be approximately equally distributed between the intervention groups randomly. However, computer-generated random numbers can also be used for simple randomization of subjects. Even though this randomization approach is simple and relatively easy to implement in clinical research, the number of participants among groups are likely to be assigned unequally if the total sample size is small (less than 100). For this reason, simple randomization is the right choice when the sample size is more than 100.[7]

Simple randomization does not guarantee equal numbers in both groups. The block randomization method is designed to randomize subjects equally to each group. The idea of block randomization is to divide potential patients into randomly selected blocks, usually of four, six, or eight patients per block. For example, an RCT with two treatment groups (treatment A and B) and a block size of four would have the blocks AABB, ABAB, ABBA, BBAA, BABA, or BAAB. The order of blocks is randomly determined, which maintains the benefits of randomization while keeping the treatment group sizes equal. However, if blocking is not masked, the investigator can predict the next assignment. In the example above, we can easily know what every fourth patient's assignment will be if we know the first three. This adds bias to the study. To avoid this bias, the allocator cannot reveal the blocking mechanism to the investigator, or they can use random block sizes, or blind treatment groups.[7,8] This is called allocation concealment.

To control and balance the possible influence of known covariates, a randomization strategy that can be applied is the stratified randomization method. This method can be used to achieve balance among groups in terms of subjects' baseline characteristics (covariates) that are known to affect the outcome of interest. Specific covariates must be identified by the researcher and require a thorough understanding of the clinical problem.[9] For example, a study of different rehabilitation methods after an injury will have a lot of covariates. The age of the subject can be highly related to how quickly a patient recovers and it could be a confounding variable and influence the outcome of study.[9] Therefore, the investigator might consider stratifying patients by age so that the groups are balanced in terms of the number of older versus younger people. A disadvantage of stratified randomization is that the stratification variable must be known before assigning patients to a group. Using this randomization method is difficult when some of these subjects' baseline characteristics are not available before randomization.[9]

6.2.4 Blinding

Human behavior is influenced by what we know or what we think we know. This human trait could lead to biased results of a clinical trial. To avoid and prevent conscious or unconscious bias in the design and execution of a clinical trial, it is recommended to use some form of blinding, also known as masking.[10] Blinding or masking is a procedure in which one or more parties in a trial are kept unaware of which treatment arms participants have been assigned to.[10]

Many groups of individuals involved in research are all possible sources of bias, including trial participants, clinical staff administering the treatment, physician assessing the treatment, the investigators, data analysts, and the study team. All these parties can be blinded to avoid bias.

There are different types of blinding: single-blind or single-masked, double-blind or double-masked, and triple blind. A clinical trial is called single-blind when only participants are unaware of the treatment they receive. If both participants and study team are blinded, it is called a double-blind study. A triple-blind study is when participants, the study team, and outcome adjudicators/data analysts are unaware of the treatment the patient receives. These terms can be misleading because there are more than three groups of people who can be blinded. Therefore, it is recommended to specify exactly who is and is not blinded in each trial.

Blinding is not always possible or feasible. For example, surgical trials are often not blinded because surgeons cannot be blinded to which surgery they are performing, and patients may be able to determine which group they are in based on surgical scars or X-ray images. Studies where all the parties are aware of the treatment participants receive are known as open-label or unblinded trials. Despite the importance of blinding, it is often poorly described in trial protocols.[11] The protocol should mention who will be blinded to the intervention groups (participants, care providers, or outcome assessors). Often the protocols lack information related to the comparability of blinded interventions such as the use of flavors to mask the taste or the use of colorants to mask the appearance.[11] Furthermore, the timing of final unblinding of the trial participants and any strategies to minimize the potential for unblinding should be described in the protocol.[12]

Apart from the importance of blinding, it is also crucial to have an emergency unblinding strategy. For example, in a situation of a medical emergency, it may be important for a patient's clinical team to know which drug a trial patient received to aid in diagnosis and treatment of the medical emergency. The patient's health always comes first. Unblinding is the disclosure of the participant, study team, and/or outcome adjudicators of which treatment the participant received during the trial. However, unblinding should not be necessarily a reason for study drug discontinuation.[11] The process of unblinding should be described in the protocol.

6.3 Outcome Measurement

An outcome (or endpoint) is a direct or an indirect result associated with individual study subjects used to assess efficacy. No matter how well designed it is, an RCT is only as good as its outcome assessment.[3]

It is very important that investigators specify in advance which outcomes they want to measure to prove whether their intervention works. Ideally, there should be one primary outcome and one or two secondary outcomes. However, most of the RCTs have more than two secondary outcomes. Either way, all the outcomes should be measured as rigorously as possible.[3]

Once the randomized trial design and the primary and secondary outcomes have been chosen, it is the time to think about how the outcomes will be measured. Just as there is a wide range of health outcomes, there is an even wider range of possible

outcome measures from which to select. Deciding which outcome measure to use can be an intimidating task. Therefore, it is important to understand the types and characteristics of outcome measures to select the measure best suited to your purpose.[13] For measurements of outcomes, it is very important to specify criteria to measure all the outcomes in a similar manner in all study groups.[14]

Once the outcomes to be measured are agreed upon and defined, it is necessary to ensure that they are assessed appropriately to reduce the risk of bias. Bias can exaggerate treatment effect, thereby making trial results unreliable and problematic when implementing for clinical practice.[15] Bias is lessened when an outcome can be measured objectively. If confounders are controlled through randomization and postrandomization bias is minimized, any observed differences in outcome between the treatment groups can theoretically be attributed to the effect of the intervention. It is also important that the tools used to assess these outcomes are developed, tested, and validated properly as the use of inappropriate tools results in unreliable or invalid data.[15]

6.3.1 Reliability and Validity of Outcomes Measures

The understanding of the measurement properties of the outcome measures is an important aspect of clinical care. Outcome measures have a crucial role in guiding clinical decision-making.

If you want to make decisions based on an outcome measure, you must be confident that, if no real change has occurred, your outcome measure will produce the same result each time you use it.[13] This is known as reliability (consistency or repeatability of a measure).

Reliability is a necessary but not sufficient characteristic of an outcome measure. If a measure does not produce consistent findings, it cannot be depended upon to measure what we want to measure.[13] The degree to which an instrument measures what we intend to measure is defined as its validity.

6.4 Quality Control and Data Collection

Data collection for clinical research involves gathering variables relevant to research hypotheses. It is important to establish a balance between comprehensiveness and practicality and collect only the variables related to the outcomes that potentially have an influence on the study intervention. Moreover, all data must be of high quality and collected in a systematic and monitored manner.

To minimize poor quality data, some actions should be taken to ensure the quality of the data such as design a comprehensive study protocol and manual of operations that guide research coordinators in implementing the study; create clear and concise study forms; pretest the forms; train research staff to standardize data collection; and be careful entering data to avoid errors.

There may be some problems that occur in data collection such as erroneous data and missing data. To detect errors and missing data in a timely manner, it is necessary to implement quality monitoring. A study data manager should review data, perform regular audits with feedback, and/or periodically perform blind reviews of data ranges to detect anomalies.[3]

RCTs often suffer from two major complications: noncompliance and missing outcomes. One potential solution to this problem is a statistical concept called intention-to-treat analysis.[16] Intention-to-treat analysis means all patients who were enrolled and randomly allocated to treatment are included in the analysis and are analyzed in the groups to which they were randomized. Inclusion occurs regardless of deviations that may happen after randomization such as protocol violations, losses to follow-up, withdrawals from the study, and noncompliance or refusal of the allocated treatment.

6.5 Recruitment of Study Participants

One of the most common challenges of RCTs is the recruitment and retention of participants. Insufficient or untimely patient recruitment into RCTs has serious consequences. The length of the trial may need to be extended, leading to increased resource use and costs. Lengthy trials delay the availability of potentially beneficial treatments to the public.[17] In addition, if there is not an adequate number of participants, the trial will not be able to answer the question of the study.

The primary reasons for recruitment failure include overoptimistic expectations, failure to start on time, inadequate planning, and insufficient

effort.[18] Good planning and close ongoing monitoring can make a difference. A good recruitment plan is detailed, includes multiple strategies, specifies interim recruitment goals, anticipates challenges and potential solutions, and remains flexible to cope with unanticipated problems.[3] Planning also involves setting up a clinic structure for recruitment with a committed investigator, involved coinvestigators, an experienced and skilled research coordinator in charge of recruitment, and other clinical or research staff required for some logistics operations. If the recruitment is slow, the problem mostly is related to protocol design, staff, site, or patient recruitment issues.

To minimize protocol recruitment issues, it is recommended to periodically review the inclusion and exclusion criteria. Sometimes they can be too strict and this makes it very difficult to recruit patients. Sometimes the investigator may find it necessary to increase the geographical catchment area, adding more sites to the study (multicenter trial), and increase the duration of recruitment or the budget for recruitment activities or the combination of some of these factors to help optimize patient recruitment.

To decrease staff and site recruitment issues, it is crucial to maintain clear and frequent communication between the sites and the sponsor. Having regular meetings is the best way to obtain information about why recruitment is low and what needs to be improved. This approach provides the sponsor with feedback and advice to enhance the numbers. The investigator also needs strong support from the institution and colleagues. As participants should generally not be in more than one trial at a time, competing studies in the same institution may decrease the participant recruitment.[18]

There are also patient-related problems. A good way to minimize them is to determine factors that encourage patients to enter in the study and to take time to answer all their questions.

6.5.1 Tips for Coordinators

Research coordinators are on the front lines of communication between everybody involved in a trial, for example, stakeholders, investigator, coinvestigators, participants, and so forth. They are the key stakeholders that make trials happen.

The trial may be inconvenient for patients because they cannot take time off work or attend follow-up visits, parking or public transport may be difficult or expensive, or they have other priorities. The study coordinator should recognize these issues and treat every patient according to their own needs. In other words, study coordinators should find the option that suits every patient best. To do this, make every attempt to bring potential subjects into your practice and have in-person conversations as they are much more personal and provide you the opportunity to get to know them better.

6.6 Participant Adherence

Many potential adherence problems can be prevented or minimized before participant enrollment. Once a participant is enrolled, taking measures to enhance and monitor participant adherence is essential.[18] There are three major considerations affecting participant adherence that investigators and study coordinators ought to consider during the planning phase.

First, an important factor in minimizing adherence problems before enrollment is the selection of appropriate participants. Ideally, only those people who are likely to follow the study protocol should be enrolled. Certain patient populations present unique challenges with adherence, for example, people with cognitive impairment, homeless patients, or mental health/substance use issues may require additional considerations when designing adherence strategies.[18] Moreover, a thorough informed consent process that makes it clear what is expected encourages participants to evaluate realistically whether they should enroll.[3] Thus, it is recommended to inform patients and family members or peers about the trial and its expectations to have their support and retain participants.

Second, the impact of design characteristics may influence the level of adherence. Shorter and simpler study protocols reduce participant dropout. Trials in which the participants are under supervision, such as hospitalized individuals, tend to have higher adherence. Whenever the study involves participants who live at their own home, the chances for low adherence increase. Studies of interventions that require participants to attend frequent visits undergo many tests or unpleasant invasive procedures are susceptible to have low adherence (▶ Table 6.2).

Third, the research setting influences participant adherence.[18] Whenever is possible, a pilot period before actual randomization may be

Table 6.2 Factors associated with low adherence

Factors associated with low adherence
• Visual, hearing, and cognitive impairment
• Knowledge about disease
• Low health literacy
• Low financial status
• Depression
• Psychotic disorders
• Personal and cultural beliefs
• Complexity of the medication regimen
• Duration of treatment
• Frequent therapy changes

recommended to identify those potential participants who will be low adherers. In addition, a positive relationship with the research team is crucial for retaining participants.

6.7 Assessing and Reporting Adverse Events (AEs)

There is no perfectly safe intervention. All treatments result in some AEs. AE severity ranges from mild symptoms to life-threatening events. Collection of AE data in RCT is a regulatory requirement and additionally can be clinically and scientifically important.[18] The protocol should be carefully designed to specify how to collect these AEs; therefore, there are no potential legal, ethical, or regulatory issues in case the AE collection is not done properly.

AEs can be classified as serious AEs (SAEs) or nonserious AEs. SAEs are defined as those events that are life-threatening, result in hospitalization, are irreversible, or are a congenital anomaly/birth defect.[18] SAEs are required to be reported to regulatory agencies (if it is a regulatory trial) within a short time period; usually, the time frame is 24 to 48 hours. Nonserious AEs are those in which participants indicate a change in their health status since baseline. AEs can be classified as mild, moderate, or severe.

The principal investigator is ultimately responsible for recognizing and reporting all AEs occurring to subjects in clinical trials, but the research coordinator is often the main person who interacts with study participants and their medical records, and is often the first to identify AEs. Often the research coordinator will also be responsible for preparing AE reports and submitting them to the ethics committee or other applicable agency. Identifying AEs is not an easy thing to do. To collect all potential AEs, a research coordinator has to do some exploration to characterize the event. When requesting AE information from the subject, it is highly recommended to ask open-ended questions to avoid leading the subject.

Once an AE is identified, the next step is to obtain as much information as possible about the event and report it to the sponsor and other applicable agencies (e.g., ethics committee and regulatory bodies). The basic information that needs to be collected about each AE is the date of the event, level of severity, relationship to the intervention if any treatment was required, the outcome of the event, and whether the AE was unexpected. Reports of AEs should be documented in the case report forms as well as reported on the subject's medical record.

It is important to consider other influences outside the study that can have an impact on the subject's health, such as other medications taken before or during the study or environmental exposures.[19] Nevertheless, what is important to keep in mind is that subject safety comes first. By remembering this and following the protocol, a research coordinator should be able to conduct a safe and accurate study.

6.7.1 Monitoring a Randomized Controlled Trial

Depending on the severity and frequency of AEs and if the data indicate that the intervention is unsafe to the participants, investigators and data safety monitors may have to decide to terminate the trial prematurely.[18] Moreover, monitoring the data can identify the need to collect more variables to clarify questions of benefit or harm that may arise during the trial.[18]

Monitoring data may be different depending on the size of the trial. For most large RCTs, monitoring is done by a data safety monitoring board (a group of people charged with monitoring participant safety and data quality), while for small RCTs, a data safety monitoring plan (one or two people or an institutional committee is designated as data safety monitors) is enough.

6.8 Ethical Considerations

There are some drawbacks to consider when conducting RCTs. The truth is that even though they are the gold standard method in clinical research, they are expensive, time-consuming, and sometimes it is not possible or ethical to randomly assign patients to groups. There are some types of research questions that cannot be answered by conducting an RCT for ethical reasons. For example, it is unethical to randomly assign patients to smoke cigarettes because there is overwhelming evidence that smoking is harmful. It may be unethical to assign patients to receive a placebo when there are known effective treatments.

There are some ethical issues about denying the control group an intervention that they believe will be helpful. However, the reason for doing the RCT is that it is not truly known whether the new treatment will help, harm, or have no effect.[3] This is called clinical equipoise.

It is important to describe what randomization is when explaining the study to participants. It is recommended not to use technical terminology and give simple examples of what randomization means, such as "like a coin flip." A research coordinator must ensure that patients are aware of what allocation to the intervention or control group involves.

In designing an RCT, investigators should consider these important ethical guidelines:
- Stage of research: RCTs are often defined by what phase of research they are in (phase I, II, III, and IV), corresponding to the stage of intervention development. Early in intervention development, potential risks associated with a new treatment may not be known.[3]
- Research with vulnerable populations: Ethical standards prohibit the exclusion of special populations without a scientifically sound reason.[3] Special populations include pregnant women, human fetuses, neonates, children, prisoners, racial minorities, and persons who are physically handicapped, mentally disabled, economically disadvantaged, educationally disadvantaged, and very sick.
- Selection of appropriate comparison groups: Ethical considerations include what the current standard-of-care is, and whether a no-treatment or wait-list control group is ethical.[3]
- Selection of assessment instruments: The instruments chosen to address the hypothesis of the study must have adequate psychometric properties.

- Institutional approval: Any research protocol must be approved by an ethics committee (also known as an Independent Research Board or Research Ethics Board). They review the proposed methods for research to ensure that they are ethical; in other words, they protect human subjects.
- Conflict of interest: This usually refers to situations in which someone has a financial or other personal interest in a company or product involved in a clinical trial. Conflicts of interest may threaten the integrity of research, give an impression of dishonesty, and negatively affect the rights and welfare of human subjects. If an ethics committee member has a conflict of interest with a research protocol under review, they must leave the room during the discussion and may not vote on that protocol.[3]

6.9 Practical Application

- Research question: Is anticoagulant agent X more effective than the standard anticoagulant agent (S) in terms of preventing venous thromboembolism (VTE)?
- Background: Procedures for trauma patients and orthopaedic lower limb surgery without trauma are much more frequent than major orthopaedic surgeries. The incidence of trauma patients requiring surgery and prolonged immobilization is rising. As a consequence, there is an increase in VTE.
- Objective: To evaluate the effectiveness of anticoagulant agent X versus agent S with respect to the occurrence of major VTE up to the end of treatment (e.g., removal of the plaster cast or brace).
- Study population: Adult subjects hospitalized for nonmajor orthopaedic surgery requiring thromboprophylaxis are eligible for this study.
- Design: Parallel design.

There are two types of treatment (agent X or S) and the treatments are randomly allocated.
- Randomization: Stratified randomization.
To balance the population within the two treatment arms, randomization will be stratified by centers and by intended treatment duration according to three options:
- From 2 weeks to 1 month.
- From >1 month to 2 months.
- Over 2 months.

The treatment duration used for the stratification is based on clinical judgment and corresponds to the planned duration of immobilization decided before randomization. These stratification factors allow population homogenization.

The randomization will be done centrally by an interactive web response system (IWRS). The IWRS will be used to assign one of the two treatment groups:
- Group 1: Anticoagulant agent X.
- Group 2: Standard anticoagulant agent.
- Blinding: The study is double-blind. Subjects, investigators, and sponsors/contract research personnel will remain blinded as to which study drug is administered. The packaging and dosages for both treatments will appear identical.
- Emergency unblinding: Unblinding of participants during the study is not allowed unless there are compelling medical or safety reasons to do so. Unblinding will be possible for the investigator only in the event of an emergency.

The main reasons are:
- Knowledge of the treatment allocation is necessary for the treatment of severe AEs.
- If a child in a participant's household accidentally takes the drug.
- Outcomes: Clinical outcomes measured to prove whether the intervention works are: pulmonary embolism, deep vein thrombosis, bleedings, and deaths.

6.10 Conclusion

In clinical research, RCTs are the best way to study the safety and efficacy of new treatments. RCTs are the gold standard in evaluating the effects of an intervention assigning participants randomly to study groups. RCTs are designed, conducted, analyzed, and reported to answer the research question. RCTs should be designed with safety in mind. It is important to ensure rigor in trial design and carefully consider ethical issues. RCTs are required to have ethics approval and sometimes regulatory approval before starting the trial.

The key for a successful RCT is the combination of all the aspects mentioned in this chapter. However, an involved research coordinator with expertise across all relevant clinical and methodological aspects is what makes the difference.

Definitions

- **Adverse event:** Is an undesirable health occurrence that occurs during the trial and that may or may not have a causal relationship to the treatment.
- **Blinding:** A procedure in which one or more parties to the trial are kept unaware of the treatment assignment. Single blinding usually refers to the participants being unaware, double blinding usually refers to the participants and investigators being unaware, and triple blinding refers to participants, investigators, monitor, and, in some cases, data analyst being unaware of the treatment assignment.
- **Emergency unblinding:** The process by which the treatment/allocation details are made available either purposefully (i.e., according to the code break procedures) or accidentally.
- **Intention-to-treat analysis:** Analysis where all patients who were enrolled and randomly allocated to treatment are included in the analysis and are analyzed in the groups to which they were randomized.
- **Open-label study:** A trial in which participants and investigators know which product each participant is receiving; opposite of a blinded study.
- **Outcome:** Is a direct or an indirect result associated with individual study subjects used to assess efficacy.
- **Randomization:** The process of assigning clinical trial participants to treatment or control groups using an element of chance to determine the assignments to reduce bias.
- **Severe adverse event:** Is defined as something life-threatening, requiring or prolonging hospitalization, and/or creating significant disability.

References

[1] Bull JP. The Historical Development of Clinical Therapeutic Trials. J Chronic Dis 1959;10:218–248

[2] Burns PB, Rohrich RJ, Chung KC. The Levels of Evidence and Their Role in Evidence-Based Medicine. Plast Reconstr Surg 2011;128(1):305–310

[3] Ebbp.org. [Internet]. Arizona: Evidence-Based Behavioral-Practice. West A, Spring B. Randomized controlled trials; c2006, https://ebbp.org/training/randomizedcontrolledtrials. Accessed May 6, 2019

[4] Houle P. An Introduction to the Fundamentals of Randomized Controlled Trials. Can J Hosp Pharm 2015; 68(1):28–32

[5] Parab S, Bhalerao S. Study Designs. Int J Ayurveda Res 2010;1(2):128–131

[6] Byron J, Kenward MG. Design and Analysis of Cross-Over Trials. 2nd ed. London: Chapman and Hall; 2003

[7] Kim J, Shin W. How to Do Random Allocation (Randomization). Clin Orthop Surg 2014;6(1):103–109

[8] Schen D. Randomization in Clinical Trial Studies [Internet]. Arizona: Lex Jansen; c2017. https://www.lexjansen.com/pharmasug/2006/Posters/PO06.pdf. Accessed May 10, 2019

[9] Suresh K. An Overview of Randomization Techniques: An Unbiased Assessment of Outcome in Clinical Research. J Hum Reprod Sci 2011;4(1):8–11

[10] Eupati.org [Internet]. California: European Patient's Academy. https://www.eupati.eu. Accessed May 9, 2019

[11] Spirit-statement.org. Utah: Standard Protocol Items: Recommendations for Interventional Trials [Internet]; c2011. http://www.spirit-statement.org. Accessed May 15, 2019

[12] Hróbjartsson A, Boutron I. Blinding in Randomized Clinical Trials: Imposed Impartiality. Clin Pharmacol Ther 2011;90(5):732–736

[13] Roach KE. Measurement of Health Outcomes: Reliability, Validity and Responsiveness. J Prosthet Orthot 2006;18(6):8–12

[14] Gordis L. Epidemiology. 5th ed. Philadelphia, PA: Elsevier Inc.; 2014

[15] Macefield RC, Boulind CE, Blazeby JM. Selecting and Measuring Optimal Outcomes for Randomised Controlled Trials in Surgery. Langenbecks Arch Surg 2014; 399(3):263–272

[16] Gupta SK. Intention-to-Treat Concept: A Review. Perspect Clin Res 2011;2(3):109–112

[17] Thoma A, Farrokhyar F, McKnight L, Bhandari M. Practical Tips for Surgical Research: How to Optimize Patient Recruitment. Can J Surg 2010;53(3):205–210

[18] Friedman LM, Furberg CD, DeMets DL, Reboussin DM, Granger CB. Fundamentals of Clinical Trials. 5th ed. New York, NY: Springer; 2015

[19] Rosenbaum D, Dresser M. Clinical Research Coordinator Handbook: GCP Tools and Techniques. 2nd ed. New York, NY: CRC Press; 2002

7 Observational Studies

Pieta Krijnen

Abstract

In observational studies, one or more groups of patients with exposure or treatment of interest are studied without randomization to an intervention. One or more outcomes are measured during follow-up. Observational studies can be performed for various reasons and may render high-quality evidence if performed properly. These nonrandomized study designs are associated with various types of bias such as selection bias and confounding. A detailed study protocol needs to be prepared before starting an observational study to lower the risk of bias. Another important consideration is the choice between retrospective and prospective study designs, as both have relevant advantages and disadvantages.

Keywords: standard care, prospective, retrospective, bias, confounding, observational studies, cohort studies, case–control studies, case series

7.1 Introduction

There are many reasons for performing observational studies. For instance, it may not be feasible or ethical to perform a randomized controlled trial. Moreover, observational studies may be performed to generate research hypotheses or as a pilot to obtain information that is needed for designing a randomized trial. Observational studies make a major contribution to the state-of-the-art evidence in medical research[1] and, if well designed, can provide valid and high-quality evidence.[2] When planning an observational study, however, one should be aware of the potential pitfalls and risks of bias that are associated with nonrandomized study designs. Types of bias associated with observational studies include selection bias and confounding.[3] Moreover, information bias may be present especially in retrospective studies. While some of these flaws can be controlled for in the data analysis, others can only be prevented by making the right choices in the design of the study. Thus, it is important to think over the study design carefully and write a detailed protocol before starting the study.

In this chapter, the adopted definitions of cohort studies, case–control studies, and case series are described and common forms of bias associated with observational studies are briefly discussed. Next, practical considerations for the design and performance of observational studies are discussed, focusing on methodological elements mentioned in guidelines for performing observational studies.[4]

7.2 Types of Observational Studies

There are three main types of observational studies: cohort studies, case–control studies, and case series. These studies include one or more groups of patients, which are followed prospectively or retrospectively.

7.2.1 Cohort Studies

Cohort studies start by identifying a population of consecutive patients and categorizing those patients into two or more groups based on a specific exposure (risk factor, diagnostic test, or treatment) of interest. These groups are naturally occurring rather than randomized. The groups (or cohorts) are followed forward in time to determine whether one or more outcomes of interest occur. Cohort studies are often used when it is impractical or unethical to randomize patients to interventions.

7.2.2 Case–Control Studies

Case–control studies are sometimes referred to as "research in reverse." They start with identifying participants who have an outcome of interest (cases). Then, another group of persons (controls) is chosen who are similar to the cases with respect to known determinants of the outcome other than the exposure(s) of interest, but who do not have the outcome of interest. Cases and controls are compared regarding one or more exposures of interest. Case–control studies are often used when the outcome of interest is rare, or when prospective studies would take too much time, for example, when the exposure happened many years before the outcome.

7.2.3 Case Series

Case series are studies including a group of consecutive patients who had a treatment of interest and are followed forward in time to determine whether they develop one or more outcomes of interest. According to a commonly used definition, the distinction between cohort studies and case series is determined by the presence (in cohort studies) or absence (in case series) of a control group.[1,5] Cohort studies are comparative and can be used to test research hypotheses, while case series are merely descriptive. For this reason, the level of evidence case series is lower than that of both case–control and cohort studies.[2,6] Case series can be useful when little is known about a new treatment, or to generate hypotheses before a higher quality study is conducted.

7.3 Pros and Cons of Observational Studies

A disadvantage of observational studies is that causal effects cannot be established because the exposure is not randomly allocated. For this reason, it cannot be ruled out that the association found in the study might be explained by other factors that are not properly controlled for. An advantage of observational studies is that results can often be generalized more readily to daily practice than those of randomized studies because the inclusion criteria in observational studies are generally broader and treatment in observational studies better reflects typical care.[3]

7.4 Types of Bias Associated with Observational Studies

Observational studies are prone to bias if not designed properly. Common forms of bias in observational studies are selection bias, information bias, and confounding.[3,7,8,9] These types of bias with examples are summarized in ▶ Table 7.1.

Selection bias occurs when the association between exposure and outcome is different between the study participants and the people who do not participate in the study. It is related to the way of selecting study participants or with factors that influence study participation.[8] Selection bias cannot be adequately controlled for after the study is performed unless information on the reason for nonparticipation or drop-out in the study is available.

Due to the nonrandomized design, the study groups in cohort studies are likely to differ with respect to variables that are associated with both exposure and outcome ("confounding variables"). A typical type of confounding in observational

Table 7.1 Types of bias and confounding associated with observational studies

Type of bias	Definition	Example
Selection bias	Selection of study participants is related to the study outcome. Thus, the study group is not a random sample from the target population	• The likelihood that patients are inclined to participate in the study depends on characteristics (e.g., disease severity and comorbidity) that are associated with the study outcome (self-selection bias) • Referral of patients to the study center is associated with the study outcome (referral bias) • Response to questionnaires is associated with the study outcome (nonresponse bias) • Loss to follow-up is associated with the study outcome (attrition bias)
Information bias	Errors in measuring exposure and/or outcome (i.e., measurement error in continuous variables; misclassification in categorical variables)	• Measuring errors are random (nondifferential misclassification) • Measuring errors are systematic (differential misclassification) • Outcome variables are measured differently in exposed and unexposed subjects (observer bias)
Confounding	Study groups differ regarding characteristics that are associated with both the exposure and the outcome	• The choice of treatment depends on prognostic factors (confounding by indication)

studies that compare different types of treatment is that the choice of treatment is often related to the patient's prognosis (confounding by indication). Confounding in observational studies can be controlled to a certain extent after the study is performed if the information on all potentially confounding variables has been collected. There are ways of controlling for confounding in the study design and in the statistical analysis (see the paragraph on data analysis).

It may be difficult to distinguish between selection bias and confounding in observational studies. The use of directed acyclic graphs may be a helpful tool to think about the risk of different types of bias in observational studies.[9,10] Moreover, different questions may be asked when assessing these types of bias.[9] Key questions for addressing selection bias are why some patients are selected for the study and others not, and why some patients have complete data and others do not. The key questions for addressing confounding are why some patients are more likely to be exposed than others or why some patients are more likely to receive a certain treatment than others.

Information bias is caused by an error in measuring exposure, outcome, or other study parameters. In the case of random measurement errors (increased variability referred to as "noise"), the misclassification is "nondifferential" and will generally lead to weakening of the study effect. If the measurement error is systematic (nonrandom), the misclassification is referred to as "differential" and may bias the study effect in either direction.[7,8,11] If study outcomes are measured differently between study groups in cohort studies, this can also introduce bias.[11] Information bias cannot be adequately controlled after the study is performed.

7.5 Designing Observational Studies

A detailed protocol is a road map for conducting the study. By writing the study protocol before the start of the study, the researcher is forced to reflect on all relevant aspects of the study, including the design, feasibility, performance, and reporting, which will improve the quality of the evidence provided by the study. Nowadays, many study protocols describing observational studies are published in peer-reviewed journals. By publishing a study protocol, readers can later evaluate whether the study was performed as was intended by the researchers. Registering a study in an (inter)national trial registry allows the scientific community to have a complete overview of ongoing studies on a specific topic.

7.5.1 General Information

General information on the study protocol should include the title and an overview of the members of the research project management team with their affiliation, role, and responsibilities in the study. It should also be mentioned in the protocol if the study is sponsored, and potential conflicts of interest of research group members should be stated. The study protocol needs to be approved by all members of the research group. The final version of the study protocol should include a version number and date.

7.5.2 Define Research Questions Based on a Literature Review

For observational studies, it might be even more important than for randomized trials to describe the study aim as exactly as possible and to formulate the research questions before designing the study. For this purpose, up-to-date knowledge on the research topic should be obtained by performing a review of the available literature. Preferably, relevant literature should be searched systematically in more than one database. For clinical research, Medline and the Cochrane Library are the most often used databases of medical literature. In addition, other databases may be worthwhile to search. For instance, Embase might be searched for studies on drugs and pharmacology, CINAHL for studies related to nursing, and PsycINFO for studies on psychological and psychiatric topics. It is recommended to ask a trained medical librarian for assistance with composing the search strategy for each literature database to ensure that no relevant publications are missed. The PICO framework is useful to define the terms in the search strategy based on specification of the patient (P), intervention (I), control (C), and outcome (O).[12] By studying the available literature, gaps in the current knowledge can be identified and a meaningful research question and hypothesis can be formulated.

7.5.3 Choose the Study Design

Retrospective or Prospective Study Design

One of the most important features of observational studies is whether the study design is prospective or retrospective. In a prospective study, the patients are actively followed during follow-up, whereas a retrospective study is started when the follow-up period of the patients is already completed and all data are already recorded. Both prospective and retrospective study designs have strengths and weaknesses, which are summarized in ▶ Table 7.2.[3]

Retrospective studies are time-efficient because they make use of existing data from sources such as registries and hospital files. Although this poses an advantage, the available dataset in such data sources is generally limited. Therefore, one has to check beforehand whether all information that is needed to answer the research question can be obtained retrospectively from available data sources. In addition, the quality of the available data depends on the type of data source. Most existing data sources are not primarily created for clinical research but can be used for this purpose. Data registries are mostly designed for policymaking or monitoring the quality of care. There are many examples of registries for different types of clinical conditions such as trauma, orthopaedic implants, and hip fracture care. The quality of registry data may be high if these data are routinely collected in a standardized way by trained staff. Population-based registries generally include unbiased datasets of large numbers of patients that may be available for research, but the available dataset is generally limited. In contrast, data in hospital files are generally not registered routinely and in a standardized manner, which may lead to information bias. Moreover,

the amount of missing data in medical files can be large and nonrandom, posing a risk of selection bias. When planning to collect data from medical files, one should consider the risk of information bias and selection bias. Based on the increased risk of bias that is associated with a retrospective study design, the level of evidence of prospective studies is considered higher than that of retrospective studies.[6] The data quality of prospective studies is generally better but data collection in prospective studies is time-consuming and costly. Given these differences, the choice between a prospective or retrospective study design is a trade-off between quality and feasibility.

Single-Center or Multicenter Study Design

A single-center study design is generally chosen for practical reasons because performing a study in only one center is much easier to organize. Another advantage is that the patient population and treatment protocols are more uniform in a single-center study. However, it may not be feasible to include the required number of patients for the study in just one center so that more centers are needed to complete the study within a reasonable amount of time. Besides feasibility, there may be other considerations for performing observational studies in more than one center. For instance, the study results may be more generalizable to clinical practice due to the fact that there is variation in patient populations and treatment protocols between centers. It may even be a study objective to assess whether differences in the setting have an influence on the study outcomes. Before starting a multicenter study, one cannot predict how many patients each participating center will include. Information on the number of patients treated for specific clinical conditions is available for most centers so that

Table 7.2 Strengths and weaknesses of prospective and retrospective designs in observational studies

Prospective	Retrospective
Data collection is time-consuming and costly	Data are retrieved from existing sources (registries and medical files)
Data quality is generally good; data are collected in a uniform way according to predefined definitions	Data quality depends on existing data sources. Data in registries are collected in a standardized way, but the dataset is generally limited. Data in medical files are often not registered routinely and in a standardized manner
Data are more complete	The amount of missing data may be high and also nonrandom

the expected number of eligible patients for the study can be assessed for each center. One has to be aware, however, that these numbers may fluctuate considerably over time. Whether most eligible patients will be identified and recruited for the study depends not only on the willingness of the hospital staff in the participating centers but also on logistics and circumstances. In daily practice, there may not be enough time or staff available to recruit all eligible patients. Moreover, the level of the commitment to a study usually varies between hospital staff. In most multicenter studies, the majority of patients are included in just a few hospitals with dedicated staff, while the other participating hospitals include only a few patients.

7.5.4 Define the Study Population

Inclusion and Exclusion Criteria

The inclusion and exclusion criteria for patients in observational studies should be described in detail. The clinical condition of the patients in the study should be well defined, for instance, in terms of classification or staging. Other relevant criteria for eligibility in the study may concern patient characteristics such as age, gender, comorbidities, cognitive status, level of consciousness, and literacy and understanding of the language (if patients have to fill out questionnaires). The study setting and study period should also be defined in the inclusion criteria. If the patients in the study undergo a diagnostic test or treatment (in epidemiological terms "exposure"), this must be described in the inclusion criteria as well.

Sample Size

The calculation of the sample size is an important aspect of designing observational studies to ensure that the study will yield reliable results, also for studies that do not involve hypothesis testing. Important decisions for planning the study depend on the required sample size, for instance, the length of the inclusion period and the number of centers that are needed to successfully complete the study (single- or multicenter study). Furthermore, it would be unethical to include more patients than needed if participation in the study involves a burden for the patients, for instance, because they have to pay extra study visits to the clinic or because they have to fill out questionnaires. The required sample size for observational studies

should, therefore, be predetermined, based on the planned statistical analysis of the primary outcome of the study. If the aim of an observational study is merely to describe a single outcome, the sample size is based on the level of precision with which the incidence is to be estimated (confidence interval).[13] If a descriptive study involves multivariable modeling, for instance, to identify risk factors or to develop a prediction rule, a rule of thumb for deriving the adequate sample size is that at least 10 events are required per independent variable in the analysis.[14] Sample size calculations for cohort studies should be based on the expected effect size and its variability (as in randomized studies) but should also take into account covariate adjustment in the statistical analysis.[15] If the effect size cannot be estimated from the literature, it may be based on what can be considered clinically relevant. For all types of studies, a certain amount of incomplete data due to loss of follow-up and other causes of missing data should be taken into account in determining the sample size. It is a good idea to consult a statistician when developing the sample size of a study.

7.5.5 Describe the Treatment and Procedures

The treatment of the patients in an observational study should be standardized as much as possible. For studies on surgical interventions, this also includes the pre- and postoperative treatment. In observational studies with a retrospective study design, patients have been treated prior to the start of the study according to the standard-of-care in a particular hospital at a particular time. As treatment protocols may differ between hospitals and may change over time, these protocols should be verified to ensure that the provided care, including the aftercare and revalidation, was comparable in the participating centers and did not change during the study period.

For prospective observational studies, it is important to standardize treatment and describe it in a treatment protocol, for both experimental treatment and standard care, and discuss the treatment protocol with the hospital staff in the participating centers. For studies involving standard care, all eligible patients in the participating hospitals should be treated according to the standardized treatment protocol throughout the study period, regardless of whether they participate in the study or not.

Are the Treatment Groups Comparable Regarding Their Prognosis?

One of the main concerns of comparative observational studies is whether the study groups are comparable at baseline. The patients included in observational studies are not randomly allocated to a treatment, which means that the choice of treatment made by the physician and/or patient might be related to the patients' likelihood of the outcome (prognosis). Then, a direct comparison of the treatment groups is likely to be biased (confounding by indication).

There are different ways of lowering the risk of confounding by indication in the study design.[7,11] One way is by restricting the study population, for example, to patients with a certain age or with a specific clinical condition (stage and classification), or to patients treated in a restricted period of time or in specific hospitals. The restriction will make the treatment groups more comparable with regard to their prognosis at baseline, which increases the internal validity. A disadvantage of the restriction of the study population is that it decreases the external validity of the study results because the results of the study are less generalizable to the target population. Another way of handling confounding in the study design is matching participants from different exposure groups with respect to characteristics at baseline. A major disadvantage of matching is that this usually is possible for only a part of the study group, especially if matching on several variables is necessary. Moreover, the effect of these variables on the outcome cannot be estimated after matching. Ways to handle confounding in the statistical analysis are described in the paragraph on "statistical considerations."

Another point of consideration is that indications for specific types of treatment and other aspects of care may also differ between hospitals and even between physicians and may change over time. When designing an observational study, one should, therefore, investigate the indications for treatment over time and—in case of a multicenter study—in the participating hospitals.

7.5.6 Describe the Study Parameters

As a rule, data collection should be limited to the variables that are needed to answer the research questions of the study. Researchers are often inclined to collect more data than are actually needed. As a result, part of the collected data remains unused in many research projects. Collecting and storing data that will not be used for research are a waste of time and money and may even be considered unethical. Data collection in well-designed studies should, therefore, be planned carefully in the study protocol.

7.5.7 Outcomes and Other Study Parameters

Besides the primary and secondary study outcomes, other study parameters that must be collected include the baseline patient characteristics that are relevant for describing the patient population and potentially confounding variables (i.e., factors that might be associated with the exposure or receiving a treatment and the outcome) that will be included in the statistical analysis as covariates. In the study protocol, all outcomes and other study parameters should be defined and the method of measuring the study parameters should be described.

Researchers who perform retrospective observational studies must depend on data that have been collected prior to the study. Data that are missing in the used data sources cannot be retrieved afterward; therefore, preferably study parameters should be chosen that are measured routinely and reliably and are recorded in a standardized manner in clinical practice. Objective ("hard") parameters are preferred over subjective ("soft") data that may be interpreted in different ways so that information bias is avoided as much as possible.

Study parameters in prospective studies are collected during patient follow-up. Outcome parameters, in particular, should be measured using valid and reliable methods or instruments. As in randomized trials, both the researcher and the study subjects are preferably blinded (i.e., unaware which treatment the latter has received) so that information bias can be avoided.

Health-related quality of life (HRQoL) is commonly measured as an outcome in clinical research, involving both general health and outcomes after specific clinical conditions, and are mostly reported by the patients themselves. Questionnaires for measuring these patient-reported outcomes (PROs) should be carefully selected. There are various general patient-reported outcome measures (PROMs) for HRQoL and disease-specific PROMs. When choosing PROMs for a study, different aspects need to be taken into consideration. First of all, the PROM should be developed and validated according to scientific standards.[16] Besides valid and reliable, the PROM should also be responsive, which means that the instrument should be able to detect clinically relevant differences between study groups and detect clinically relevant changes within patient groups over time. If the PROM will be used in another language than the original language, the PROM should be cross-culturally translated, adapted, and validated.[17] The PROM should preferably be commonly used in other research so that the study results can be compared to those of other studies in the literature. Moreover, the length of the PROM should be considered carefully. A questionnaire should also be as short as possible, as patients will then be more willing to fill them out completely. Especially patients who have fully recovered and those who are too sick may be less inclined to fill out long questionnaires, which may increase the risk of (mostly selective) loss to follow-up and selection bias. On the other hand, the questionnaire should cover all relevant aspects of what it is intended to measure. As HRQoL is a multidimensional concept, the researcher should consider whether a short PROM such as the EQ-5D is sufficient or whether a more detailed and thus longer PROM such as the SF-36 that can measure specific dimensions of HRQoL on separate subscales should be chosen. If no questionnaires are available for measuring a study outcome or other parameter, the researcher can design a self-made questionnaire. However, one has to bear in mind that it is a research project in itself to properly develop and validate a new questionnaire, which involves several studies. If this is not feasible, as is most often the case, the researcher should at least test whether the self-made questionnaire is understandable and appropriate for patients and whether the questions and answering options are formulated unequivocally by performing a pilot, including a few patients of different ages and educational levels.

7.5.8 Study Procedure

To avoid selection bias in observational studies, it is important to identify all consecutive patients that are eligible for the study. For retrospective studies, various data sources may be used to identify all eligible patients during a calendar period, including registries and patient listings such as surgical planning lists, medication lists, and hospital billing lists, as long as these are complete. To identify eligible patients for prospective studies, patients' lists of specific departments such as the emergency and radiology departments might be checked, and team meetings might be attended to ensure that no patients are missed.

Informed consent of participating patients may be needed for the use of routinely collected data in observational studies and for active participation in studies, for instance, when patients have to fill out questionnaires or pay extra visits to the hospital. In the study protocol, it should be described how and by whom eligible patients are informed about the study and how informed consent will be obtained.

Data collection forms ("case record forms" or "CRFs") should be designed and tested before starting the study. Moreover, it should be described who will collect the data and, for prospective studies, if this will be performed by blinded observers. The study protocol should also describe how the data will be stored and checked for accuracy (for instance, by double data entry). For prospective studies, a table presenting the timeline of the study with the scheduled study visits and assessments can be included in the study protocol to provide a clear overview of all study procedures.

7.5.9 Statistical Analysis Plan

The study protocol should include a detailed statistical analysis plan. For observational studies, it is of particular interest to describe how potential confounding bias will be dealt with and how missing data will be handled. These issues are discussed in the paragraph on data analysis.

7.5.10 Ethical Considerations/ Data Handling

Ethical requirements for observational studies are generally less strict than for experimental research with humans in most countries. Still, observational studies also need to be approved by an ethics committee by law before the study is allowed to be started in most countries. Although regulations and review procedures for obtaining ethics approval for observational studies may differ between and even within countries, as a rule, the ethics paragraph of the study protocol should describe if and how patients will be informed about the study, whether informed consent will be obtained, how the collected data will be handled and stored, how the confidentiality of included patients will be guaranteed, which research group members will have access to which part of the data, and for how long the data will be stored.

7.6 Performing the Study

7.6.1 Initiation Phase

Once the study protocol is finalized and approved by all members of the research group, realistic planning of all activities that have to be performed before the actual start of the study is needed. It is important to realize that some of these activities, such as obtaining required approvals or obtaining funding for the study, may take several months to achieve. Moreover, the organization of study logistics may take some time to realize, especially for multicenter studies. For sponsored and multi-center studies, it is necessary to draft and sign a clinical trial agreement, which is a legally binding agreement between the study sponsor and a participating center so that the responsibilities, terms of collaboration, financial aspects and reimbursements, indemnification and insurance, publication and other study-related rights, and obligations of both parties are documented.

For prospective studies performed in the clinic to be successful, it is important to obtain the cooperation of the hospital staff. Before the start of the study, the researcher needs to inform the staff that will be involved in the study in all participating centers, for instance, by presenting and discussing the study during staff meetings. Staff members who are asked to perform certain activities for the study, such as collecting data on CRFs or measuring study parameters, should be individually informed and trained so that they know what is expected of them. After setting up the study logistics, it is worthwhile to test these thoroughly in a number of patients in a pilot so that these can be adjusted if necessary. If the study logistics are set up properly and the workload for the staff is minimized as much as possible, this will increase the probability that the study will be performed successfully.

If data are to be collected from medical files, obtaining permission for and actually gaining access to medical files or other data sources for researchers can pose a challenge due to privacy regulations. Application procedures for data from existing data registries may also take considerable time as most registries require that a scientific review board must approve data requests before the data are provided.

Other activities that have to be undertaken before the start of the study include developing and testing the CRFs and the database. Preferably, medical research data should not be stored in applications such as Excel or Statistical Package for Social Sciences as these applications do not meet the current standards for medical research data storage and privacy assurance. Several online data management systems are available that do meet all requirements for this purpose. Online data management systems are especially useful for multicenter studies because the online database can be accessed and data can be entered from different geographical locations at the same time by researchers that are assigned access to specific data in the database. When choosing a data management system, it should be verified that the system is compliant with the requirements regarding privacy regulations as laid down by national law.

7.6.2 Data Collection

When the study preparations are finished, the data collection can be started. In the case of retrospective studies, all study subjects have already completed the follow-up and their data are retrieved from existing data sources. As the data are generally not registered in a standardized manner, it is preferable that only one researcher collects the data to avoid interobserver variability. If more than one researcher collects data, some of the data might be scored by both so that the interobserver agreement can be evaluated.

Data collection in prospective studies should be standardized as much as possible to avoid information bias. Monitoring the data collection by checking the collected data with the data source by an independent assessor during the study will improve the quality of the data, and thus of the study. Paperwork such as completed informed consent forms and questionnaires should be stored in the study center in a locked cupboard. It should be recorded in the patient file that the patient participates in the study and has provided informed consent. If the study involved repeated study visits, the researcher should keep track of when patients are due for study visits or questionnaires. CRFs and questionnaires should be checked for completeness timely so that missing data and questionnaires can be retrieved if possible. Maximum effort to contact study participants is important to avoid missing data as much as possible as these increase the risk of bias that is hard to adjust for.

7.6.3 Patient Inclusion in Prospective Studies

When conducting a prospective study, all eligible patients should be identified to avoid selection bias. It pays off to check department's lists of new patients and to attend daily staff meetings where patients are discussed. Patients may also be made aware of the study by hanging posters with study information in the waiting room.

Preferably, a list of all potentially eligible patients should be kept, and relevant characteristics of the patients that do not participate in your study should be recorded. In this way, the risk of selection bias and generalizability of the study results can be assessed and reported on. For this purpose, it is also useful to record the reason for nonparticipation of eligible patients.[9] It is important that the recorded information of nonparticipants is anonymous because nonparticipants do not provide consent for the use of their data for study purposes.

7.6.4 Keep the Staff Informed and Committed during the Study

Prospective clinical studies cannot be successfully completed without the help of residents and staff on the work floor. Hospital staff usually have a role in the actual performance of a study. They are usually relied on for specific activities such as identifying eligible patients, informing patients about the study by providing oral and written information, and including patients in the study by obtaining informed consent. Moreover, during the course of the study, hospital staff may be relied on for collecting data, performing measurements, and handing out questionnaires to participating patients. The trick is to keep the hospital staff in each participating center informed and to obtain their commitment to perform these tasks. This may be challenging as hospital staff work in shifts and residents come and go. Residents can be kept informed about the study and what is expected

of them throughout the study period by presenting the study on a regular basis, for instance, the morning staff meetings. Another way of providing study information is by handing out pocket maps with concise study information and by hanging posters with study information in staff rooms and near the coffee machines. To promote active collaboration in the study by residents and staff, it may be worthwhile to add a competitive element by awarding a prize to the staff member or to the participating center that contributes the most patients every month or so. Moreover, (digital) newsletters could be sent ever so often informing the participating centers on the study progress.

7.7 Data Analysis

If observational studies involve the comparison of study groups, the characteristics of these groups should be described in detail so that the difference regarding prognostic factors at baseline can be assessed. The data analysis should be performed according to the statistical analysis plan described in the study protocol. The main concerns of observational studies (e.g., confounding and missing data) should be addressed in the statistical analysis.

7.7.1 Dealing with Confounding

Several ways of dealing with confounding in the statistical analysis have been described. Stratification implies that the study subjects are analyzed in strata (i.e., within groups of subjects with similar characteristics such as age groups). An adjusted effect is then estimated by combining the stratum-specific estimates using the Mantel–Haenszel procedure or a similar method. A disadvantage of stratification is that a large sample size is needed to provide conclusive results if more than a few confounders have to be taken into account so that the study group must be divided into several strata.[7,11] Alternatively, one can adjust for confounding variables using multivariable regression techniques.[7,9,11] Multivariable regression analysis allows for controlling more confounders than can be controlled with stratification. Although this is an advantage, it can also be considered a disadvantage if many potential confounders are included in the analysis, leading to large models with wide confidence intervals that are hard to interpret.

Nowadays, more advanced statistical techniques such as the use of propensity scores are increasingly used for adjusting confounding by indication in observational studies.[9,18,19] Propensity scores are derived from statistical modeling and reflect the probability that a subject receives a certain treatment given all confounders. There are different approaches to use propensity scores (matching, weighting, stratification, and regression adjustment) that result in different estimates and involve different assumptions (for instance, regarding the homogeneity of the treatment effect). Moreover, various strategies for selecting variables for propensity score estimation have been proposed.[19] Obtaining unbiased estimates for treatment effects using propensity scores in observational studies is complex[20] and should preferably be performed with the help of a statistician.

Despite all these available techniques, the risk of confounding cannot be completely ruled out in observational studies. Residual confounding is likely to remain present due to prognostic parameters that are not measured or unknown. In particular, confounding by indication is difficult to adjust for because the exact reasons for assigning treatment in clinical practice cannot be measured.[18]

7.7.2 Handling Missing Outcome Data

Missing outcome data in observational studies should be avoided as much as possible during data collection as these can lead to biased effect estimates if undealt with and can be difficult to handle properly. Unfortunately, missing data occur in all clinical research. Naive but commonly used approaches to deal with missing data should be avoided because these generally lead to biased estimates. These approaches include replacing the missing value with the mean of the observed values, creating an additional category for missing values, and for repeated outcomes, replacing the missing value with the previously measured value ("last value carried forward").[21] The three types of missing data have to be considered that require a different statistical approach.[21,22,23] If the data of patients are missing completely at random (MCAR), the patients with missing outcome data are a random sample of the study population. Consequently, an analysis of only the patients with complete data (complete case analysis) will render unbiased results, but the decreased sample size will lead to less precise estimates. If the missingness of the outcome data is related to unknown

patient data or on the value of the unobserved outcome, the data are classified as missing not at random (MNAR). If data are MNAR, there are no proper statistical methods to assess unbiased estimates for the association under study. In most clinical research, however, missing data are neither MCAR nor MNAR. The reason for the missingness of data is usually related to other measured variables in the dataset, which is referred to as missing at random (MAR).[23] Several valid methods for dealing with MCAR and MAR data in the statistical analysis that lead to unbiased effect estimates are described. A relatively easy and transparent method is to perform complete case analysis with covariate adjustment where all variables associated with missingness are included in the regression model.[22] A more statistically advanced and more powerful method for dealing with MAR data is multiple imputation where multiple alternative datasets are generated in which the missing data are replaced (imputed) by sampling from their predictive distribution obtained from modeling the observed data.[21] By pooling estimates derived from analysis of the separate imputed datasets, an unbiased and more precise estimate of the study effect is obtained.[21,23] Although multiple imputation is nowadays available in standard statistical software, a thorough understanding of the assumptions and potential pitfalls is needed to obtain valid estimates when using this technique. For this reason, consulting a statistician is advisable for multiple imputation of missing data.[21]

7.8 Reporting

The readers of observational study reports should be provided with detailed information on all aspects of the study to be able to appreciate the strengths and weaknesses of the study design and conduct, to interpret the results of the study, and to form an opinion about the conclusions that were drawn by the researchers. It is strongly recommended and nowadays demanded by most medical journals that observational studies are reported according to the Strengthening of Reporting of Observational Studies in Epidemiology (STROBE) Statement.[24] These guidelines include a checklist of 22 items that should be addressed in the report of an observational study. Recommendations for the reporting of each item are provided.

As the length of study reports in medical journals is restricted, there may not be enough space to describe relevant aspects of the study in detail. Detailed information, for instance, on the technical aspects of the applied advanced statistical techniques for handling missing data or adjusting for confounding, should nevertheless be provided in a supplement.

7.9 Practical Application

A step-by-step plan for performing observational studies presented in ▶Table 7.3 is illustrated by describing aspects of a prospective cohort study that is currently being performed in the Netherlands. In this study, the outcomes of two surgical approaches for hemiarthroplasty in elderly patients with a femoral neck fracture are compared. The study protocol was published in an open-access, peer-reviewed journal so that a more detailed description of all aspects of the study can be found elsewhere.[25] The study was also registered in the Dutch Trial Registry.

Table 7.3 Step-by-step plan for performing observational studies

Study phase	Activity
Study protocol	Perform a systematic review of the literature
	Define research questions
	Choose the study design: retrospective/prospective and single-/multicenter
	Define the study population: inclusion/exclusion criteria and sample size
	Describe study procedures and treatment protocols
	Describe study parameters: exposure, outcome(s), and confounders
	Describe the statistical plan after consulting a statistician about handling confounding and missing data
	Describe ethical aspects and data handling
	Write study information and informed consent form for patients
	Obtain approval of study group members
Initiation phase	Obtain approval of institutional review board(s)
	Obtain funding
	Draft and sign a clinical trial agreement with participating center(s)
	Inform and discuss the study with staff in participating center(s)
	Set up and test study logistics in participating center(s)
	Obtain access to data sources in the participating center(s)
	Develop and test case record forms and database
	Publish the study protocol
Data collection	Keep lists of all eligible patients
	Register reasons for nonparticipation
	Collect the data on case records forms
	Store and check the data in the database
	Keep the staff in participating center(s) informed and committed
Data analysis	Perform the analysis according to the statistical plan
	Consult a statistician when applying advanced statistical techniques
Reporting	Report the study according to the STROBE guidelines in a peer-reviewed journal

Abbreviation: STROBE, Strengthening of Reporting of Observational Studies in Epidemiology.

7.9.1 Background

At present, the lateral approach is mostly used for hemiarthroplasty in the Netherlands. An alternative approach is an anterior approach, which minimizes soft tissue damage and may, therefore, facilitate early and improved postoperative mobility, leading to better functional outcomes. An extensive literature search showed no conclusive evidence for this hypothesis.[26]

7.9.2 Study Objective

The aim of the study is to compare hip function, postoperative complications, and patient mobility after hemiarthroplasty via the anterior or lateral approach for a displaced femoral neck fracture in elderly patients.

7.9.3 Study Design

The study is designed as a single-center prospective comparative cohort study in a large teaching hospital in the Netherlands where annually more than 500 patients with femoral neck fractures are treated. In this center, the multidisciplinary hip fracture care is standardized and data on patient characteristics and outcomes are prospectively and routinely documented of all consecutive admitted hip fracture patients.

7.9.4 Patients

In the present study, all consecutive patients aged 70 years or older admitted to the study hospital with an X-ray proven displaced femoral neck fracture (AO type 31 B1–B3), treated with a cemented hemiarthroplasty, and considered able to rehabilitate are included. Eligibility for rehabilitation is determined during hospitalization twice weekly by a multidisciplinary team. Patients are considered fit for rehabilitation when they can participate in physiotherapy by being physically and mentally able to follow instructions adequately. Patients fit for rehabilitation are either discharged home with ambulatory physiotherapy or to a geriatric rehabilitation care institute. Patients with an active lifestyle and unrestricted mobilization without walking aids are considered eligible for total hip arthroplasty and excluded from the study.

7.9.5 Treatment

Admitted patients are treated according to the treatment guidelines for proximal femoral fracture in the elderly of the Dutch Surgical Society. Surgical procedures as well as pre- and postoperative treatment are standardized and are described in detail in the study protocol.[25] Both the lateral approach and the anterior approach are used standardly for hemiarthroplasty in the study hospital. The choice of a specific surgical approach depends on the experience of the surgeon on call: all surgeons use the approach they are most familiar with.

7.9.6 Study Outcomes and Other Parameters

The primary outcome is the patients' functionality in daily life measured with the validated Dutch version of the Harris Hip Score, a patient-reported questionnaire. Secondary outcomes include clinical outcomes (surgical parameters and complications, nonsurgical complications, cognitive status, readmission, operative revision, and 1-year mortality) and PROs (functionality, pain, performance of daily activities, and general HRQoL). Other study parameters described in the study protocol included general patient characteristics, medication use preoperative nutritional status, and prefracture functional and cognitive status. In the published study protocol,[25] it is described in detail how and at which follow-up moments the study outcomes and other study parameters are measured.

7.9.7 Sample Size

Only two studies reported estimates for 1-year postoperative results for the Harris Hip Score in hemiarthroplasty patients, and estimates for specific surgical approaches are lacking in the literature. Therefore, the sample size was based on a difference in functionality of 10 points as this is considered as a clinically relevant difference in scores according to the literature. We calculated that at least 41 patients with complete 1-year follow-up in two equally sized cohorts are needed to detect such a difference (with $\alpha = 0.05$, power = 80%). Anticipating failure to follow up of 40%, the sample size of the study was increased to 69 patients in each group (138 patients in total).

7.9.8 Statistical Analysis

As the choice for surgical approach is not randomized in the study but at the discretion of the treating surgeon, there might be a risk of confounding. Therefore, potential confounding will be adjusted for by including propensity scores in the analysis.

7.9.9 Ethical Considerations

The study was approved by the ethics committee. The data are coded in the database to ensure confidentiality.

7.10 Conclusion

Observational studies are associated with a risk of various types of bias but can provide valid results if planned and performed carefully. Transparent and detailed reporting of the study protocol and results are essential to appreciate the quality of an observational study and the validity of its conclusions.

References

[1] Hoppe DJ, Schemitsch EH, Morshed S, Tornetta P III, Bhandari M. Hierarchy of Evidence: Where Observational Studies Fit in and Why We Need Them. J Bone Joint Surg Am 2009;91(Suppl 3):2–9

[2] Concato J, Shah N, Horwitz RI. Randomized Controlled Trials, Observational Studies, and the Hierarchy of Research Designs. N Engl J Med 2000;342(25):1887–1892

[3] Euser AM, Zoccali C, Jager KJ, Dekker FW. Cohort Studies: Prospective Versus Retrospective. Nephron Clin Pract 2009;113(3):c214–c217

[4] Morton SC, Costlow MR, Graff JS, Dubois RW. Standards and Guidelines for Observational Studies: Quality is in the Eye of the Beholder. J Clin Epidemiol 2016;71:3–10

[5] Kooistra B, Dijkman B, Einhorn TA, Bhandari M. How to Design a Good Case Series. J Bone Joint Surg Am 2009;91(Suppl 3):21–26

[6] Marx RG, Wilson SM, Swiontkowski MF. Updating the Assignment of Levels of Evidence. J Bone Joint Surg Am 2015;97(1):1–2

[7] Jepsen P, Johnsen SP, Gillman MW, Sorensen HT. IInterpretation of Observational Studies. Heart 2004;90(8):956–960

[8] Rothman KJ. Dealing with biases. Epidemiology: An Introduction 2nd ed. New York, NY: Oxford University Press, Inc.; 2012

[9] Haneuse S. Distinguishing Selection Bias and Confounding Bias in Comparative Effectiveness Research. Med Care 2016;54(4):e23–e29

[10] Shrier I, Platt RW. RReducing Bias through Directed Acyclic Graphs. BMC Med Res Methodol 2008;8:70

[11] Grimes DA, Schulz KF. Bias and Causal Associations in Observational Research. Lancet 2002;359(9302):248–252

[12] Schardt C, Adams MB, Owens T, Keitz S, Fontelo P. Utilization of the PICO Framework to Improve Searching PubMed for Clinical Questions. BMC Med Inform Decis Mak 2007;7:16

[13] Sedgwick P. Sample Size: How Many Participants are Needed in a Cohort Study? BMJ 2014;349:g6557

[14] Steyerberg EW, Eijkemans MJ, Harrell FE Jr, Habbema JD. Prognostic Modeling with Logistic Regression Analysis: In Search of a Sensible Strategy in Small Data Sets. Med Decis Making 2001;21(1):45–56

[15] Greene T. Randomized Controlled Trials 5: Determining the Sample Size and Power for Clinical Trials and Cohort Studies. Methods Mol Biol 2015;1281:225–247

[16] Boynton PM, Greenhalgh T. Selecting, Designing, and Developing your Questionnaire. BMJ 2004;328(7451):1312–1315

[17] Sousa VD, Rojjanasrirat W. Translation, Adaptation and Validation of Instruments or Scales for Use in Cross-Cultural Health Care Research: A Clear and User-Friendly Guideline. J Eval Clin Pract 2011;17(2):268–274

[18] Bosco JL, Silliman RA, Thwin SS, et al. A Most Stubborn Bias: No Adjustment Method Fully Resolves Confounding by Indication in Observational Studies. J Clin Epidemiol 2010;63(1):64–74

[19] Brookhart MA, Wyss R, Layton JB, Stürmer T. Propensity Score Methods for Confounding Control in Non-Experimental Research. Circ Cardiovasc Qual Outcomes 2013;6(5):604–611

[20] Freemantle N, Marston L, Walters K, Wood J, Reynolds MR, Petersen I. Making Inferences on Treatment Effects from Real World Data: Propensity Scores, Confounding by Indication, and Other Perils for the Unwary in Observational Research. BMJ 2013;347:f6409

[21] Sterne JA, White IR, Carlin JB, et al. Multiple Imputation for Missing Data in Epidemiological and Clinical Research: Potential and Pitfalls. BMJ 2009;338:b2393

[22] Groenwold RH, Donders AR, Roes KC, Harrell FE Jr, Moons KG. Dealing with Missing Outcome Data in Randomized Trials and Observational Studies. Am J Epidemiol 2012;175(3):210–217

[23] Donders AR, van der Heijden GJ, Stijnen T, Moons KG. Review: A Gentle Introduction to Imputation of Missing Values. J Clin Epidemiol 2006;59(10):1087–1091

[24] von Elm E, Altman DG, Egger M, Pocock SJ, Gotzsche PC, Vandenbroucke JP; STROBE Initiative. The Strengthening the Reporting of Observational Studies in Epidemiology (STROBE) Statement: Guidelines for Reporting Observational Studies. Int J Surg 2014;12(12):1495–1499

[25] van der Sijp MPL, Schipper IB, Keizer SB, Krijnen P, Niggebrugge AHP. Prospective Comparison of the Anterior and Lateral Approach in Hemiarthroplasty for Hip Fractures: A Study Protocol. BMC Musculoskelet Disord 2017;18(1):361

[26] van der Sijp MPL, van Delft D, Krijnen P, Niggebrugge AHP, Schipper IB. Surgical Approaches and Hemiarthroplasty Outcomes for Femoral Neck Fractures: A Meta-Analysis. J Arthroplasty 2018;33(5):1617–1627.e9

8 Surveys

Miriam Garrido Clua

Abstract

The purpose of this chapter is to describe survey research as one approach to the conduct of research so that the reader can understand and conduct studies employing survey research. At the end of this chapter, the research coordinator should have a better idea of what is a survey, and how to administer it and select the right method considering all the factors.

Keywords: survey, questionnaire, postal mail, interviews

8.1 Introduction

There are several methodological approaches in conducting research. Selection of a research approach depends on the purpose of the research, the type of research questions to be answered, and the availability of resources. Survey research is a commonly used method of collecting information about a population of interest. This type of research can use quantitative research strategies (e.g., using questionnaires with numerically rated items), qualitative research strategies (e.g., using open-ended questions), or both strategies (i.e., mixed methods).[1] Survey research has been used to obtain information from individuals and groups for decades. It can range from asking a few targeted questions to some individuals on a street corner to obtain information related to behaviors and preferences to a more rigorous study using multiple valid and reliable instruments.[1] Common examples of less rigorous surveys include market research and election polling.

More recently, surveys have been applied in health research, with scientifically tested strategies describing who to include (population of interest), what to measure (research question), and how to measure (instrument/tool), to ensure a high-quality research process and outcome. Survey research, like any other type of research, involves research aims, sampling and recruitment strategies, data collection instruments, and methods of survey administration. Given this, it is important to consider any potential bias as well as techniques for reducing bias to report accurate conclusions.[1]

8.1.1 What Is a Survey Study?

Survey studies may have roots in English and American "social surveys" conducted in the 20th century by researchers and reformers who wanted to document the extent of social problems such as poverty. By the 1930s, the US government was conducting surveys to document economic and social conditions in the country.[2] As survey research is often used to describe and explore human behavior, surveys are therefore frequently used in social and psychological research. Understanding and evaluating survey research are also used in several academic fields, including political science and public health—where it continues to be one of the primary types of research for collecting new data.

Survey research is a quantitative and qualitative method with the primary purpose of obtaining information describing characteristics of a relatively large sample of individuals from a predetermined population known as the population of interest (i.e., the group of people whom the researcher is interested in to consider sample). The researcher administers (in person, by telephone, through the mail, or over the internet) a standardized form to the participants, who are often called respondents in survey research. This form is usually, but not necessarily, a questionnaire or interview where participants report directly on their thoughts, preferences, or behaviors. Using surveys, it is possible to collect data from large or small populations. Large random samples provide the most accurate estimates of what is true in the population.[2]

There is much variety when it comes to surveys; they can take many forms. In terms of time, there are two main types of surveys: cross-sectional and longitudinal.

Cross-Sectional Survey

Cross-sectional surveys are those that are administered at just one point in time. These surveys offer researchers a snapshot of what is happening in that group at that particular time. They usually give us an idea about how things are for our respondents and describe behavior or attitudes.

Longitudinal Survey

Longitudinal surveys, rather than taking a snapshot, enable the researcher to make observations over an extended period of time (usually months or years). This means that if whatever behavior or other phenomena the researcher is interested in changes, either because of some event or people age, the researcher will be able to capture those changes.

There are several types of longitudinal surveys but they usually take one of two forms:

- **Cohort studies:** The researcher identifies a category of people (e.g., people of particular generations and people who have had a particular medical treatment) that are of interest and then regularly surveys the same people over time.
- **Trend studies:** The researcher takes repeated samples of different people each time but always using the same questions. They are interested in how people's inclinations change over time.

8.2 Research Methods

It is important to remember that a survey is a type of research design. In contrast, an interview or a postal questionnaire is a method of data collection. There is a wide range of methods available for collecting data, but the three main methods of collecting survey data are: questionnaires, telephone interviews, and face-to-face interviews (▶ Table 8.1).

8.2.1 Questionnaires

Questionnaires are usually paper-and-pencil instruments that the respondent completes, whereas interviews are completed by the interviewer based on the respondent says. It is believed that questionnaires ask short closed-ended questions, while interviews always ask broad open-ended ones. However, there are questionnaires with open-ended questions (although they still are shorter than interviews) and there will often be a series of closed-ended questions asked in an interview.[3]

One of the common questionnaire types is postal questionnaire, also known as mail survey. All of us have, at one time or another, received a questionnaire in the mail. Mail surveys are relatively cheaper than personal interviews and require less involvement from both subject and researcher than many other forms of surveys. This method involves sending the exact same instrument to a large sample of people covering a wide geographical area

Table 8.1 Advantages and disadvantages of survey methods

Survey Type	Advantages	Disadvantages
Postal questionnaires	Ease of administration and cost-efficient No interviewer and respondents may be more willing to share information	Response rates are low (possibility of bias) Need for translation for people who do not understand the language False respondent
Online questionnaires	Low costs Relative speed and flexibility Automation and real-time access Less time needed Easy access to large (worldwide) population No interviewer and respondents may be more willing to share information	Technical skills and time required to develop the questionnaire Limited sampling and respondent availability Possible cooperation problems (computer illiteracy) False respondent
Telephone interviews	Large-scale accessibility in many countries Rapid data collection Anonymity Flexibility People are used to telephone calls from strangers	False respondent Lack of visual materials Interview length must be limited No facial expressions
Face-to-face interviews	Higher response rates Better quality and quantity of data Identify respondent Attitude can be observed Use of visual materials	Expensive Time-consuming Interviewer bias Anonymity not maintained May produce a nonrepresentative sample

and it gives subjects the time to think about the questions, and if necessary, obtain further information from elsewhere. However, there are some disadvantages as well. This method requires a valid address of the subject; otherwise, the subject may not receive it, leading to a lower response rate.[4] The response rate for this type of method is usually low, around 20%, depending on the content and length of the questionnaire. As response rate is low, a large sample is required to ensure that the demographic profile of survey respondents reflects that of the population of interest and to provide a sufficiently large dataset for analysis.[5] Another disadvantage is that if they do not understand the question, there is no one to ask unless a helpline has been set up. Besides, mailed out questionnaires can be easily forgotten or thrown away.[4]

It is recommended not to administer long questionnaires as this is likely to decrease the response and completion rate. The respondents need to be able to complete the questionnaire in as little time as possible while gaining the most information as possible. The questions need to be straightforward and easy to answer, otherwise, lack of understanding by the respondent may result in low completion rate or inappropriate answers.[4]

All mailed questionnaires should be accompanied by a covering letter. Questionnaires sent to populations with a covering letter from their general practitioner tend to have very high response rates. A cover letter should include information such as the organization behind the study, including the contact name and address of the researcher, details of how and why the respondent was selected, the aims of the study, and potential benefits and harms resulting from the study, and what will happen to the information provided.[5]

The past decade has seen a tremendous increase in internet use. Studies of online populations have led to an increase in the use of online surveys. Some advantages include access to individuals in distant locations, the ability to reach difficult to contact participants, and the convenience of having automated data collection, which reduces researcher time and effort. However, some disadvantages of online survey research include uncertainty over the validity of the data and sampling issues and concerns surrounding the design, implementation, and evaluation of an online survey.[6]

A less familiar type of questionnaire is the household drop-off survey. It has been presented as an alternative for reducing noncoverage error associated with the mail method at a lower cost than face-to-face interviews. In this approach, a researcher goes to the respondent's home or business and hands the respondent the questionnaire. In some cases, the respondent is asked to mail it back or the interviewer returns to pick it up. Like the mail survey, the respondent can work on the instrument in private and fill it out at their own convenience. Besides, the interviewer makes personal contact with the respondent and the respondent can ask questions about the study and get clarification on what is to be done. Generally, this would be expected to increase the percentage of people who are willing to respond.[3]

8.2.2 Face-to-Face Interviews

Face-to-face interviews can take both qualitative and quantitative approaches but surveys tend to take a quantitative approach.[7] Interviews are a more personal form of research than questionnaires. This type of interview involves the researcher approaching respondents personally and working directly with them.

As the researcher has the opportunity to explain the research to potential respondents, the response rate is typically higher than the postal questionnaires. The researcher asks the respondent some questions and notes their responses. Unlike with mail surveys, the interviewer can explain questions and explore the answers in more detail, if necessary.

Face-to-face interviews are time-consuming, costly, and logistically more difficult, however, the researcher can select the sample of respondents to balance the demographic profile of the sample.[5] Interviewers carrying out face-to-face interviews for a quantitative study will use a highly structured interview schedule.[7] Face-to-face interviews are appropriate if you need to show and explain complex examples or diagrams, or where certain disabilities may make completing a questionnaire in another fashion prohibitive.[7]

8.2.3 Telephone Interviews

Telephone interviews, like face-to-face interviews, are a two-way interaction between the researcher and the respondent and allow the interviewer to ask follow-up questions. Telephone interviews are cheaper and enable a researcher to gather information quicker than face-to-face interviews. However, they also have some major disadvantages.

This may not be an appropriate method for a study population where telephone ownership is likely to be low. Besides, people often do not like the intrusion of a call to their homes.

Telephone interviews are particularly useful when the respondents to be interviewed are widely geographically distributed, but the complexity of the interview is limited without the use of visual aids and prompts.[7] The length of a telephone interview is also limited; interviews should be relatively short or people will feel imposed upon.

The advantage of telephone interviews compared to face-to-face interviews is that they are easier to organize and carry out as no visits are required. The duration of telephone interviews should not be more than around 30 to 45 minutes, while face-to-face interviews can be longer than some of the other methods (1–2 h).[4]

Both facilitate entry directly into an electronic database, which reduces the data entry effort. Sometimes the answers can be typed directly into a computer as the interview is being conducted. When it comes to quality control, interviews may need to be recorded for quality control purposes and some measures are recommended to avoid data entry mistakes. When doing a face-to-face or telephone survey of respondents in their own homes, it is important to do some evening calls, otherwise, the survey may be restricted to those who are at home during the day.[7]

8.3 Selecting the Survey Method

Selecting the type of survey is one of the most critical decisions in many research contexts. It is recommended to use your own judgment to balance the advantages and disadvantages of different survey types to select the right method.

The selection of the appropriate method depends upon a number of factors related to the population, research question, content of the study, bias issues, and resources.

8.3.1 Population

Access to Potential Participants/ Respondents

For some populations, it is difficult or impossible to have a list or a register of all the potential respondents. For instance, if you are doing a study that requires input from homeless persons, you are very likely going to need to go and find the respondents personally because no one keeps a complete and accurate list of homeless people. In this case, postal questionnaires or telephone interviews are not the appropriate method.

The Literacy Level of Respondents

Questionnaires require that your respondents can read. Clearly, there are some populations that you would expect to be illiterate, such as young children. Additionally, there are many adult populations who have a low reading level or have a language barrier. These populations would not be good targets for written questionnaires.

Geographic Restrictions

Sometimes the population of interest is dispersed over too broad a geographic range. This makes it difficult to conduct a personal interview. It may be feasible to select postal questionnaires or telephone interviews as a research method.

8.3.2 Research Question

Sometimes the nature of the question will determine the selection of the survey.

The Subject Matter

If there are personal questions, respondents might feel more comfortable filling out an anonymous questionnaire, whereas if lots of details in the responses are needed, it is preferable to conduct an interview; therefore, the researcher can extract more information of one question.

Complexity of the Questions

Sometimes the subject or topic of interest is complex and the questions are going to have multiple parts or require skip logic. This should be taken into consideration when selecting a survey method.

Screening Questions

A screening question may be needed to determine whether the respondent is eligible for the study. Sometimes it is recommended to screen on several variables (e.g., age, gender, experience).

The more complicated the screening, the less likely it is that the researcher can rely on paper-and-pencil instruments without confusing the respondent.[3]

Lengthy Questions

If the subject matter is complicated, the researcher may need to give the respondent some detailed background for a question and the respondent might not sit long enough in a phone interview.

8.3.3 Content of the Study

The content of the study can also pose challenges for different survey types.

Knowledge about the Question

If the respondent does not keep up with the news (e.g., by reading the newspaper, watching television news, or talking with others), they may not know about current events issues included in the study.[3]

The Need to Consult Records

Even if the respondent understands what the researcher is asking about, they may need to consult their records to get an accurate answer. In this case, an interview is not the best option. They would have to go look things up while the researcher is waiting (this could be uncomfortable for participants).

8.3.4 Bias Issues

People have their own sets of biases and prejudices. This may affect survey results.

Social Desirability

If the researcher asks respondents about the information that may put them in an embarrassing position, they may not tell the truth, or they may "spin" the response so that it makes them look better. This may be more of a problem in an interview situation where they are face to face or on the phone with a live interviewer.[3]

Interviewer Bias

Interviewers may distort an interview as well. They may not ask questions that make them uncomfortable. They may not listen carefully to respondents on topics for which they have strong opinions. They may make the judgment that they already know what the respondent would say to a question based on their prior responses, even though that may not be true.[3]

Respondent Identity

With mail surveys or phone interviews, it may be difficult to know who actually responded. However, with personal interviews, there is a reasonable chance of knowing who the interviewer is speaking with.

8.3.5 Resources

Cost

Sometimes it is preferable to do personal interviews but it may be difficult to fund the high cost of training and paying for the interviewers or to send out an extensive mail survey with its associated printing and mailing costs.

Facilities

Before selecting the type of survey, it is important to think about the required facilities to conduct the study. For phone interviews, researchers should have well-equipped phone surveying facilities, or for face-to-face interviews, researchers must have a comfortable and accessible room and equipment to record and transcribe responses.

Personnel

Different types of surveys make different demands of personnel. Interviews require interviewers who are motivated and well trained. Some studies may be in a technical area that requires some degree of interviewer expertise also.[3]

8.4 Sample and Sampling

One of the primary strengths of having a proper sampling strategy is that accurate estimates of a population's characteristics can be obtained by surveying a small proportion of the population. If the participants in the study are very rare, then the researcher might decide to study every case. However, usually, it is more likely to be in a situation where the potential participants (sampling frame) in the study are much more common and you cannot practically include everybody.[7] The survey methods described below influence how a sample is selected and the sample size. There are two categories of sampling: random and nonrandom sampling.

8.4.1 Random Sampling

Random sampling is employed when quantitative methods are used to collect data (e.g., questionnaires).[5] Sometimes it is necessary to reduce the number of participants included in the survey without biasing the findings in any way. Random sampling is one way of achieving this.

Random sampling techniques can be split into simple random sampling, cluster sampling, and stratifies sampling.

Simple Random Sampling

Simple random sampling is the most basic form of sampling. Using this technique, every member of the chosen population has an equal chance of being selected. This sampling process is random, like flipping a coin. Researchers often use a random number table, which can be generated using computer software.

Cluster Sampling

Cluster sampling is generally used when it is geographically impossible to undertake a simple random sample. Cluster sampling allows individuals to be selected in geographical batches. This technique randomly assigns groups from a large population and then surveys everyone within the groups.[5] Cluster sampling requires that adjustments are made in statistical analyses.

Stratified Sampling

Stratified samples are used when a researcher wants to ensure that there are enough respondents with certain characteristics in the sample. The researcher first identifies the people in the population who have the desired characteristics and then randomly selects a sample of them. Stratified sampling requires that adjustments are made in statistical analyses.[8]

For example, a researcher may want to compare survey responses of Asian and Caucasians. To ensure that there are enough Asians in the survey,

the researcher will first identify the Asians in the population and then randomly select a sample of Asians.

8.4.2 Nonrandom Sampling

Nonrandom sampling is applied when qualitative methods (e.g., interviews) are used to collect data. Nonrandom sampling deliberately targets individuals within a population.[5] Common nonrandom sampling techniques include quota sampling, convenience sampling, and snowball sampling.

Quota sampling is a technique for sampling where a specific population is identified and only its members are included in the survey. On the other hand, selecting respondents purely because they are easily accessible is known as convenience sampling. Finally, snowball sampling involves identifying participants as the survey progresses.

Nonrandom samples cannot be generalized to the population of interest. For this reason, in survey research, random, cluster, or stratified samples are preferable.[8]

8.5 Research Tool Design

The objective of questionnaire design is to minimize error in exposure measures while creating an instrument that is easy for the interviewer and subject to use and easy to process.[9]

Whether using a postal questionnaire or interview method, the questions asked should be carefully planned and piloted (►Fig. 8.1). Questionnaires can only produce valid and meaningful results if the questions are clear and precise and if they are asked consistently across all respondents.[7] The right design can minimize bias in results.

When designing a questionnaire or question route for interviewing, the following issues need to be considered: types of questions, questionnaire layout, question wording, question order, interview questions, and pilot testing.

8.5.1 Types of Questions

Survey questions can be divided into two types: open-ended questions and closed-ended questions.

Open-ended questions offer participants a space into which they can answer by writing text. These can be used when there are a large number of possible answers to precode or possible replies are unknown. Open-ended

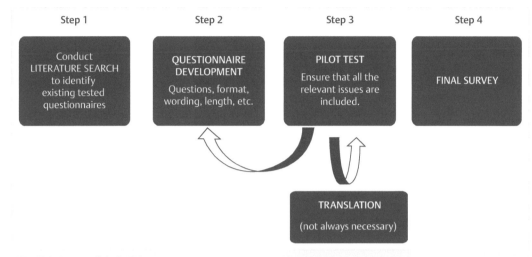

Fig. 8.1 Process of designing a survey.

questions are questions without restrictions on the answers of the subjects. Open-ended questions are generally used to record simple factual information such as name, weight, height, date, age, and occupational title.[4]

Open questions are more demanding for respondents but if well answered, the researcher can capture all of the details in the information provided. However, this type of question can be time-consuming to administer and difficult to analyze. Besides, the text responses will need to be reviewed by one member of the research team (blinded to treatment allocation), who will assign one or more codes that categorize the response before analysis; this may take a lot of time and careful interpretation of some of the answers and may itself introduce bias.[4]

Closed-ended questions have restrictions in the form of a limited number of possible answers. The responses are precoded, for example, multiple-choice questions. Closed questions may contain mutually exclusive response option only (make sure to avoid potential overlap) or a clear instruction that participants may select more than one response option (e.g., "tick all that apply").

There is some evidence that answers from closed questions are influenced by the values chosen by investigators for each response category offered and that respondents may avoid extreme categories.[10] Besides, the answer may differ depending on the number of categories that are provided as a possible answer. However, the

effect of the category definition can be reduced by knowledge of the expected frequencies of the responses.

Whether using open or closed questions, researchers should plan clearly how answers will be analyzed.

8.5.2 Questionnaire Layout

Questionnaires used in survey research should be clear and well presented. The format of the questionnaire is as important as the actual questions. The researcher must do as much as possible to encourage respondents to answer the questionnaire.

In the case of paper questionnaires, long and complex-looking questionnaires do not encourage the subject to start filling them out. A nice and tidy questionnaire is more appealing.[4] Font size and color may further affect the legibility of a questionnaire, which may also impact on data quality and completeness.[10] Sometimes it is important to consider who the respondent is to design a questionnaire. For instance, questionnaires answered by older participants may require the use of a larger font than those answered younger participants.

Some other recommendations to increase the response rate are: place clear instructions and headings to make the questionnaire easier to follow; avoid using all caps (this format is hard to read); and, questions should be numbered and clearly grouped by subject. Besides, the use of the visual elements of brightness, color, shape, and location in a consistent manner defines the path for respondents to follow when answering the questionnaire.[10]

Branching off (or question skipping)—that is, going into more detail for particular questions depending on a response to previous questions, is not easy with self-administered paper questionnaires as it will take up a lot of space on a page and a respondent may get confused about what to answer. To avoid this, arrows or color coding may help.[4] For some open questions, the use of matrices can be very helpful at times. For example, when asking for a job history having rows for each job and columns for job title, industry, tasks, and start and finishing date can be helpful.[4]

Following these recommendations may help to ensure that when participants complete a questionnaire, they understand what is being asked, how to give their response, and which question to answer next.

The legibility and comprehension of the questionnaire can be assessed during the pilot phase.

8.5.3 Question Wording

The wording of the questions is very important as it has a direct impact on the outcome. The words used in the questionnaire should be understood by the respondents and they should meet the reading level of the target audience. The participant should not have to figure out what is actually being asked. There should be no unexplained or vague terms, jargon, or abbreviations, although, at times, jargon may be needed for specialized jobs or tasks.[4]

The questions should be clear, short, and to the point. It is recommended to avoid using ambiguous words and questions; leading questions; two or more questions in one; and questions containing double negative.

Only one question at a time should be asked and the questions should be unbiased. Questions cannot be too precise and the subject needs to be familiar with them. The answers should be able to be linked to the aims and objectives of the questionnaire.[4]

8.5.4 Question Order

The order of the questions is a particularly important issue to consider when planning a survey. It is highly recommended to use a logical order for the questions and start with some general questions first to get the respondent going. Starting with general fact-finding questions, which are easily understood and will apply to everyone, helps getting the respondents to ease themselves into the questionnaire. Then move onto more specific questions, which may filter people into different questions. Certain personal questions, such as age, social class, and ethnicity, may be left until later, near the end of the questionnaire, when a level of rapport has been established.[7] Likewise, embarrassing or sensitive questions may be best left until nearer the end. Use the order in such a way that the respondents keep an interest and that there is a natural flow.[7]

It may be difficult at times to ask many specific questions to control groups, particularly when the participant does not know about the topic. For this reason, the response rate among controls often tends to be lower compared to the response rate among cases.

8.6 Training the Interviewers

The interviewer is considered a part of the measurement instrument and interviewers have to be well trained in how to respond to any contingency. In many ways, the interviewers are the "measurers," and the quality of the results is totally in their hands. Even in small studies involving only a single researcher-interviewer, it is important to organize in detail and rehearse the interviewing process before beginning the formal study.

Sometimes a research coordinator is an interviewer, but other times, he/she is the one who trains the interviewer. For this reason, it is crucial to know some of the major topics that should be included in interviewer training. Here, there are some considerations[3]:

- **Describe the entire study:** Interviewers should learn about the background for the study; it will help them to understand why the study is important.
- **State who is the sponsor of the research:** Interviewers and respondents have a right to know what company is conducting the research and paying for the research (if applicable).
- **Teach about survey research:** Interviewers will need to understand the rationale for how the instrument was constructed.

- **Explain the sampling:** Interviewers need to know the importance of the sampling strategy. They may wonder why it is necessary to go through all the difficulties of selecting the sample so carefully. You will have to explain that sampling is the basis for the conclusions that will be reached and for the degree to which your study will be useful.
- **Explain interviewer bias:** Interviewers need to know many ways that they can inadvertently bias the results. Moreover, they need to understand why it is important that they not bias the study.
- **Introduce the interview:** It is recommended to walk through the entire interview so that the interviewers can get an idea of the various parts and how they interrelate.
- **Teach how to identify respondents.**
- **Rehearse interview:** Have several rehearsal sessions with the interviewer team.
- **Explain timing schedules:** In some studies, it will be imperative to conduct the entire set of interviews within a certain time period. In most studies, it is important to have the interviewers available when it is convenient for the respondents, not necessarily the interviewer.

Interviewer training helps improve the quality of survey data by reducing missing data, increase the data accuracy, and increase survey participation by teaching interviewers how to identify and respond to respondents' concerns.[11,12]

8.7 Pilot Testing

Once a completed survey has been compiled, it needs to be tested. A pilot stage will ensure that all the relevant issues are included, the order and the flow of the questions are correct, ambiguous or leading questions are identified, the flow of the question, and whether the questions are interpreted similarly. This at times may be difficult to establish and it may need some more discussion with the pilot subjects to determine how they interpreted the question and what they thought when giving an answer.[4] This process is known as cognitive interviewing.

The ideal situation is to test the questionnaire on a small number of respondents who are the same type as those in the sampling frame. However, this is not always possible and the questionnaire may have to be tested with slightly different participants. At the very minimum, it should be evaluated by a number of other researchers, particularly those who have used similar questionnaires and the answers in an epidemiological study.[7] After this, the questionnaire should be tested on a small sample of the target population in a controlled setting, which may highlight areas in which work still needs to be done.

Where possible, being present while the pilot is going on will allow a focus group-type atmosphere in which you can discuss aspects of the survey with those who are going to be filling it in. This step may seem nonessential but detecting previously unconsidered difficulties needs to happen as early as possible and it is important to use your participants' time wisely as they are unlikely to give it again.[13]

8.8 Translation

The globalization of research sometimes means that we do research in different countries. We live in a multilingual world and there are some countries that are officially multilingual. More and more, international multicenter studies are conducted, for example, in Europe, and this may require translation of questionnaires into different languages. Furthermore, immigrants in the country are being studied and this requires translation of the questionnaire into other languages as they may not be familiar with their new language to be able to answer any questions satisfactorily.[4] Although a simple translation to and translation back from the second language (back translation) might be enough, further piloting and cognitive interviews may be required to identify and correct for any cultural differences in interpretation of the translated questionnaire.[10] Translators should be experts, familiar with the language and the topic.

After the translation has been done, the questionnaire should be pilot tested again to make sure that no information has been lost in the process and the questions are interpreted in the same way as in the original questionnaire.[4]

Translation into other languages may alter the layout and formatting of words on the page from the original design. For this reason, it is important to consider further redesign of the questionnaire after the translation is done.[10]

8.9 Reliability and Validity

The most important consideration in the design and administration of a questionnaire is that it must be able to measure accurately what it is designed to measure.[14] The accuracy of the data obtained from a questionnaire has two components: reliability and validity.

When the questionnaire actual measures what it needs to measure, it is known as validity. For example, do people who report smoking 10 cigarettes per day actually smoke 10 cigarettes per day? Ideally, all questions and answers should be validated, compared to the gold standard. However, selecting a gold standard is not always easy. Sometimes there is no way to measure the subject of interest. It is very important not to select a poor gold standard to avoid misleading information about the questionnaire.[4]

The sensitivity, specificity, positive predictive (PPV), and negative predictive value (NPV) are the most common indices of validity of the information of the questionnaire. Sensitivity is defined as the probability that the individual with the trait is correctly identified by the questionnaire as having the trait.[14] For example, a questionnaire on drinking habits is sensitive if individuals who drink are correctly identified by the questionnaire as drinkers. Specificity is the probability that the individuals without the trait are correctly identified by the questionnaire that the trait is not present.[14] Thus, for the same questionnaire on drinking habits, the specificity is high for those who do not drink. The PPV is the probability that a positive test will correctly identify individuals with a specified trait.[14] NPV, on the other hand, is the probability that a negative test will accurately identify people without the trait.[14] For further reading on this complex topic, please see the Users Guides to the Medical Literature reference in the Further Reading section of this chapter.

Besides the validity, there is the repeatability of the questionnaire (known as reliability or reproducibility). The reliability of a questionnaire may be assessed by administering the questionnaire to a proportion of subjects in the target population at two different points of time. The interval between the two occasions should be long enough to provide independent observations but not too long to avoid true variation in exposure.[4] It is crucial to administer the questionnaire using the same method to avoid additional variation into the process.

The validity of an instrument is affected by reliability. If there is poor reliability, validity will be reduced.[14]

8.10 Analysis of Survey Data

It is all too easy to busy oneself with the questionnaire design and data collection and forget about the analysis. It is very crucial to think about the analysis very early on to establish the data type of the main outcome measure. The data type determines which type of statistical test is most appropriate, and this has implications for the required sample size.[7]

The method of data analysis will depend on the design of the survey and should have been carefully considered in the planning stages of the survey. Data collected by qualitative methods should be analyzed and establish methods such as content analysis, and where quantitative methods have been used, appropriate statistical test can be applied. For advanced analysis, a statistician should be consulted.[5]

The collected data will come in a number of forms, depending on the method of collection. Data from telephone, personal interviews, or electronic questionnaires can be directly entered into a computer database, whereas postal data can be entered at a later time. Problems appear at the time of data entry when questionnaires are returned with missing data fields. As mentioned earlier, it is essential to have a statistician involved from the beginning for help with data analysis. The statistician can help to determine the sample size required to ensure that your study has enough power.[13]

8.11 Ethics of Survey Research

Concerns over ethical considerations in survey research can be traced to reported abuses of human subjects during World War II. In response to these and other mistreatments of study participants, the research community developed a set of basic ethical principles related to investigations involving human subjects, the core of which are respect for persons, beneficence, and justice.[15] Basically, the ethical principles are the standards for conduct that distinguish between right and wrong. They help to determine the difference between acceptable and unacceptable behaviors on the part of the researcher.

In addition to the treatment of human subjects, ethical concerns in survey research involve designing studies ensuring ethical practice. The research protocol must be reviewed by an ethics committee and the informed consent from subjects should be obtained, except where the research is judged to present no more than minimal risk.[9] The ethical principles also ensure confidentiality of personally identifiable data. It is crucial that researchers keep respondents' identities confidential. To ensure confidentiality, research coordinators should not link respondents' identifiers to their survey responses when using data.

Survey researchers face a number of choices in conducting any study, from the mode of data collection to sample selection, questionnaire construction, and the amount of resources devoted to collecting information from selected respondents. All these procedures should be done under ethical principles. In reporting survey results, researchers should be transparent and fully disclose their methods and conclusions so that they can be evaluated and replicated by other researchers.[15]

8.12 Practical Application

- **Research question:** Do health professionals who work in the intensive care unit (ICU) have burnout?
- **Background:** Burnout has been described as a prolonged response to chronic emotional and interpersonal stress on the job that is often the result of a period of expending excessive effort at work while having too little recovery time. An ICU is a continuously busy, high-stress, complex, and multidisciplinary environment in which critically ill patients are on life-support treatment under intensive monitoring and healthcare professionals routinely provide numerous forms of advanced life-support and life-sustaining measures. Healthcare workers who work in a stressful medical environment, especially in an ICU, may be particularly susceptible to burnout. In healthcare workers, burnout may affect their well-being and the quality of professional care they provide and can, therefore, be detrimental to patient safety.
- **Objective:** To determine the prevalence of burnout in the ICU setting and to identify factors associated with burnout in ICU professionals.

- **Methods:** Web-based survey of health professionals working in an ICU. The survey captured sociodemographic data and integrated the validated Maslach Burnout Inventory (MBI).
- **Survey design:** It is a prospective cross-sectional survey.
- **Study population:** All healthcare professionals working in the ICU. The survey targeted all registered nurses, nurse practitioners, registered respiratory therapies, allied health professionals (i.e., dietitians, pharmacists, physiotherapists, and social workers), and critical care physicians (MD).
- **Administration mode:** It is a self-administered questionnaire. The survey is distributed using SurveyMonkey.com, a secure web-based electronic tool.
- **Pilot:** The survey underwent pre-, pilot, and clinical sensibility testing for clarity, comprehension, face validity, and administrative ease. Pilot testing was also performed on the connectivity and online form of the survey to assess functionality and flow.
- **Survey content:** The survey integrated selected sociodemographic factors (eight questions) included: age, sex, marital status, religiosity, provider type, experience (years of practice), duration in ICU (years), and current position (full-time and part-time); and a validated tool to screen and evaluate for burnout syndrome (MBI for Human Services Survey [MBI-HSS]).

The MBI is a 22-item questionnaire asking respondents on a 7-point Likert scale the frequency with which they have experienced recent feelings related to their work.

The MBI evaluates three subscale domains:
- **Emotional exhaustion:** Measures feelings of being emotionally overextended and exhausted by one's work (nine items).
- **Depersonalization:** Measures an unfeeling and impersonal response toward recipients of one's service, care, or treatment (five items).
- **Personal accomplishment:** Measures the feelings of competence and successful achievement in one's work with people (eight items).

The MBI-HSS has been reliable and valid and is easy to administer.
- **Survey instrument:** MBI-HSS.

Instructions: On the following pages are 22 statements of job-related feelings. Please read each statement carefully and decide if you ever feel this way about *your* job.

If you have *never* had this feeling, select the button under the Never column. If you have had this feeling, indicate *how often* you feel it by selecting the phrase that best describes how frequently you feel that way.

The phrases describing the frequency are:

Never (0)
A few times a year or less (1)
Once a month or less (2)
A few times a month (3)
Once a week (4)
A few times a week (5)
Every day (6)

1. I feel emotionally drained from my work.
2. I feel used up at the end of the day.
3. I feel fatigued when I get up in the morning and have to face another day on the job.
4. I can easily understand how my recipients feel about things.
5. I feel treat some recipients as if they were impersonal objects.
6. Working with people all day is really a strain for me.
7. I deal very effectively with the problems of my recipients.
8. I feel burned out from my work.
9. I feel I am positively influencing other people's lives through my work.
10. I have become more callous toward people since I took this job.
11. I worry that this job is hardening me emotionally.
12. I feel very energetic.
13. I feel frustrated by my job.
14. I feel I am working too hard on my job.
15. I do not really care what happens to some recipients.
16. Working with people directly puts too much stress on me.
17. I can easily create a relaxed atmosphere with my recipients.
18. I feel exhilarated after working closely with my recipients.
19. I have accomplished many worthwhile things in this job.
20. I feel like I am at the end of my rope.
21. In my work, I deal with emotional problems very calmly.
22. I feel recipients blame me for some of their problems.

- **Survey interpretation:** Three levels of burnout: high level of burnout (−8 to +34); a moderate level (−21 to −9); and a low level (−45 to −22).
- **Type of questions:** Closed-ended questions. There is a limited number of possible answers, including questions related to demographics. For instance, age is categorized into four options: less than 25 years; 26 to 34 years; 35 to 50 years; and more than 51 years.

8.13 Conclusion

Survey research is a type of research of gathering information from a large cohort. Survey research has the ability to collect large amounts of information and consequently having greater statistical power and validated models. However, to yield meaningful results, conducting a survey requires money, time, and effort. Often having a high response rate to a survey can be hard to control.

The key of a successful survey research study is proper design, implementation, analysis, and pilot testing, always having in mind that the topic of interest should be carefully planned and relate clearly to the research question.

Definitions

- **Household drop-off survey:** A survey technique in which a researcher drops off questionnaires for respondents to complete in their own time; the completed forms are mailed back to the researcher or picked up again some time later.
- **Questionnaire:** Is a set of questions used to collect data. Questionnaires can be administered face to face, over a telephone, on the web or by self-completion. Questionnaires can include closed- and open-ended questions.
- **Response rate:** Is the proportion of people who have participated in a study or completed a questionnaire. It is calculated by dividing the total number of people who have participated by those who were approached or asked to participate.
- **Sampling frame:** Are the potential participants for entry into a study. The sampling frame is also known as the "population of interest."
- **Survey:** Is a method of collecting large-scale quantitative data but does not use an experimental design. With a survey, there is no control over who receives the intervention or when. Instead, a survey design can examine the real world and describe existing relationships.

References

[1] Ponto J. Understanding and Evaluating Survey Research. J Adv Pract Oncol 2015;6(2):168–171

[2] Paul CP, Rajiv SJ. I–Chant AC. Research Methods in Psychology. 2nd ed. BC Open Text Project; 2016. https://opentextbc.ca. Accessed June 8, 2019

[3] socialresearchmethods.net. [Internet]. California: Web Center for Social Research Methods; c2004. https://socialresearchmethods.net/kb/index.php. Accessed June 10, 2019

[4] Nieuwenhuijsen MJ. Design of Exposure Questionnaires for Epidemiological Studies. Occup Environ Med 2005;62(4):272–280, 212–214

[5] Kelley K, Clark B, Brown V, Sitzia J. Good Practice in the Conduct and Reporting of Survey Research. Int J Qual Health Care 2003;15(3):261–266

[6] Wright KB. Researching Internet-Based Populations: Advantages and Disadvantages of Online Survey Research, Online Questionnaire Authoring Software Packages, and Web Survey Services. J Comput Mediat Commun 2005;10(3)

[7] Mathers N, Fox N, Hunn A. Surveys and Questionnaires. East Midlands/Yorkshire and Humber: NIHR RDS; 2007

[8] researchconnections.org. [Internet]. Michigan: Child and Care Early Education Research Connections; c2004. https://www.researchconnections.org/childcare/datamethods/survey.jsp. Accessed June 8, 2019

[9] Armstrong BK, White E, Saracci R. Principles of Exposure Measurement in Epidemiology: Monographs in Epidemiology and Biostatistics. New York, NY: Oxford University Press; 1995

[10] Edwards P. Questionnaires in Clinical Trials: Guidelines for Optimal Design and Administration. Trials 2010;11(2):2

[11] Billiet J, Loosveldt G. Improvement of the Quality of Responses to Factual Survey Questions by Interviewer Training. Public Opin Q 1998;52(5):190–211

[12] O'Brien EM, Mayer TS, Groves RM, O'Neill GE. Interviewer Training to Increase Survey Participation. Proceedings of the Section on Survey Research Methods. Alexandria, VA: American Statistical Association; 2002

[13] Jones TL, Baxter MAJ, Khanduja V. A Quick Guide to Survey Research. Ann R Coll Surg Engl 2013;95(1):5–7

[14] Saw SM, Ng TP. The design and assessment of questionnaires in clinical research. Singapore Med J 2001;42(3):131–135

[15] Gideon L. Handbook of Survey Methodology for the Social Sciences. New York, NY: Springer; 2012

Further Reading

Guyatt GH, Rennie D, Meade MO, Cook DJ, eds. Users' Guides to the Medical Literature: A Manual for Evidence-Based Clinical Practice. 3rd Edition. McGraw-Hill Education; 2015. ISBN 978-0-07-179071-0

9 Qualitative Studies

Patricia Schneider

Abstract

Qualitative research methods are robust tools for health researchers. They are selected as the study method of choice when the objectives of the research are to examine, understand, or describe a specific phenomenon, beliefs, or behaviors that cannot be quantified. Unlike quantitative studies, qualitative studies are subject to inherent biases as the researcher plays an important role within the study, and sampling strategies are often deliberately selective; however, when conducted properly and with the proper management of these biases, qualitative research can produce high-quality, information-rich data. This chapter provides details on how to properly plan for and execute a qualitative study.

Keywords: interview, focus group, observation, sampling strategies

9.1 Objectives

This chapter is intended to provide research personnel with an overview of qualitative research concepts and study design. We will discuss the different types of qualitative studies and provide some practical considerations for the design, implementation, and conduct of qualitative studies in health research.

9.2 Introduction

9.2.1 Why Qualitative Research?

Qualitative research is a form of inquiry that can help us analyze invaluable information conveyed through language so that we can understand the underlying behaviors, attitudes, and perceptions that determine health outcomes. Qualitative methods can also help understand the health care system, and the complex relationships between individuals, groups, and institutions within them. While there is no universal method or plan, there are a few basic concepts and principles that are common to most approaches to the conduct of qualitative research.

9.2.2 What is Qualitative Research?

Originating from the social sciences, qualitative research methods provide a systematic approach to gathering non-numerical data, and are used to understand people's beliefs, experiences, attitudes, behaviors, and interactions. It requires the reflection on the part of researchers throughout the duration of the research process. Although qualitative research encompasses a broad range of study methods, most qualitative studies in health research utilize interviews and focus groups.

9.2.3 Qualitative versus Quantitative Research

Since a qualitative researcher does not set out to measure, it is often seen as the exact opposite of quantitative research. In quantitative research, data are facts that should remain separate from their personal and subjective values as subjectivity can mean bias. Quantitative research is deductive. However, in qualitative research, it is accepted that the world is perceived only partially by any one individual and the many aspects of reality should be described. To the qualitative researcher, subjectivity is an essential element of the research process as accessing these multiple worldviews is through the subjective experiences and understandings of study participants. Qualitative research is inductive.

In reality, qualitative and quantitative research are complementary to each other, and each can offer a compelling view of a problem. Therefore, it is important to determine which method is the most appropriate to effectively and efficiently answer the research question.

9.2.4 Advantages of Qualitative Research

Once thought to be incompatible with experimental research, qualitative research is now recognized for its ability to add a new dimension to interventional studies that cannot be obtained through the measurement of variables and outcomes alone.

Qualitative research generates rich, detailed data and leaves the perspectives of participants intact in order to obtain a more realistic view of the world that cannot be understood in numerical data. It is appropriate when you want to understand the perspectives of participants, explore the meaning they give to an event or phenomena, or observe a process in depth.

9.3 Designing and Conducting the Study

Before conducting a study, it is important to prepare a detailed study protocol as it will force you to consider all major aspects of the study, such as those detailed below. This, in turn, should improve the overall quality of the study. Once prepared, the study protocol should be approved by all members of the research team.

9.3.1 General Study Details

Like all study protocols, a qualitative study protocol should include the study title, an overview of the research team with academic affiliations, and any study funding.

9.3.2 Research Question

It is important to first define the research problem in order to lay the foundation for the research question and study objectives. To do so, a systematic review should be conducted to evaluate the current literature. It is best to conduct the search in multiple databases, such as EMBASE, MEDLINE, and the Cochrane Library, and then delete any duplicates to ensure a comprehensive search of all available literature. Consulting with the appropriate librarian to develop your search strategy is advised. From here, knowledge gaps can be identified so that a meaningful question can be developed. In the case of qualitative studies, the PICO (Population, Intervention, Comparison, and Outcome) framework is not applicable.

9.3.3 Research Objectives

In a study protocol, the research objectives provide a map of the overall purpose or your study. They tend to use words such as "to explore," "to examine," or "to describe."

9.4 Study Methods

It is important to determine which methodology will best answer your research question. There are many schools of thought among qualitative researchers on matters of the methods to be used. There are several different qualitative methodologies; this section provides a brief overview of the three most common methodologies: ethnography, grounded theory, and phenomenology.

9.4.1 Ethnography

Ethnography involves researchers using direct observation to study participants in their natural environments ("real lives") over time.[1] The natural environment is as important as the participants because it acknowledges that the environment and context can influence participants' behaviors and outcomes.[1]

9.4.2 Grounded Theory

Grounded theory is a framework for qualitative research that suggests that theory should derive from data, rather than other forms of inquiry that suggest the exact opposite.[2] This study methodology involves the interaction of researchers with participants, such as in-person interviews and focus groups, to explore a research phenomenon to help clarify a problem when little to nothing is known or understood, and any attempt to start with a theory is, at best, speculation.

9.4.3 Phenomenology

Phenomenology involves the study of human experiences in their own world and provides researchers with a tool to understand subjective experiences.[3,4] It attempts to understand problems or opinions for the perspective of common understanding (rather than differences).[3] Phenomenological studies often utilize participant observation.

9.5 Sampling

Like all clinical research, it is not possible for you to collect data from all individuals in a given area or population. Therefore, you must collect data from a subset, or sample, of the overall study population.

In quantitative research, the objective would be to obtain a random sampling that was representative of the overall population. However, the objective of qualitative research is to provide an in-depth understanding of a given group, individual, or problem. To do so, qualitative research utilizes several different sampling strategies to reach their target sample. The three most common sampling strategies are purposive, quota, and chain-referral (snowball) sampling.

9.5.1 Purposive Sampling

Purposive sampling is one of the most common sampling strategies in qualitative research. This sampling strategy relies on participants being grouped according to preselected criteria.[5] This allows for the inclusion of "information-rich" cases, which often enables a more thorough analysis of data and reaching more relevant conclusions.[6] For example, if a researcher wants to elucidate the views and opinions of stay-at-home mothers, the researchers can knock on doors during the day when children are likely to be at school to identify their target population. Purposive sample sizes are often determined on the basis of theoretical saturation (i.e., the point in data collection when new data no longer bring additional insights to the research question). Therefore, this sampling strategy is most successful when data collection and analysis are simultaneously conducted. There are several different techniques to purposively sample a population, including maximal variation, extreme case, typical, homogenous, and opportunistic.

9.5.2 Quota Sampling

Another common sampling strategy is quota sampling, which is often considered a subtype of purposive sampling. This strategy requires the study team to determine the number of participants that fit each specific preselected criterion to be included.[5] This is typically decided on during the design phase of the study. For example, if gender were hypothesized to have an effect on participation in the workforce, a quota sample would seek an equal number of male and female participants (assuming a 1:1 gender ratio in your population of interest).

9.5.3 Chain-Referral (Snowball) Sampling

Chain-referral sampling, also known as snowball sampling, utilizes existing study participants to refer individuals from their social networks to contribute to the study.[7] This sampling strategy is often used to find hidden populations (i.e., groups that are not easily accessible using conventional sampling strategies).[7] For example, if a researcher is interested in obtaining the views and insights of sex trade workers on sexually transmitted disease testing, he/she may ask participants to refer their colleagues to participate in the study.

▶ Table 9.1 shows some advantages and disadvantages of each sampling method.

9.6 Sample Size

Once a sampling strategy has been chosen, you must consider your study's sample size. Sample sizes in qualitative research are not determined by fixed rules, but by factors such as depth and feasibility. Larger sample sizes do not necessarily produce greater applicability of the findings.[8] In fact, larger samples may exchange depth of the data for range of information.[8] Moreover, too much data

Table 9.1 Advantages and disadvantages of qualitative sampling strategies

Sampling strategy	When to use	Advantage(s)	Disadvantage(s)
Purposive	When proportionality with the overall population is not a concern	Flexible	Highly prone to selection bias
Quota	When strata are present and stratified sampling is impossible	Ensures some degree of representativeness of all individuals within a population	External validity is questionable
Chain referral	When subjects are hard to locate	Allows for studies to be conducted where it might otherwise prove impossible due to a lack of participants	Difficult to make inferences about the overall population

may be also be produced, which may overwhelm the analysis stage.[8] Therefore, the sample size depends on the study's aims, feasibility, resources, and saturation. In reality, the sample sizes of qualitative research studies tend to not exceed 50 participants.

9.7 Qualitative Data Collection

Primarily, three categories of qualitative research are of interest to clinical researchers—observation, interviews, and focus groups. It is important to determine which is best for your specific research study.

9.7.1 Observation

Observation is the earliest and most rudimentary source of human knowledge. Studying actual behavior can be helpful to evaluate how long individuals spend on various activities, witness nonverbal communication, and determine who interacts with whom. Depending on the purpose of your research, you will have to recognize whether you should observe individuals from an insider's or outsider's perspective. There are two general types of observation—outside and inside. Outside observation, such as **direct observation**, requires that the observers maintain a greater distance in order to view events from their own perspectives.[9] Inside observation, such as **participant observation**, on the other hand, requires that observers interact with the individuals they are observing in order to view events from the perspectives of the participants.[10]

Once you have selected a site to observe and determined your role as an observer (outside or inside), ease into the site by slowly looking around to obtain a general sense of the site. Once you have settled into the site, identify the individuals or events to observe, as well as when and for how long observations should take place. Also, consider the information that is important for you to record during your observation sessions, including both descriptive and reflective field notes. Conduct multiple observations on multiple occasions to obtain a thorough understanding of the site and the individuals there. Ensure that your note-taking is as discreet as possible. ▶ Box 9.1 provides other suggestions for taking detailed field notes. Once you have concluded your observation, slowly withdraw yourself from your observation site.

9.7.2 Interview

In-depth interviews explore the experiences of participants and the meanings they attribute to them.[9] Researchers encourage participants to talk about issues pertinent to the research question by asking open-ended questions, usually in one-on-one interviews. The interviewer might reword, reorder, or clarify the questions asked to further investigate topics introduced by the interviewee. In qualitative research, interviews are often used to study the experiences and meaning of disease, and to explore personal and sensitive themes.[9] They are appropriate when the topics of a discussion are highly sensitive and argue for a discussion format that maximizes confidentiality.

9.7.3 Focus Group

Focus groups are semistructured discussions with small groups (5–15 individuals) that aim to explore a specific set of issues.[11] Discussion facilitators often begin by asking broad questions about the topic of interest, before asking more focused questions.[11] Although participants individually answer the facilitator's questions, they are encouraged to discuss and interact with other group participants.[11] This qualitative technique assumes that the group environment encourages participants to explore and clarify individual and shared perspectives.[12] Focus groups are often used to explore views on health issues, services, interventions, and research. They are appropriate when the topics of discussion focus on cultural norms, attitudes, or reactions of a group, and when individuals feel comfortable disclosing specific relevant information in front of their peers.

9.7.4 Discussion Guide/Interview Script Development

When designing a discussion guide or interview script, it is imperative to ask questions that are likely to yield as much useful data as possible in order to address the research objectives. As such, most researchers prefer a semistructured discussion guide/interview script that contains questions that reflect on the initial themes of the basic research problem. This tool serves as a framework for the material that should be covered during the discussion, and often contains a set of standardized open-ended questions with examples of multiple ways the questions can be worded. Typically, a discussion guide/interview script will start with questions that are easily answered, before advancing to more difficult or sensitive topics. This will help build a rapport with participants, which is likely to generate information-rich data later on in the discussion. A discussion guide/interview script will also often contain possible probes to prompt discussion with greater depth and follow-up questions for a number of possible responses. ▶ Box 9.2 shows some common errors to avoid when facilitating interviews and discussion groups.

The typical structure of a discussion guide is as follows:

1. Welcome

Welcome participants to the focus group. Review what the focus group is trying to accomplish, what will be done with the information collected, and why the participants were asked to participate.

2. Consent Process

Review the Participant Information Sheet and Consent Form with participants. Inform participants that the information provided is completely confidential, and their names will never be associated with anything said during the focus group. Explain to participants that they can refuse to answer any questions.

3. Explanation of the Focus Group Process

Ask the participants if anyone has participated in a focus group before. Explain that the intent of a focus group is not to achieve consensus—it is merely to collect data. Inform participants of the approximate length of time the discussion will last. Explain any "ground rules" for the discussion period. Finally, inform participants that they should say their names prior to answering any question during the discussion. Turn on your voice recorder at this point.

4. Introductions

Introduce yourself and the remainder of your study team. Ask participants to go around and introduce themselves.

5. Discussion

Ask participants if they have any questions before the discussion period begins. If not, begin working through your discussion guide at this point. Make sure to give participants sufficient time to think before answering the questions, and refrain

---

Box 9.2: Common Errors to Avoid while Facilitating Interview/Focus Groups

- Asking "leading" questions that might influence the responses of participants, such as:
  - Would you agree that ... ?
  - Do you mean ... ?
  - Don't you think that ... ?
- Repeating the original question you asked rather than rephrasing.
- Allowing only a few individuals to dominate a discussion rather than trying to engage quieter participants.
- Remaining too long on a topic, especially when saturation has already been reached.
- Interrupting, or allowing other participants to interrupt, individuals who disclose different points of view.
- Using technical or overly complicated language, rather than lay terms.
- Letting an important question go unanswered.
- Not asking for clarification of unfamiliar and/or vague terms.
- Not probing a question further if the opportunity presents itself.
- Being afraid of silence and nonverbal prompts.
- Presenting your own perspective.
- Conducting the interview or focus group in a location prone to interruptions.

from moving on too quickly. Use the discussion guide's question probes to ensure that all issues are addressed, but move on when the discussion begins to reach saturation (a situation where participants are reiterating what others have mentioned and new ideas cease to be discussed).

6. Closing Remarks

Inform participants that the focus group has now concluded. Thank participants for taking the time to attend and for contributing to the discussion. Inform participants of any next steps at this point.

It is suggested that you first pilot a discussion guide/interview script to test its face validity before you begin formally using it to collect data. This will provide you with the opportunity to reword any questions that were unclear or restructure the script/guide if the ordering was illogical.

9.7.5 Interview/Focus Group Question Development

When developing the questions to ask in an interview or focus group, first identify topic domains and any subtopics that pertain to your research objectives. Then arrange them in a logical sequence to ensure flow, beginning with general questions to orient your participant(s) and gain his/her/their trust. Develop specific questions for each topic domain, ensuring that each domain contains a main question to introduce the topic, follow-up questions that take the discussion to a deeper level and probe/seek clarification and ask for greater detail. Place more sensitive questions toward the end, which you can tackle once you have established a rapport with your participant(s).

9.7.6 Collecting Initial Demographic Details

Obtaining a brief demographic overview of each participant can provide valuable information for the analysis phase of the research study as it may assist you in the interpretation of the discussion, as well as help you describe your sample as you report your study.

The demographic data you collect should be succinct and relevant to the research study. Typically, age, sex/gender, level of education, marital status, and occupation are considered essential demographic questions that should be asked. When conducting an interview, it is acceptable to directly ask these questions to the participant; however, when conducting a focus group, the questions should be administered via a form for participants to individually complete in order to maintain confidentiality.

9.7.7 Obtaining Adequate Responses

Interviewing or facilitating a focus group requires interpersonal skills to quickly develop a nonjudgmental conversation while also maintaining the progress of a discussion. It is important to be responsive to interviewees/meeting participants by demonstrating an interest or curiosity in what they say. Similarly, it is also crucial that an interviewer/facilitator is flexible and responsive in order to quickly react to the responses of interviewees/meeting participants. This will ensure that the responses to your questions are adequate for analysis. ▶ Box 9.3 describes some other important characteristics of a good qualitative interviewer/facilitator.

Box 9.3: The Makings of a Good Interviewer and Focus Group Facilitator

- Good verbal and listening skills.
- Good sense of timing.
- Able to create a safe environment so that others feel comfortable engaging in thoughtful discussion.
- Able to maintain neutrality, thereby preventing personal biases from impacting others.
- Empathetic and enthusiastic.
- Able to quickly build rapport and demonstrate acceptance of participants.
- Able to put others at ease.
- Patient.
- Responsive (not reactive).
- Sensitive.
- Intuitive to the overall feelings/mood of the group.
- Able to quickly interpret the responses of participants in order to further explore research problem.

9.7.8 Transcription of Interviews and Focus Groups

For the purposes of this chapter, we have assumed that all interviews and focus groups have been digitally recorded. Best practice dictates that you should transcribe your recordings from discussions or focus groups as soon as possible. If left to be reviewed until all fieldwork is complete, you will miss the opportunity to add nonverbal points, as well as the opportunity to follow-up on emerging hypotheses. Thankfully, transcription services exist to transcribe the conversation, but only you can add important nonverbal information. Recordings should be transcribed verbatim, irrespective of how comprehensible the dialogue may be when read back. Lines of text should be numbered for easy identification. Once the transcription process is complete, read the transcript while listening to the recording as a final review. Then remove any identifying names, places, or noteworthy events to anonymize the data.

Managing the transcriptions of focus groups is slightly more challenging as multiple voices are involved. Labeling each individual voice (such as Voice A, Voice B, etc., or Participant 1, Participant 2, etc.) is the most common way of handling this issue. If a second facilitator was present during the focus group and took field notes regarding participants, you may be able to cross-reference the transcript with the field notes to ensure that you are accurately labeling each voice.

9.8 Data Analysis and Interpretation

9.8.1 Qualitative Data Analysis Approaches

The type of analysis approach you choose is typically related to the purpose and intentions of your study. As such, the approach to your analysis is typically decided on before you begin conducting your study. Some brief explanations of four common analysis approaches are presented in the following sections. For further information on data analysis approaches, please consult:

Formative Approach

A form of exploratory research, the formative approach is used to better understand a specific population or problem so that a larger investigation is relevant and acceptable.[13]

Descriptive Approach

The qualitative descriptive approach is an appropriate analysis approach when a straightforward description of a particular phenomenon or event is the objective of a study.[13]

Explanatory Approach

While most often a quantitative analysis approach is used to establish a cause-and-effect relationship among variables and outcomes in clinical research, incorporating qualitative methods in mixed-methods study designs can produce convincing new insights that can help clarify patterns and relationships observed in data.[13]

Transformative Approach

A transformative approach typically involves the engagement and empowerment of participants in order to understand not only the group but also their individual needs.[13]

9.8.2 Qualitative Data Coding

Once your data collection period is complete, you will be left with copious amounts of data that include observation journal entries, interview transcriptions, or open-ended questionnaire responses. You will likely already, intuitively, have developed answers to your research questions. However, you now need to analyze your data as objectively as possible. To do so, you will first need to review your data and assign a code—a process called **open coding**.[14] Then, you will need to organize these codes into themes, patterns, or categories—a process called **axial coding**.[14] This process is often nonlinear as you will often analyze data while you are collecting data, as well as notice new concepts in data that you have already analyzed as you continue to develop your analysis (see ▶ Fig. 9.1).

Step 1: Breaking Down Data

The first step is to break down the data into parts that are manageable for analysis. Typically, qualitative researchers will divide interview responses into sections that represent complete thoughts. For focus group transcriptions, responses will be separated by participants.

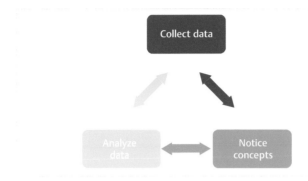

Fig. 9.1 Qualitative data analysis process.

Step 2: Initial Review of Data—Coding

Once the transcription has been broken down into manageable sections, your initial review of the data should begin. Tag (code) different sections of the data with labels appropriate to represent the concepts they signify. These labels will be used later to identify the concepts for further analysis.

Step 3: Second Review of Data—Categorizing

As the analysis phase continues, you may begin to notice common characteristics and group them into categories. These categories can be given names derived directly from the data itself, also known as "in vivo" names. Some categories may contain clusters of coded data that require further refinement into subcategories.

Step 4: Developing Theories

When major categories are compared with each other, they can be merged under a theme or concept.

9.8.3 Data Management Software

Since qualitative analysis can produce large quantities of textual data, qualitative data management software can help efficiently store and retrieve data. NVivo is one of the most popular data management programs as it is possible to import large transcription documents and code or write memos in the margins of the document. It is important to note that while software such as NVivo can help organize data, it will not code the data for you. However, the investment of time required to learn how to operate software such as NVivo is substantial and not always worth it (especially for smaller studies). However, if you will be generating a large dataset and multiple researchers will be working on it, software may facilitate easier retrieval and management of data.

9.9 Reporting and Disseminating the Study

Determining the dissemination format that you choose to disseminate your research findings depends on the primary audience you intend to inform, your purpose for disseminating the findings, the study's characteristics, and any obligations to the study participants. Irrespective of how you intend to disseminate the results, the nature of qualitative research has important implications for how study findings are reported. Qualitative reporting conventions dictate that you keep the following four principles in mind:

1. **Balance and accuracy, not neutrality.**
Accurately present all sides of the research problem and the insights of participants.

2. **No harm.**
Ensure that no harm comes to the participants as a result of the dissemination of their opinions or experiences, which includes not only maintaining confidentiality at all times but also ensuring that any information you disclose in the manuscript does not reveal the identity of participants.

3. **A public voice for participants.**
Including quotes of the participants maintains the authenticity of the data and helps convey important contextual information to readers.

4. **Context of interactions and role.**
In order for your audience to judge the quality of the research, they must have adequate, forthright information regarding your relationship with the participants.

If your purpose is to further academic discussion with your colleagues, writing a manuscript for publication in a peer-reviewed journal would be appropriate. Publications usually state conceptual frameworks or theories for better understanding an issue, describe the methodologies used, present the results, interpret the data, and then relate the findings to other studies. Publications intended to reach your colleagues also often includes suggestions for better practices (if applicable) and policy recommendations. It is also strongly recommended that qualitative studies are reported according to the Consolidated Criteria for Reporting Qualitative Research (COREQ), a set of guidelines established by the Enhancing the QUAlity and Transparency Of health Research (EQUATOR) network. Included in these guidelines is a 32-item checklist with recommendations for each item to be reported.

If your purpose is to reach policymakers, reports/briefs are typically used, which typically include a summary of the most important points and recommendations for courses of action. Some approaches, such as analytic, narrative, policy, and problem-solving approaches, are widely used to organize these reports.

When disseminating study results to participants, it is important to, again, consider maintaining confidentiality. This is tremendously important because others may be unaware of an individual's participation in the research study. Some appropriate ways include announcing key study findings in a public setting or on social media.

9.9.1 Where to Publish?

If you have decided on publishing in a peer-reviewed journal, it is important to consider the subject matter of your study when determining what journal is appropriate. While numerous journals focus on particular diseases or populations, others focus on other aspects of a study, such as certain methodologies, including qualitative studies. Another important consideration is the audience that you intend to reach.

9.9.2 Authorship

According to the International Committee of Medical Journal Editors (ICMJE), coauthors should meet all of the following criteria:
- Substantial contributions to the conception or design of the study, or the collection, analysis, and interpretation of the data.

- Drafting the manuscript or critically revising the manuscript for important intellectual content.
- Final approval of the manuscript.
- Agreement to be accountable for the accuracy and integrity of all aspects of the manuscript.

See the following recommendations for further details: http://www.icmje.org/recommendations/browse/roles-and-responsibilities/defining-the-role-of-authors-and-contributors.html.

9.10 Ethical Implications

Asking individuals to discuss experiences can induce or exacerbate anxiety. It may cause distress not only during the data collection phase but may also afterward. Therefore, qualitative researchers—like any other individuals involved in human research—should undergo formal research ethics training.

9.10.1 Informed Consent

Typically, formal informed consent is required for all qualitative research except participant observation, irrespective of the sampling method used to identify potential participants and the strategies used to recruit them.

9.10.2 Protecting Confidentiality

It is not always possible to understand the dangers that exist for your participants. It is, therefore, imperative to protect the identity of the individuals from whom you collect data. If collected, identities must be protected at all times and not left out in the open for others outside of the research team to see.

9.11 Other Considerations

Several limitations in the design and conduct of qualitative research exist.

9.11.1 Generalizability

The findings of qualitative research cannot be extended to wider populations with the same degree of certainty as quantitative research, as the findings are not tested to determine whether they are statistically significant.

9.11.2 Ambiguities

Because of the multiple meanings that words or phrases can take on, qualitative data can often be ambiguous and may be interpreted differently by different coders or data analyzers.

9.11.3 Frequency

Because the aim of the qualitative research is to provide a detailed description of the opinions and experiences of the study participants, no attempt is made to assign frequencies to categories and themes that are identified. This means that a view that is identified once will receive the same amount of attention as those more frequently discussed.

9.12 Types of Bias Associated with Qualitative Studies

The very nature of qualitative research entails subjective interpretation and, therefore, the potential for bias to influence the conclusions reached. However, the tests and measures used to establish validity and reliability in quantitative research, such as p-values and confidence intervals to estimate the size of error, cannot be applied to qualitative research. Below are several categories of bias that can influence qualitative research that the researcher should be aware of, including sampling bias, moderator bias, question bias, and reporting bias.

- *Facilitator bias:* The facilitator's tone, body language, and facial expressions may compromise the neutrality of the interview/focus group and, therefore, may influence the responses obtained and produce bias.
- *Observer bias:* When a researcher observes a specific group, he/she usually has prior knowledge (and, therefore, subjective thoughts) of the group, which can influence what the researcher observes (i.e., we see what we want/expect to see).
- *Question bias:* Biased questions, such as leading questions, may suggest what the correct response is and, therefore, may influence a participant's responses.
- *Reporting bias:* When a participant is selective in disclosing information regarding their views, thoughts, or experiences, it can distort data interpretation and, therefore, the study's conclusions.
- *Sampling bias:* When a sample consists of participants that are not representative of the overall group of interest, it can compromise the generalizability of the study results with the overall population.

9.12.1 Strategies for Managing Bias

Because of the inherent subjectivity (and, therefore, the risk of bias) in qualitative studies, it is important to keep the subjectivity in check to maximize the study's rigor. Bias in qualitative research can be minimized if you know how to manage it. Below are several suggestions for how you can adequately manage bias.

1. **Maintain a careful researcher/participant boundary.**
When conducting qualitative research, it is important to become a part of the group. However, for the safety of both researchers and participants, as well as the integrity of the data, it is important to maintain a boundary.

2. **Carefully document your experiences/data.**
Lost data can have profound consequences on the interpretation of other data, which can result in reaching erroneous or incomplete conclusions.

3. **Use multiple coders to analyze the data.**
The greater the consistency between your interpretation of the data and the interpretation of others, the more likely there is some validity to your interpretations. Discrepant interpretations, however, are not always a methodological weakness—multiple realities may result in contradictory but valid perspectives.

4. **Verify your interpretations with other data sources.**
If you can find other sources of data that support your interpretations of the data, the greater the confidence you can have in your interpretations.

9.13 Practical Application

In this section, a step-by-step approach for conducting a qualitative study is provided, using a qualitative descriptive study as an example. In this study, we aimed to identify barriers and facilitators to participating in collaborative research by orthopaedic oncology surgeons. A more detailed description of this project can be found in the study's final publication.[15]

9.13.1 Background

Extremity sarcomas are rare tumors, accounting for less than 1% of all malignancies. As such, sarcoma centers do not treat enough patients to conduct single-center prospective comparative trials. Therefore, multicenter collaboration is essential to the conduct of meaningful research that will result in evidence-based advances in sarcoma patient care. Given that there is now some experience of international collaboration in orthopaedic oncology, we thought it would be beneficial for posterity to understand what drives individuals to participate in collaborative clinical research and any issues with participating they have encountered.

9.13.2 Study Objective

The aim of this study was to identify facilitators and barriers encountered in large-scale collaborative research by surgeons currently involved, or interested, in the Prophylactic Antibiotic Regimens In Tumor SurgerY (PARITY) trial, the first multicenter randomized controlled trial in the field of orthopaedic oncology.

9.13.3 Study Design

The qualitative study was designed as a focus group. All members of the PARITY collaborative network, including surgeons at active sites and those at sites that were not enrolling patients, were invited via email to participate in a focus group discussion on their involvement in the trial. The participants met in person at a single venue. The discussion was digitally recorded and transcribed verbatim by an independent transcriptionist. One member of the research team was also present to take field notes.

9.13.4 Participants

The most important eligibility criteria were being an orthopaedic oncologist and having expressed an interest in participating in collaborative, large-scale research in the field. A total of 13 surgeons confirmed their voluntary participation and attended the focus group.

9.13.5 Discussion Guide

The research team, which included three orthopaedic surgeons, one qualitative researcher, the PARITY project manager, and an orthopaedic research program manager, developed and refined the questions in the semistructured discussion guide. The questions were vetted within this team for clarity and face validity. Questions were worded in a neutral manner in order to ensure that

they do not lead the study participants. The team knew that being involved (in some capacity) in the PARITY trial was common to all participants. In addition, most were familiar with each other, and all were highly educated; therefore, the team was confident in their ability to cover a number of different topics pertaining to their experiences. The team also prioritized questions so that if there was insufficient time, the most important topics would be covered. This study's discussion guide can be found in Appendix A.

9.13.6 Sample Size

A convenience sample with the goal of using purposeful sampling of the variable of experience with the PARITY collaborative network was utilized. It was expected that 10 to 20 individuals would participate, which would provide enough redundancy in the data to adequately describe the perceptions about incentives, facilitators, and barriers to prospective collaborative orthopaedic oncology research.

9.13.7 Ethical Considerations

Prior to the conduct of any research, the study received ethical approval from the appropriate institutional ethics board. The transcription of the discussion was anonymized by the qualitative researcher who led the discussion to ensure complete confidentiality of the participants' responses.

Data Collection

Focus Group Set-Up

We booked a meeting room in Orlando, Florida, United States, to correspond with the Musculoskeletal Tumor Society (MSTS) 2015 Annual Meeting. We arrived early before the focus group began to set up the room. We set up the chairs in a circle and set up the refreshments off to the side of the room. We tested the recorder and then placed it in the center of the discussion circle.

The Consent Process and Initial Data Collection

Upon arrival, we greeted the participants and then directed them to the refreshments. We then introduced ourselves, described our roles, reviewed the Informed Consent Form, acknowledged the digital recorder, and explained that it was there to ensure that all discussion contributions were documented. We assured participants that the recording would not be shared outside the research team and no written reports would identify them. After the consent process was completed, we individually collected demographic details by administering a short participant questionnaire.

Focus Group Discussion

We then described the focus group discussion process and the "ground rules." We emphasized that the opinions of all participants should be respected, that all participants should participate, and that there were no incorrect responses. We asked participants to silence their cellphones. We then began working through our discussion guide.

Conclusion

We finished the focus group by thanking participants and informing them of the next steps in the project.

Transcription

After the conclusion of the focus group, we hired a transcription service to transcribe the digital recording.

9.13.8 Analysis

The qualitative descriptive approach was utilized. Transcripts and field notes from the discussion were analyzed using conventional qualitative analysis, with codes being derived directly from the data rather than using preconceived categories. Within 6 weeks of the focus group, four members of the research team independently undertook line-by-line open and axial coding of the transcript and held a consensus meeting to develop the list of codes. They also assessed the level of data saturation. The research team then conducted axial coding of the data (i.e., reviewed the list of codes, discussed the relationship between them, and organized them into categories). NVivo Version 10.0 (QSR International | Doncaster, Australia), a qualitative software program, was used for data management and analysis. Demographic data were analyzed using descriptive statistics.

9.13.9 Reporting

Writing of the final report extended over 4 months after the completion of the final analysis. Reporting of the study followed the guidelines ascribed by the COREQ Checklist for Interviews and Focus Groups.

9.14 Conclusion

In conclusion, qualitative research can have important implications in the understanding of health outcomes and the health care system. Qualitative research is an accessible way for researchers to (1) provide insight into the underlying behaviors, attitudes, and perceptions of individuals that determine health outcomes; (2) identify the social and structural facilitators and barriers to the using the health services; and (3) clarify how to design a new intervention so that it has a greater potential for adoption/success. However, qualitative research is not easy and requires careful planning, consideration, and resources to conduct and produce quality findings. There are several ways to conduct qualitative research. This chapter has provided an introduction to several methodologies, concepts, and practical considerations. Further reading on the subject is essential to your true understanding of the concepts introduced.

Definitions

- **Analytic approach:** A method of report organization that involves describing what has been learned and how it fits or changes the larger framework.
- **Bias:** Any influence that provides a distortion in the results of a study.
- **Descriptive field notes:** A record of the events, activities, and individuals during an observation/focus group.
- **Direct observation:** A method of qualitative research that involves watching individuals and events in an unobtrusive manner (without interacting with research participants).
- **Discussion guide:** A set of guidelines that includes a list of topics, specific questions, and probes to cover during the interview/focus group.
- **Dissemination:** The act of circulating study data to stakeholders and other individuals who are interested in the research.

- **Dissemination format:** The style for the presentation of study findings.
- **Extreme case sampling:** A purposive sampling technique in which the researcher studies an outlier of a given population.
- **Facilitator:** The researcher who leads the focus group discussion with participants.
- **Follow-up question:** A question that directs the discussion to a deeper level by asking for further details.
- **Homogenous sampling:** A purposive sampling technique that involves the researcher sampling individuals based on specific, defining characteristic(s).
- **Main question:** A question that begins the discussion.
- **Maximal variation sampling:** A purposive sampling technique in which the researcher samples individuals who differ on a distinct characteristic.
- **Narrative approach:** A method of report organization that explains the problem in a chronological narrative from multiple perspectives.
- **Opportunistic sampling:** A purposive sampling technique in which the researcher takes advantage of events as they unfold to help answer the research question.
- **Participant observation:** A qualitative method that requires interacting with research participants so that you can learn about their lives.
- **Policy approach:** A method of report organization that presents a conclusion as to why a problem occurs.
- **Probes:** A type of follow-up question that directs the discussion to a deeper level but does not necessarily reference the topic of interest. Some examples of probes include "I don't think I understand what you mean. Can you clarify?" or "Please tell me more about that" or "What happened next?".
- **Problem-solving approach:** A method of report organization that states the problem and describes its importance and its implications.
- **Reflective field notes:** A record of the researcher's personal views and insights that emerge during an observation session.

- **Saturation:** A point in data collection where sampling will not lead to anymore new information or insights.
- **Typical sampling:** A purposive sampling technique in which the researcher is interested in typical individuals within a given population.

References

[1] Fetterman DM. Ethnography: Step-by-Step. Thousand Oaks, CA: Sage Publications, Inc.; 2010

[2] Strauss A, Corbin JM. Basics of Qualitative Research: Grounded Theory Procedures and Techniques. Thousand Oaks, CA: Sage Publications, Inc.; 1990

[3] Baker C, Wuest J, Stern PN. Method Slurring: The Grounded Theory/Phenomenology Example. J Adv Nurs 1992;17(11):1355–1360

[4] Dahl CM, Boss P. The Use of Phenomenology for Family Therapy Research: The Search for Meaning. In: Sprenkle DH, Piercy FP, eds. Research Methods in Family Therapy. New York, NY: The Guilford Press; 2005:63–84

[5] Robinson OC. Sampling in Interview-Based Qualitative Research: A Theoretical and Practical Guide. Qual Res Psychol 2014;11(1):25–41

[6] Palinkas LA, Horwitz SM, Green CA, Wisdom JP, Duan N, Hoagwood K. Purposeful Sampling for Qualitative Data Collection and Analysis in Mixed Method Implementation Research. Adm Policy Ment Health 2015;42(5):533–544

[7] Sadler GR, Lee H-C, Lim RS, Fullerton J. Recruitment of Hard-To-Reach Population Subgroups via Adaptations of the Snowball Sampling Strategy. Nurs Health Sci 2010;12(3):369–374

[8] Sandelowski M. Sample Size in Qualitative Research. Res Nurs Health 1995;18(2):179–183

[9] Patton MQ. How to Use Qualitative Methods in Evaluation. Thousand Oaks, CA: Sage Publications, Inc.; 1987

[10] Jorgensen DL. Participant Observation. In: Emerging Trends in the Social and Behavioral Sciences. Atlanta, GA: American Cancer Society; 2015:1–15

[11] Ritchie J, Lewis J, Nicholls CM, Ormston R. Qualitative Research Practice: A Guide for Social Science Students and Researchers. Los Angeles, CA: Sage Publications, Inc.; 2013

[12] Asbury J-E. Overview of Focus Group Research. Qual Health Res 1995;5(4):414–420

[13] Thorne P. Data Analysis in Qualitative Research. Evid Based Nurs 2000;3(3):68–70

[14] Saldana J. The Coding Manual for Qualitative Researchers. Los Angeles, CA: Sage Publications, Inc.; 2015

[15] Rendon JS, Swinton M, Bernthal N, et al. Barriers and Facilitators Experienced in Collaborative Prospective Research in Orthopaedic Oncology: A Qualitative Study. Bone Joint Res 2017;6(5):307–314

9.15 Appendix A: Collaborative Research Focus Group Discussion Guide

The following is a discussion guide for a focus group exploring orthopaedic surgeons' perspectives on collaborative research, as well as investigating the facilitators and barriers to participating in collaborative research in the field. This discussion guide can be used as a template from which you can develop your own guide for your study.

9.15.1 Welcome, Introductions, and Informed Consent

The focus group will begin with the facilitator introducing himself/herself, and welcoming individuals to the focus group.

The facilitator will review the Participant Information Sheet and Consent Form, provide an opportunity for questions about the Participant Information Sheet and/or Consent Form, and then obtain written informed consent from all participants.

The facilitator will then ask the focus group participants to briefly introduce themselves and to describe their stake/role in collaborative research and how long they have been interested/invested/involved.

The facilitator will review a few "ground rules" for the focus group discussion including the following:

- Ask participants to speak one at a time.
- Ask participants to respect the confidentiality of each other's participation in the research study and the confidentiality of the discussion.
- Ask participants to respect views that may be different from their own—the purpose of the focus group discussion is to explore perceptions and experiences of the individuals in the room.

○ "We expect that there will be differing perspective and it is important for us to capture and explore as many perceptions and experiences as we can."

9.15.2 Discussion Topics

1. Please describe your initial thoughts when you hear the phrase "collaborative research."
   - Probe: Where do you think these thoughts come from?
   - Probe: Does the idea of collaborating on a study where you are not the overall Principal Investigator evoke any particular reaction—positive? Negative? Neutral?

   Collaborative research is described as multiple researchers/institutions partnering together to advance scientific knowledge, enrich processes, and/or develop new products.

2. Please describe what you think are some of the most common types of research collaboration opportunities available to orthopaedic surgeons and their research teams.
3. How important do you think collaboration is in orthopaedic surgery research?
   - Do you think all orthopaedic surgeons should participate in collaborative research?
4. Does your institution have any policies related to recognition for participation in multicenter prospective research?
   - If yes, what are the policies? Are they used? If used, how are they used? If not, why do you think they aren't used?
   - If no, why do you think your institution does not have policies related to recognition for participation in multicenter prospective research?
5. How many prospective collaborative research studies are you involved in?

   If participants describe other collaborative studies, or just the clinical trial:
   - What has led you to participate in these studies?

- What is your experience with participating in these studies?

If participants describe not participating in other studies:
- What is the main reason you do not participate in other prospective collaborative studies?
- What are other reasons you do not participate in other prospective collaborative studies?
  - Probes: Time constraints, lack of resources, lack of interest, lack of institutional recognition?

6. In addition to factors that have already been discussed, what do you think are the barriers to prospective collaborative research in orthopaedic surgery?
   - Probes: Barriers at the individual level, at the institutional level, and in the field of orthopaedic surgery.
7. So far, we have discussed the following barriers to participating in prospective collaborative research in orthopaedic surgery (facilitator to summarize the barriers discussed).
   - Which of these barriers do you think have the most influence on your behavior/decision around prospective collaborative research?
   - Which of these barriers do you believe are amenable to change (i.e., could be overcome)? Why do you believe these barriers are amenable to change?
   - Which of these barriers do you believe are not amenable to change (i.e., cannot be overcome)? Why do you believe these barriers are not amenable to change?
8. Thinking about the barriers that have been described as amenable to change, what resources or strategies do you think could diminish or overcome these barriers (facilitator to summarize these barriers)?
9. Are there other factors, processes, or resources that you think would facilitate participation in prospective collaborative research in orthopaedic surgery?
10. Would having access to a full-time research staff member facilitate participation in prospective collaborative research? Why or why not? If yes, describe what that access could look like.
11. What do you think orthopaedic surgeons and their research staff can do to overcome barriers to prospective collaborative research in orthopaedic surgery?
    - Probe: Different professions (surgeons, allied health professionals, and residents).
12. Is there anything that we haven't discussed related to prospective collaborative research in orthopaedic surgery?
Review of Next Steps in the Research

10 Principles of Good Clinical Practice and Research Conduct

Naveen Khan

Abstract

Good clinical practices (GCP) are the internationally recognized standards governing the conduct of clinical studies. Over the years, the principles outlining GCP have been outlined in documents and guidelines ranging from the Declaration of Helsinki to the current ICH-GCP guidelines. GCP ensures that clinical research procedures protect the participating study subjects in addition to ensuring that the studies meet international standards of quality and are universally accepted. The ICH-GCP guidelines outline specific and practical principles for research conduct in addition to providing a detailed description of the roles and responsibilities of major parties involved in clinical research. As progress is made in the field of medical research, these guidelines will need to be continuously revised to remain current and relevant.

Keywords: good clinical practice, international standards, quality, protection, ethics

10.1 Introduction

Many clinical studies include the involvement of human subjects, making it extremely important that ethical standards are set to protect participants from harm and to ensure their rights and interests are safeguarded. Good Clinical Practices (GCP) are a number of internationally recognized principles that outline specific facets of clinical study development including designing, running, and closing a research study that involves human subjects.[1] The purpose of these guidelines is to protect human subjects involved in medical research and to ensure that high-quality data are obtained from such studies.

This section will delve into the subject of GCP by first providing readers with some background on the development of ethical guidelines in health research throughout history. We will then turn our focus to the current internationally recognized GCP guidelines developed by the International Council for Harmonisation of Technical Requirements for Pharmaceuticals for Human Use (ICH).

Here, we will review the principles and major topics presented in the document. We will then discuss future directions and upcoming challenges that the current GCP guidelines will face in the years to come. Finally, we will close by providing a practical application of the chapter where we will discuss some helpful tips to help you ensure clinical studies that you are managing are meeting GCP requirements.

10.2 History of Good Clinical Practice

10.2.1 Revisiting a Drastically Different Era of Clinical Studies

With the increasing regulations and ethical guidelines present today, we may find ourselves forgetting a time when those who managed clinical studies did not ensure the rights and safety of human subjects. There are multiple components of present-day GCP that protect human participants including informed consent, confidentiality, and documented paper trails. However, this was not always the case. For much of history, medical research has been at odds with human rights. As we go back in time, we are reminded of how far we have come in the area of research ethics and clinical study conduct.

A prominent example includes the 1932 study conducted by the United States Public Health Service called the "Tuskegee Study of Untreated Syphilis in the Negro Male." Six hundred black men were recruited for the study, of which 399 men had syphilis. It is important to mention that the participants of this study were not approached to obtain their informed consent and were not aware that they were even involved in the research. In addition, the treatment that could potentially cure them was deliberately withheld from them. This study continued for almost 40 years and is a clear example demonstrating the integral need for ethical standards to be set in place within the field of medical research.[2] A number of such studies were conducted in the early 20th century. Fortunately, as the years went by, internationally recognized guidelines and regulations we developed. We will review these historical documents in the upcoming section.

10.3 The History of GCP Guidelines

Major advancements have been made in the area of health research ethics since the Tuskegee study. In this section, we will summarize some key milestones in the journey to achieving the current ethical standards in medical research.

Nuremberg Code (1947): The Nuremberg Code was the initial universally accepted guideline for the ethical conduct of research involving human participants. The Nuremberg Code was created during the trial against Nazi physicians who had conducted terrible studies on people imprisoned at Nazi war camps throughout World War II.[3] A central principle outlined in the code was the need to obtain voluntary informed consent from research participants.[4] In addition, the Nuremberg Code explicitly stated the requirement for sound scientific support as the basis for development of a clinical study.[2] The code is often referred to as one of the original documents outlining the principles of ethical medical research.

Declaration of Helsinki (1964): The World Medical Association (WMA) developed the Declaration of Helsinki to provide further guidance to health care providers on ethical research conduct.[4] Within the document, it reiterated the need for doctors involved in clinical research to protect the rights and safety of human participants.[3] However, the Declaration of Helsinki also provided physicians with greater flexibility with obtaining informed consent from participants. In particular, the requirement could be omitted in "special situations."[2] In 1975, the Declaration of Helsinki was revised to include the principle that clinical study protocols were to be reviewed and approved by an independent research ethics committee.[2] In addition, the declaration clearly defined the expectation that study subjects are assured access to the best treatment identified in the research.[5] The revised version of the declaration rectified shortcomings in the prior version to become a universally accepted document summarizing research ethics and conduct.

Belmont Report (1979): An additional document that paved the way for the current GCP guidelines is the Belmont Report that was established by the National Commission for the Protection of Human Subjects of Biomedical and Behavioral Research.[3] There are three major principles that are outlined in the report. The first is the "Respect for Persons," which states that all individuals are to be treated with dignity and respect.[3] To extrapolate that notion to the realm of medical research, it is crucial to obtain voluntary informed consent from all participants. The second tenet is "Beneficence," which acknowledges the need to have clinical studies that protect participants by maximizing benefits and minimizing harm. The final principle is "Justice," which establishes the requirement of fair recruitment procedures and the just treatment of study subjects.[3]

International Ethical Guidelines for Biomedical Research Involving Human Subjects (1982): This document was developed by the World Health Organization along with the Council for International Organizations of Medical Sciences (CIOMS). Its purpose was to assist developing countries in applying the same standards and principles to medical research as outlined in the Nuremberg Code and the Declaration of Helsinki.

International Conference on Harmonisation of Technical Requirements for Pharmaceuticals for Human Use—Good Clinic Practice (1996): Over time, numerous groups and committees established their own set of criteria outlining the ethics governing medical research. The need for a consistent and globally recognized GCP guideline overcoming international discrepancies was clear.[3] This goal was achieved with the advent of the Good Clinical Practice guidelines developed by the ICH, which we will now refer to as ICH-GCP. The ICH-GCP guidelines were approved on July 17, 1996, and were implemented throughout the world on January 7, 1997.[3] Its predominant function was to provide internationally recognized principles aimed at protecting clinical study participants and ensuring quality data were obtained from medical research studies.[1] Currently, this document is the most widely accepted guideline outlining GCP in the world. It covers numerous elements of clinical research including ethical research conduct from initiation to closure of the study. In addition, it thoroughly outlines the role played by all parties involved throughout the study and identifies the essential documents that are to be created during the study.[1] As a result, the ICH-GCP allows for the acceptance and exchange of clinical research internationally.[1] We will discuss these guidelines in greater detail in the next section.

10.4 The ICH-GCP Guidelines

10.4.1 Introduction and Major Principles

As previously mentioned, the initial version of the GCP guidelines by the ICH was developed in 1996 and was implemented in early 1997. This document specified the role and the expectations of all participants (i.e., investigators, regulatory bodies, and sponsors) involved in conducting a clinical study. In addition, the document outlined the various steps of conducting a medical study to ensure that the data obtained are of high quality. The guidelines also included sections describing the essential documents needed when conducting a clinical study such as the study protocol and the investigator's brochure (IB).[6] The ICH-GCP guidelines provided a unified standard for the European Union (EU), Japan, and the United States enabling joint acceptance of clinical research data by the respective regulatory bodies of each state.[7] The existing GCP principles of Australia, Canada, the Nordic countries, and the World Health Organization (WHO) were also taken into account during development of the ICH-GCP guidelines.[7]

In 2016, the ICH-GCP guidelines were amended to promote adoption of the guidelines and to incorporate more streamlined approaches to clinical study design, conduct, monitoring, and reporting while still ensuring that the rights of study subjects were safeguarded and the data obtained from the research were reliable. Revisions were also made to integrate the increasing use of electronic records and newer technologies.[6]

There are 13 major principles present in the ICH-GCP guidelines. They are summarized in ▶ Table 10.1. Overall, the principles state the need for all clinical studies to be conducted in accordance with ethical principles, sound scientific evidence and a detailed protocol to protect the rights and freedoms of human subjects and generate quality data.[3]

In this section, we provided some background on the ICH-GCP guidelines and its development for the purpose of protecting research participants and ensuring quality data are obtained from clinical studies for universal acceptance. In the next section, we will outline the ways in which the document does so through its detailed explanations of the roles and responsibilities of all involved parties during a clinical study.

10.4.2 Roles and Responsibilities of Involved Parties

The ICH-GCP guidelines outline a number of participants that are involved in conducting a clinical study. These include the study sponsor, the investigators, the ethics committee, the regulatory authorities, and the patients. The roles and responsibilities of some major participants are highlighted in the following sections.

The Ethics Committee

The ethics committee plays a central role in developing and conducting a clinical study. It is one of the major figures responsible for ensuring the protection of all study subjects as per the ICH-GCP guidelines. As per the document, the ethics committee should consist of at least one independent member from the study site and at least one nonscientist member.[1] Only committee members who are independent of the study sponsor and the study investigator can vote during key decisions. Such a structure enables the ethics committee to maintain their impartiality and avoid possible conflicts of interest during the evaluation of a clinical study and when providing a judgment.[1] In addition, the involvement of a nonscientist in the ethics committee provides an exclusive viewpoint to the discussion that will largely be aligned with the average person's thoughts.[1]

The ethics committee is responsible for the study protocol and for providing a detailed opinion on it. In addition to the protocol, the committee should review all documents and materials presented to research participants including study information, informed consent forms (ICFs), data collection forms, and marketing strategies.[1] When evaluating the documents, the committee should ensure that the information is fair and allows the prospective subject to best understand the research, its outcomes, and what is expected of the participants. In addition, it will ensure that they have the freedom to choose to participate without coercion and withdraw for the study if need be.

Table 10.1 The principles of ICH-GCP

Principle number	Principle
1.	Clinical studies should be managed in a manner that they are aligned with the GCP and the necessary regulatory requirement(s) in addition to being based on the ethical values rooted in the Declaration of Helsinki.
2.	Before beginning a clinical study, the benefits and risks to the study subject and to society should be valuated. The study should only proceed if the advantages of conducting the study warrant the adverse outcomes.
3.	The health and security of study participants are of utmost importance during the clinical study. It is given precedence over all other interests including those in the name of science.
4.	The proposed research study should be sufficiently supported by the presented information on the investigational product (clinical and nonclinical).
5.	A comprehensive protocol should be developed to describe the research and to demonstrate that the study is supported by sound scientific methodology.
6.	Only those protocols that are reviewed and approved by an institutional review board (IRB) or an independent ethics committee (IEC) should be used in conducting the study.
7.	A licensed and qualified health care provider should be responsible for the clinical care of the study participant and any medical decisions made on their behalf.
8.	All clinical study personnel should be qualified based on their knowledge and expertise in conducting their designated tasks.
9.	All study participants are required to freely provide their informed consent to participate in the clinical study.
10.	To ensure precise reporting, analysis, and review, the information from the research study should be captured and stored in a suitable manner regardless of the type of media used.
11.	Any documents identifying participating individuals will need to be managed in a manner that the confidentiality of those subjects is protected.
12.	The relevant principles of good manufacturing practice (GMP) as outlined in the approved protocol should be used to develop, transport, and store investigational products used in the clinical study.
13.	It is necessary to implement practices and procedures that ensure that all areas of the research study are of the highest standard.

Source: Adapted from ICH 2016.[6]

Principal Investigator

The principal investigator at the clinical site plays a significant role in both the protecting study participants and ensuring quality data are obtained from the research. In order to safeguard the rights and safeties of the study participants, the principal investigator needs to be well informed and should have a thorough understanding of the study protocol and all information related to the research and the investigational product. He/she should also monitor the product to make sure it is being stored, handled, and administered as per the protocol and IB. This will allow him/her to confirm that only consented study subjects are using it.[1] The principal investigator is also required to ensure that a signed and dated consent form is received from each participant prior to beginning of the study. Further details regarding the consent form and other documentation collected from study subjects will be outlined in future chapters (see Chapter 18 on patient consent).

The principal investigator is not specifically required to be a medical doctor as per the ICH-GCP guidelines.[1] Nonetheless, the principal investigator should ensure that all medical decisions that are study related are made by a qualified medical doctor. If a subject develops any complications or adverse events as a result of participation in the study, the principal investigator is responsible for making sure that sufficient medical care is provided to them.[1] No deviation from the study protocol should be made without communication with the ethics committee, unless there is an urgency to protect the patient.

Along with safeguarding the rights of study participants, the principal investigator plays a crucial role in protecting the credibility and quality of the clinical study data. This includes ensuring that adequate time to properly complete the study is given and that clinical research staff that are delegated any study-related responsibilities are correctly trained and well informed of all study specificities.[1]

Proper documentation is a central tenet in the ICH-GCP guidelines and it plays a crucial role in ensuring data obtained from the study are of a high standard. The principal investigator is responsible for ensuring that the data collected and recorded on all source documents (i.e., medical records, X-rays) are consistent with the information provided to the sponsor.[1] Any changes made to the data will need to be accounted for with documentation explaining the deviation and should be signed by the individual making the correction. A paper trail outlining the course of the study for each study subject is required.[1] Finally, the principal investigator plays a role in facilitating the sponsor or associated regulatory bodies with any monitoring or auditing of the study by providing access to all documentation to the auditing or regulating party.[1]

Study Sponsor

Along with the ethics committee and the principal investigator, there are a number of responsibilities that the study sponsor has in order to protect the study participants from harm. First, prior to initiation of the study, the sponsor is required to provide all data (clinical and preclinical) related to the investigational product in addition to all information justifying the study for a particular population group.[1] In addition, the sponsor is responsible for ensuring that the drug used in the study is developed and manufactured in accordance with GMP. The product should be packaged to ensure that there is no contamination or degradation throughout storage and transportations. The study drug must be evaluated on an ongoing basis throughout the study to ensure safety.[1]

The study sponsor has many key responsibilities to ensure that study participants are safe from harm. In double-blind studies, which are studies where neither the participant nor the investigator knows whether the study drug or placebo are being administered, the sponsor is required to provide a mechanism by which emergency unblinding can be done quickly so that the investigator can gather crucial, and potentially life-saving, information regarding the drug that a participant was taking.[1] The sponsor is also responsible for ensuring that any new data that could negatively impact patient safety or alter their decision to participate is disseminated to all involved parties as soon as possible.[1]

In addition to safeguarding patients, the study sponsor also plays a key role in protecting the data obtained from the study and ensuring that they are of high quality. It is essential for the sponsor to develop a system of both quality control (QC) and quality assurance (QA) to ensure the integrity of research data. Some mechanisms should be integrated into the process itself such as proofreading and routine checking of the data in clinical research forms (CRFs) and in the database. Other processes should be performed by external staff or an organization as an independent function outside of the study procedures. This would provide an independent evaluation of the study processes and functions.

10.4.3 Essential Documents

The ICH-GCP guidelines outline a variety of essential documents required throughout the clinical study process. They define these essential documents as those documents that can allow for the audit and evaluation of study conduct and data quality. These documents also validate the fact that the sponsor and investigator complied with the GCP standards when conducting the study. Other purposes of the essential documents include assisting those involved in the study with managing its various components and providing reviewers with clearly documented information regarding the study.

A number of essential documents are required throughout the study process. The ICH-GCP guidelines differentiate them based on whether they should be created before, during, and after the study process. ▶ Table 10.2 outlines the major documents outlined in the guidelines. Some of these documents will be further described later in this chapter.

The documents outlined in ▶ Table 10.2 should be collected and filed within the Trial Master File (TMF). The TMF should contain all essential documents that

Table 10.2 Essential documents outlined in the ICH-GCP guidelines

Before the study begins	During the study	After the study concludes
• Investigator's brochure	• Updates to investigator's brochure	• Documentation accounting for study drug/investigation product at sites
• Signed protocol (with amendments) and sample CRFs	• Any revisions to study-related documents	
• Information given to study subjects (i.e., ICF)	• Documented and signed approval for any changes or revisions to study-related documents by the ethics committee and/or regulatory body	• Documentation of destruction of investigational product
• Financial aspects of the study; insurance statement (if necessary)	• CV for new investigators	• Completed subject identification code list
• Signed agreements between involved parties	• Updates to normal value(s) for medical/laboratory/technical procedure(s)/test(s) in protocol	• Audit certificate
• Document of approval of protocol and major documents from the ethics committee	• Updates to medical/laboratory/technical procedure(s)/test(s)	• Final study closeout monitoring report
• Ethics committee composition details	• Documentation of shipments of study-related materials and the study drug	• Treatment allocation and decoding documentation
• Approval from regulatory authority	• Analysis certificates for new batches of investigational products	• Final report by investigator to ethics committee (if required) and to regulatory bodies (if required)
• Curriculum vitae (CV) and other documents outlining qualifications of investigators	• Monitoring visit reports	• Clinical study report
• Normal value(s)/range(s) for medical/laboratory/technical procedures and/or tests in the protocol	• Other communications between parties beyond site visits	
• Medical/laboratory/technical procedures and/or tests	• Signed ICFs	
• Label sample(s) attached to study drug or investigational product	• Source documents	
• Instructions for handling of investigational product	• All completed CRFs (signed and dated)	
• Shipping records for all study-related materials and study drug	• Documentation outlining corrections in CRFs	
• Analysis certificate(s) of investigational product(s)	• Notifications regarding an unexpected serious adverse events or safety information	
• Decoding procedures for blinded studies (if applicable)	• Subject screening log	
• Master randomization list	• Subject identification code list	
• Prestudy monitoring report and study initiation monitoring report	• Subject enrolment log	
	• Documentation accounting for study drug or investigational product at sites	
	• Signature sheet	
	• Records of retained body fluids/tissue samples (if necessary)	

Source: Adapted from ICH 2016.[6]

may be reviewed by a regulatory authority and/or by the ethics committee. It should be created during study initiation and documents should be continually added as the study proceeds. Final closeout of the study cannot be done unless the documents present in the TMF are complete and up-to-date and reviewed by the monitoring body.[8]

Protocol

The study protocol is a document outlining how the study will be conducted in a detailed and clear format. As per the ICH-GCP guidelines, the study protocol should include the following topics:
• General information regarding the study.
• Background information.
• Study objectives and purpose.
• Study design.
• Information on the selection and withdrawal of subjects.
• Treatment of subjects.
• Assessment of efficacy.
• Assessment of safety.
• Statistics.

- Direct access to source data/documents.
- Quality control and quality assurance.
- Ethics; data handling and record keeping.
- Financing and insurance.
- The publication policy.[6]

There may be some sections that are present in other essential documents such as the IB that should be referenced within the protocol. Details regarding the protocol and its various components are provided in the ICH-GCP guidelines.

Investigator's Brochure

Among the essential documents listed in the ICH-GCP guidelines is the IB. The IB is a collection of all data regarding the study drug or product that are important to the clinical study.[6] It provides all the contextual information for study personnel to better understand the product and the reasons behind its specific features such as dosage and mode of administration. As a result, it facilitates clinical management of the study participants throughout the study. The ICH-GCP guidelines outline the various components and sections that should be included within the IB. These include a summary and introduction of the product; its physical, chemical, and pharmaceutical properties and formulations; and information on the effects on humans, among others.[6] As per the guidelines, the IB should be reviewed on an annual basis at minimum and should be revised as needed throughout the course of the study. Any new information that is received will need to be added to the IB on an ongoing basis. However, it is important to keep in mind that some new information may be so significant and vital to the protection of participants that it should be communicated to those involved with the clinical study prior to being included in a revised IB.[6]

10.4.4 Advantages of the ICH-GCP Guidelines

There are a number of advantages of the ICH-GCP guidelines. Two major advantages are harmonization and credibility. Prior to the development of the document, different countries and jurisdictions had their own set of principles governing conduct during clinical studies. With the advent of the ICH-GCP guidelines, the principles governing such conduct have become more consistent and universally applicable.[9] This has allowed for greater coordination and collaboration between nation states. In addition, the ICH-GCP guidelines outline specific instructions and procedures that should be followed when conducting a clinical study. As a result, this significantly reduces the chance that medical research is unethical or of poor quality as a detailed and clear clinical study process is outlined.[1]

10.5 Future Directions and Challenges

GCP provides a guideline by which clinical studies should be conducted in order to ensure the quality of medical research and safety of all involved human participants. Therefore, it is a practical tool that should be used regularly by all individuals and organizations involved throughout the clinical study process. Despite this, there are some challenges the GCP guidelines will face in the coming years, which will have to be addressed in the future.

10.5.1 Globalization and the Universal Adoption of GCP

Clinical studies are becoming increasingly globalized with various components of the studies occurring in multiple regions throughout the world. Although the GCP guidelines define universally accepted procedures for the conduct of clinical studies, there are some differences in its adoption in some localities. For example, the Declaration of Helsinki's position that placebo-controlled studies, in general, should only be used in the absence of existing proven therapy is not entirely followed by the United States. In April 2008, the U.S. Food and Drug Administration (FDA) abandoned the need for clinical studies outside of the United States to comply with the Declaration of Helsinki. In effect, the FDA would allow placebo-controlled studies to be run internationally even if existing treatment was present.[10] In addition, new legislation and regulations governing privacy in the EU and financial disclosure in the United States complicate the universality of the GCP guidelines.[9]

There are also key differences in the implementation of GCP between developing and developed countries. This causes obstacles with respect to the quality of the data produced and the protection of the study participants. Particular issues such as the lack of a regulatory framework and poor financial conditions can make the adoption of ICH-GCP guidelines increasingly difficult in developing nations.[11] In order to deal with this, the GCP guidelines will have to take the specific situations of these nations into account and provide guidance and facilitation to help them adopt the GCP standards. For example, to ensure that all human subjects are given the choice to consent or decline participation for a study, an independent observer may need to be present. This will minimize any exploitation of poor individuals who are largely vulnerable due to lack of education or access to basic resources in developing nations.[11]

In addition to variations in the adoption of GCP standards, clinical studies are becoming more global as sponsors from wealthy nations shift studies to developing countries.[5] Though the ICH-GCP document is effective in outlining the procedures necessary to ensure safe and high-quality clinical studies, the guidelines are only as effective as they are understood and executed properly. In the years to come, measures should be taken to allow for greater flexibility to ensure that research procedures are compatible with the requirements of society and the specific research objectives.[5]

10.5.2 Technological Advancements

With the advent of new and improved technology, the landscape of medical research has become increasingly different from that witnessed in the past. As new tools are designed and incorporated into clinical studies, there will be a need for the GCP guidelines to integrate such changes into its standards. One major advancement has been the rising use of the electronic health record (EHR), which is playing a key role in altering research conduct. For instance, the abundance of such detailed clinical data in the EHR has paved the way for more streamlined pragmatic clinical trials (PCTs).[12] PCTs are designed to focus on the effectiveness of a treatment or intervention in real-world settings rather than in a "controlled" situation. Changes such as entrenching randomization at point of care and utilizing EHRs as case report forms have been proposed as the potential direction clinical research is heading in.[13] PCTs have broad eligibility criteria to allow for a diverse

population to be recruited enhancing the generalizability of the results. They aim to improve study efficiency by streamlining the screening and recruitment of participants.[12] As a result, PCTs can be directly opposed to some of the central aims of GCP such as rigorous quality. With respect to patient enrollment, GCP guidelines outline the requirement of screening and obtaining written informed consent by clinical study staff. In contrast, PCTs focus on recognizing eligible subjects through the use of EHRs and incorporating them in the study through mass enrollment.[12] In addition, GCP outlines that all medical decisions that are related to the study are to be made by a qualified physician who has a thorough understanding of the study. PCTs consider involving health practitioners from a broad range of backgrounds and experiences who may have minimal study-related training.[12] Although the amendments made to the ICH-GCP guidelines in 2016 worked to incorporate some of these streamlined approaches, the GCP standards will need to be continually revised over the years to remain current and to better align with greater efficiencies in clinical study procedures.

Living in an increasingly digital age will lead to further progress in the field of clinical research. It will be absolutely imperative for future GCP guidelines to incorporate emerging technologies and their usage in conducting medical studies. The standards for the conduct of clinical studies will need to evolve to keep up with and benefit from current technologies.[13]

10.6 Practical Application

In my experience working in clinical research, knowledge of GCP and research conduct is extremely important. By being aware of the relevant guidelines, you can ensure the quality and safety of your medical research. Clinical research coordinators should have thorough knowledge of many aspects of the study including the clinical study protocol, the investigational products, and the essential documents.

Many issues can arise from not following GCP standards during clinical studies. Common issues include problems with obtaining informed consent, incorrect screening procedures, source data problems, errors related to randomization, and unreported serious adverse events.

Below is a checklist tool outlining major responsibilities that clinical research coordinators should ensure are complete throughout the study process. These will ensure that many issues mentioned earlier are avoided.

10.6.1 Good Clinical Practice Checklist for Clinical Research Coordinators

Before Study Begins:
- Become well acquainted with GCP by reviewing the relevant GCP guidelines.
- Familiarize yourself with the investigational product by reading the IB and ensure proper handling and storage of the product.
- Read and become well acquainted with the study protocol.
- If necessary, contact your ethics committee to determine the documents required for review and obtain an approval letter.
- Become familiar with the randomization procedures of the study and any necessary unblinding procedures.
- Review the process of obtaining informed consent.
- Review the CRFs and practice completing the form to determine if any issues arise.
- Review your responsibilities with respect to safety reporting as per the study protocol.

During the Study:
- Enroll study participants strictly in adherence with the protocol after obtaining informed consent.
- Ensure that the investigational product is administered as per the randomization scheme.
- Complete CRFs clearly and carefully and retain all source documents.
- Report serious adverse events immediately to the sponsor as per the study protocol.
- Ensure that all CRFs are complete and signed, and any corrections have been documented.

After the Study is Complete:
- Once the study has been completed, inform the ethics committee.
- Store all files related to the study carefully and arrange for archiving as outlined in the protocol or as discussed with the study sponsor.

This checklist was adapted from Forwengel 2003.[14]

10.7 Conclusion

To conclude, GCP is a practical standard that ensures ethical and scientific quality of clinical studies throughout the world. The latest ICH-GCP guidelines have allowed for a universally accepted set of rules and procedures to be adopted in the realm of medical research. In addition to outlining specific principles for research conduct, the guidelines summarized specific roles and responsibilities of the participating groups and the essential documents required to ensure data integrity and quality. After the initial development of the ICH-GCP guidelines in 1996, they were reformed in 2016 to incorporate changes in the medical research and to facilitate adoption of its practices. As the landscape of medical research changes with increased globalization and the advent of new technologies, GCP will need to be continuously revised in the future.

Definitions

- **Good Manufacturing Practice:** A set of guidelines and principles that have to be followed by manufacturers of medical devices and pharmaceutical products in order to meet regulatory standards of regulatory agencies.
- **Placebo:** A treatment administered to patients without a therapeutic effect. It is used as a control during clinical studies.
- **Pragmatic trials:** A type of clinical study that is streamlined in nature and focuses on providing evidence of the effectiveness of the intervention in "real-world" settings.
- **Double-blind studies:** Studies where neither the participant nor the investigator knows whether the study drug or placebo is being administered to the patient.

References

[1]   Switula D. Principles of Good Clinical Practice (GCP) in Clinical Research. Sci Eng Ethics 2000;6(1):71–77
[2]   Guraya SY, London NJM, Guraya SS. Ethics in Medical Research. J Microsc Ultrastruct. 2014;2(3):121–126
[3]   Vijayananthan A, Nawawi O. The Importance of Good Clinical Practice Guidelines and its Role in Clinical Trials. Biomed Imaging Interv J 2008;4(1):e5
[4]   Bhatt A. Evolution of Clinical Research: A History Before and Beyond James Lind. Perspect Clin Res 2010; 1(1):6–10
[5]   Glickman SW, McHutchison JG, Peterson ED, et al. Ethical and Scientific Implications of the Globalization of Clinical Research N Engl J Med 2009;360(8):816–823

[6]   International Council for Harmonisation of Technical Requirements for Pharmaceuticals for Human Use. Integrated Addendum to ICH E6(R1): Guideline for Good Clinical Practice. November 6, 2016. Available from: https://www.ich.org/fileadmin/Public_Web_Site/ICH_Products/Guidelines/Efficacy/E6/E6_R2__Step_4_2016_1109.pdf

[7]   Verma K. Base of a Research: Good Clinical Practice in Clinical Trials J Clin Trials 2013;3(1):128

[8]   National Institute for Health Research. Good Clinical Practice (GCP) Reference Guide. 2016. Available from: https://www.nihr.ac.uk/our-faculty/documents/GCP%20Reference%20Guide.pdf

[9]   MaRS Discovery District. Clinical trials and Good Clinical Practice (GCP). Toronto, ON: MaRS. November 6, 2012. Available from: https://www.marsdd.com/mars-library/clinical-trials-and-good-clinical-practice-gcp/

[10] Burgess LJ, Pretorius D. FDA Abandons the Declaration of Helsinki: The Effect on the Ethics of Clinical Trial Conduct in South Africa and Other Developing Countries. S Afr J Bioeth Law 2012;5(2):87–90

[11] Caballero B. Ethical Issues for Collaborative Research in Developing Countries. Am J Clin Nutr 2002;76(4):717–720

[12] Mentz RJ, Hernandez AF, Berdan LG, et al. Good Clinical Practice Guidance and Pragmatic Clinical Trials: Balancing the Best of Both Worlds. Circulation 2016;133(9):872–880

[13] Antman EM, Bierer BE. Standards for Clinical Research: Keeping Pace with the Technology of the Future. Circulation 2016;133(9):823–825

[14] Forwengel G. Guide for Clinical Trial Staff: Implementing Good Clinical Practice. Basel, Switzerland: Karger Publishers; 2003

Part III

From Idea to Study Start-Up

11 Principles of Grant Writing:
   Tips for a Successful
   Experience   *120*

12 Dollars and "Sense":
   A Guide to Research
   Finances   *130*

13 Maintaining Records and
   the Trial Master File   *143*

14 Ethics Submissions   *155*

15 The Basics of Research
   Contracts   *161*

16 How to Start Up a Study   *169*

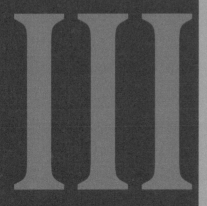

11 Principles of Grant Writing: Tips for a Successful Experience

Milena R. Vicente, Sarah Desjardins

Abstract

Writing a compelling grant application in the current environment of fierce competition for scarce research dollars requires a significant amount of time and planning. This chapter reviews the critical components of a successful grant application and provides tips on how to manage the application process from planning stages to submission. Advice on identifying potential funding sources, organizing your grant proposal, and understanding the review process will be provided. Specific details on writing the basic sections of a grant application and resubmissions will also be discussed.

Keywords: grant writing, research funding, grant review, principals, guide, proposal

11.1 Introduction

Considerable planning and development of research grant application projects is vital to secure funding for any project. An effective grant application should be easy to read, concise, attractive, and tell a compelling story.[1] In preparing to apply for a research grant, you should already have a preliminary project proposal or a research study idea that can help determine what type of granting agency you should be aiming for, and in what types of competitions you are most likely to be successful. Discuss your project with others, foster potential collaborations, and put together a multidisciplinary team to support your proposal. Consider the size and scope of your study and have a general estimate of how much funding should be secured. Fine tuning your plan and formal writing of your proposal are best left until a grant competition has been found and decided upon, as the direction of your research may change slightly to fit the specific needs of the granting agency.

11.2 Getting Started

11.2.1 Start Early

Research teams often underestimate the amount of time required to complete a grant application. It is not unreasonable to allocate 6 to 8 months of preparation for most clinical research grant applications,

factoring in time to prepare preliminary data, develop key elements of the proposal, and to have the application reviewed internally by subject experts and peers. Some larger grants may require a year or more of preparatory work (▶ Table 11.1). Sufficient time must be given to establish collaborations with local coinvestigators and external institutions and to liaise with internal departments and stakeholders. Formal letters of support from collaborators may be required by some grant agencies, and will most certainly strengthen the application. Allow sufficient time to review and refine the grant and to incorporate feedback received. Contact experienced investigators with a successful track record in securing grants and consider adding them as coinvestigators or collaborators to the project. Successful grant holders can also act as consultants or mentors to the project, and can provide guidance and sound advice to newer applicants. Most academic institutions also offer a grant review service, either free or pay-per-use, with experienced grant reviewers or previously successful grantees who can offer valuable feedback on the proposal. Recognize that these reviews take time, and require that the bulk of the grant application be prepared well before the granting agency's submission deadline. Note your institution's individual policies on grant submissions; some organizations require that the fully completed grant be submitted for full institutional internal review, or internal budget review, prior to submitting to a granting agency. Depending on the degree of review, this internal submission process may need to be started weeks or months prior to the granting agency's submission deadlines. Verify the required timeline with your institution. This is especially important if institutional signatures are required for your specific grant. Any opportunity to strengthen the application should be embraced, as it will ultimately improve your chances for successful funding.

Identify Funding Agencies and Resources

There are thousands of both public and private granting agencies and organizations. Funding opportunities are available from federal bureaus,

Table 11.1 Grant preparation timeline

Time	Tasks
1 y before deadline	Think of an interesting research question. Review the literature for existing gaps in knowledge. Discuss your idea with others. Determine the best granting agency to fund your project.
9 mo prior to deadline	Develop pilot projects or preliminary studies to support your main project. Continue to network with investigators/collaborators. Create a draft project. Have your project reviewed by peers and collaborators. Make revisions as required.
8 mo prior to deadline	Collect and analyze preliminary data from pilot projects. Review the funding agency specifications and timeline and contact the program officer to clarify any issues. Contact your institution and inform them of your interest to apply for the grant; verify any conditions required by your institution. Revise your draft based on collaborators' reviews and granting agency specification.
6 mo prior to deadline	Obtain quotes for equipment, supplies, or material required. Collect signed letters of collaboration and letters of support. Submit your study to your ethics board for review.
3 mo prior to deadline	Create a budget. Submit your study to your institution's peer review/budget review. Notify granting agency of intention to apply (LOI as required)
8 wk prior to deadline	Revise your proposal based on your institution's peer review process and ethics committee. Create final draft of the proposal. Obtain final ethics committee approvals.
2–4 wk prior to deadline	Collect required signatures from collaborators and institution. Collect and organize required supporting documentation.
2 wk to deadline date	Review your application for grammar typos and paragraph structure. Have a second person review the final draft.
2 d before deadline	Submit the application.

Abbreviation: LOI, letter of intent.

government agencies, private foundations, and industry/pharmaceutical companies.[2] Teams can search for funding opportunities online, through their institutional grants departments or through professional associations. A successful research team regularly reviews all available resources for grant announcements that could potentially support their research projects. Since the type of available grants varies greatly, consider the following characteristics when searching for opportunities:

1. The source of funds (e.g., federal, provincial, private, corporate).
2. The activity proposed (e.g., clinical study, infrastructure, pilot project).
3. The research subject area (e.g., osteoporosis, diabetes, cardiovascular).
4. The geographic area (e.g., the PSI Foundation in Ontario).
5. The investigator's career level (e.g., junior vs. senior investigator grants).
6. The investigator's affiliation with a specific professional society (e.g., Hip Society, Orthopaedic Trauma Association).
7. The size of the grant.

These factors are not mutually exclusive, and several characteristics may apply for any given grant.[2] It is important to obtain specific information related to the priorities of each grant and ensure that your proposal is consistent with the funding agency's priorities, mission, and language, and that the proposed research aligns well with the specific grant announcement.[3]

With continuous decreases in research funding and intense competition for large grants, teams should consider other options. For example, you may be more successful applying for numerous smaller grants, dividing the total required funding for the project over multiple sources of funding. The complete research proposal may also be split into several smaller projects in order to qualify for grant competitions that are of a shorter duration and have lower funding maximums. You may also find success in funding a start-up or pilot project through private donations from an interested philanthropist or an "angel investor." Since few government agencies are offering grants that are able to fully fund a clinical study from start to finish, some ingenuity is required for success.

Review the Funding Agency Specifications

Once you have decided on the appropriate granting agency and reviewed the information available on the organization's website, the next step should be to contact the organization's program officer or grant administrator to ensure that your proposed research project really does fall within the scope of the particular funding competition. The program officer is usually the person within the funding agency that will be responsible for the management and administration of the grant application and review process and can be a great source of information. They will have thorough knowledge of the grant announcement, funding details, applicant eligibility, and specific aims of the opportunity and scientific and/or technical aspects of the grant competition.[4] The program officer may also be able to provide information regarding previous successful applications, or previous reviewer criteria that could prove useful when formulating your own grant proposal. Many agencies make available online a list of successful grant proposals from previous competitions; review these to get a general sense of what types of proposals are typically funded by the agency to which you are applying. If you personally know any of the successful applicants listed, you may wish to contact them about their experience.

Understand How Grant Applications are Reviewed

The process by which reviewers evaluate or "grade" grant applications is often included in the funding announcement. For example, the Canadian Institutes of Health Research (CIHR) Adjudication Criteria and Interpretation Guidelines assign a percentage value for each of the following sections of the grant: concept (25%); approaches and methods (50%); and expertise, experience, and resources (25%).[5] The National Institutes of Health (NIH) indicates that reviewers determine the scientific and technical merit for each grant application and assign a separate score for each of the following criteria: significance, investigator(s), innovation, approach, and environment.[4] It is essential that your grant proposal addresses each criterion that reviewers are expected to evaluate. Understand what benchmark the reviewers will be seeking and highlight these specific aspects of your proposal to give your application an advantage over a competitor's (▶ Table 11.2). Reviewers typically review and grade a large number of applications, which can be a long and arduous process. Providing a compelling proposal that is easily understood, meets the graded criterion, and aligns with the agencies' aims is essential.

The composition of reviewing panels tasked with evaluating all the submitted applications will vary slightly depending on the granting agency and specific competition that you are applying for. All review panels consist of numerous scientists, surgeons, or field experts that either jointly or individually have the expertise required to judge and grade the proposal fairly. It is not uncommon for review panels to seek additional expertise if a particular proposal is outside the realm of the panel's knowledge. Review panel members who have a stake in any of the grant proposals (i.e., they are coinvestigators or collaborators on a proposed project) must disclose this information to the review committee and are excused from reviewing that particular application. Review panels may also contain community representatives from the patient population relevant to the proposal (e.g., patient representatives from the Canadian Cancer Society). This community representative typically does not score or grade the grant application; however, they provide feedback on the perceived significance of the proposed research, clarity of the application, and potential benefit to the community and/or patient population.

Applications are typically assigned to one or two individual reviewers, who are tasked with reading through the entire application, and scoring it based on their defined set of criteria. The review panel will then meet in person, and the individual reviewer (or reviewers) will present to the panel a brief synopsis of the proposal, as well as their score, highlighting what the reviewer(s) felt were

Table 11.2 Potential reviewer questions

Criteria	Reviewer questions
Background	Has the current body of knowledge been described? Does the published literature support the project? Is there a need for the project?
Significance	Does the project address a critical problem? Will results of the study change practice?
Innovation	Is the project original? Does the project involve development of innovative concepts or methods? Are there new data being created?
Methodology	Are the research methods clearly described? Is the research design appropriate to accomplish the aims of the project? Are the inclusion/exclusion criteria justified? Is the study statistically sound? Is the analysis plan appropriate? Has the research team thought of potential pitfalls and limitations and described how these may be addressed?
Feasibility	Do the investigators and collaborators have adequate knowledge, experience, and training to carry out the project? Is the timeline appropriate to carry out the proposed project? Are there adequate resources and is the proposed research environment appropriate to ensure success of the project? Does the research institution support the project and does it have a respectable track record in conducting clinical research?

the strengths and weaknesses of the application. Grants are then ranked from highest to lowest score, and depending on the amount of funding available, the top few proposals are awarded funding. The granting agency will then notify all applicants whether their proposal was successful or not, and often will provide the individual reviewer(s) comments. These can highlight areas of your proposal that may need to be strengthened to be successful in the future, and should be carefully considered. Reviewer comments may suggest potential clarifications, protocol modifications, alternative statistical considerations, or the addition of an area expert to the research team.

Follow Instructions

Granting agencies often have very detailed and specific instructions on grant application length, content, format, as well as precise criteria for applicant eligibility. Yet invariably, many proposals submitted do not follow the guidelines provided or fail to meet minimum standards as described in the funding announcement. Failure to adhere to the agencies' guidelines is a quick way to sabotage any chance for funding even before the proposal gets to the reviewer. Failing to observe and follow

instructions will result in an incredible level of frustration for all stakeholders upon discovering that the application is ineligible for that particular grant competition, especially when you consider the time and personal effort spent on preparing the application.

Make note of prerequisites; some grants require a preproposal or a letter of intent (LOI) to be submitted prior to the actual grant application. Specific submission timelines for LOI and final submissions of grant applications must be observed; requests for submission deadline extensions are typically not granted.

Funding announcements that allow a single submission per institution will necessitate an internal competition within the institutions applying for the grant, prior to submitting to the granting agency. Contact your institution and inform them of your intention to apply for the competition, and follow the processes to determine whether your proposal may be submitted.

Verify the submission process and obtain information on whether the application is to be submitted to the agency using a courier service, via electronic submission, or through an online portal system. Do not wait for the last minute to submit your application; allow time to create an account on the online submission system, if required, and allocate extra time for potential delivery delays or online glitches.

Follow the specific directions for each individual section within the grant application and pay close attention to length as some online portals will only allow sufficient space for a predetermined number of words. If your section is too lengthy, you run the risk of having sentences cut off. Read all of the instructions on required font, size, margins, subject headings, and number of figures and/or tables allowed in your proposal. Confirm that references are formatted according to the specifications provided, and do not exceed stated limits. If you require clarification, contact the program office of the granting agency.

Obtain Ethics Approval

If your proposal requires human or animal ethics approval, these should be obtained prior to submission of your grant application to the granting agency. Agencies may require approval before accepting a submission, or at the very least, will require full approval before disbursing grant funds. The ethics approval process and timeline vary by institution, ranging from 6 weeks to up to 4 months or longer, depending on the complexity of the project and the number of revision required. Most clinical studies require either a full ethics review (full board) or delegated review (for minimal risk studies), involving submission of a detailed application package containing the research protocol, patient information, study instruments, recruitment information, and signatures, all of which will be reviewed during an ethics committee meeting. For research involving animals, animal ethics committees typically follow a similar procedure to the human ethics committees. If your grant application is successfully funded, having ethics approvals already in place will allow for a quicker start to your research project, making adhering to your proposed timeline more manageable. Additionally, the ethics review committees typically consist of highly qualified individuals with expertise in methodology and statistics that provide feedback and critiques on the proposal being presented. Undergoing an ethics review process and addressing any shortfalls at this time may further strengthen your proposal.

Writing a Compelling Research Proposal

Once you have collected all the information required, you are ready to put your grant application together. Although there is some variation between granting agencies depending on the complexity and size of the project, most grant applications can be divided into separate sections:
- The summary or abstract.
- Background and significance (often these are two separate sections).
- Methods or study design (often includes subsections).
- Investigators, research team, environment.
- Budget.
- Supporting documentation.

Study Summary

The summary should be a clear, succinct outline of your proposal containing few words and no jargon. The reviewer should be able to understand immediately what you are trying to accomplish, even if they are not knowledgeable on the specific subject matter. This is your chance to make a significant first impression, to convince the reviewer that your proposal is exciting and novel, to draw to their attention the current gaps in knowledge, and to demonstrate how your proposed project will bridge that gap. Where possible, reference how the application is directly related to the mission of the granting agency. It is not an easy task to say so much in such limited space, so pay special attention to your research question: Is the question simple to understand, unique, and important? Does it compare controversial treatment strategies to current relevant standards of care? Does it match both the funding source and the intended audience? Research grant proposals should boil down to specific, testable questions. Several templates are available to assist in developing and framing a testable research question. One of the most popular templates for research question development is the PICOT format, developed in 2006.[6] PICOT stands for population (or patient, or problem), intervention, comparator intervention, outcome, and timeline (▶Table 11.3). Ensure that your application starts with a well-framed research question by addressing all five of these criteria and reviewers will know exactly what you are trying to accomplish.

Table 11.3 PICOT criteria

Acronym	Element definition	Description
P	Population, or patient, or problem	What specific patient populations are you investigating? Ensure you have a clearly defined patient population.
I	Intervention or exposure	What is your investigational intervention? Is it novel or an old intervention being used in a novel way?
C	Comparison	What is the main alternative to compare? Does it reflect "standard-of-care"?
O	Outcome	What do you intend to measure? What are your primary endpoints versus secondary endpoints?
T	Time	What is the time frame? (not always included)

Briefly describe the process by which the project will address the research question, and identify the expected impact of the study results. Aim to convince the reviewer within the span of the abstract that it is indeed feasible to fully answer the research question by completing the project as proposed, and how these outcomes may shape the current knowledge in the field.

Background

In this section, provide context and make a case for the need of the project by describing the current state of knowledge on the topic. Grant applications typically limit the space allocated for this section; however, it is important to demonstrate understanding of the current evidence, highlight gaps in the current literature, identify the most logical step for research, and describe how your proposal will expand that knowledge.[7] Reviewers will use this section to become more familiar with the specific subject of your grant. Include any preliminary studies or pilot data related to the project and indicate whether they were completed by members of the research team, to indicate to the reviewer that the hypothesis is testable and that

the project is feasible.[6] Discuss the published literature and current controversy on the topic, and demonstrate that the research team has sufficient understanding and expertise to improve upon the current state of knowledge. This section is where you set up the basis to make a compelling case as to the absolute necessity of completing the research project and the potential impact to patient care. Statements regarding the advancement of evidence-based medicine in this field can also act as a bridge to the significance and innovation section of the grant application.

Significance

This section of the application should justify the research question by clearly articulating why the question is important, how the study is unique, the relevance of the project to the current literature, and what impact the results may have on patients, policy, etc. Highlight innovative aspects of your project by describing original ideas on how to address the knowledge gap. This section should be as short and succinct as possible but very well referenced. Emphasize the relevance of your proposal by relating your specific aims to the previously discussed background. Use this section to convince the reviewers that your project can have a significant impact and potentially change the current standard-of-care or that the manner in which the problem is currently being addressed can be significantly improved by your proposal.

Methodology

The purpose of the methods section is to describe the proposed project. This section is typically extensive, detailed, and arguably the most substantial piece of the grant application. It is the methods section that garners the most critiques from reviewers and often what leads to an unsuccessful application. This section is often easy to understand if you are closely involved with the project, so the objective of a well-written methodology section is to formulate and provide enough detailed information to also allow reviewers to comprehend exactly what approach will be taken to answer the research question.

Clinical research can be categorized into experimental or observational. In experimental studies, the investigator assigns the exposure, whereas in observational studies, participants are observed either at a specific time point (cross-sectional studies) or over time (longitudinal studies), with no exposure assigned.[8] Observational studies are further categorized into those with and without a comparison group (▶ Fig. 11.1).[9]

The methods sections for most studies include a description of study design, interventions, randomization (allocation of treatment groups, as applicable), inclusion and exclusion criteria, study duration, expected recruitment rate, frequency of follow-up, primary and secondary outcomes, sample size and justification, and analysis plan. Often you will also need to describe the roles of each member of the research team and include information on the Data Safety Monitoring Board (DSMB) and Steering Committee (SC), if any.

Organize the methods section starting with study design, ensuring that it is logical and appropriate for the research question as this is crucial in convincing reviewers that your study is feasible. Describe recruitment activities, including how potential participants will be identified and how

they will be informed about the study (e.g., direct recruitment, use of recruitment letters, advertising, referrals, etc.). Justify your inclusion and exclusion criteria. To demonstrate that the study is viable within the established timeline, include information on how many centers will be involved in the study and the expected recruitment rate for each center. If applicable, include detailed information on randomization methods and what steps will be taken to minimize bias. Provide details on the outcomes being measured, including a description of the primary outcome and why it was chosen as the most important outcome for the study. Include a sample size determination and a rigorous statistical analysis. Consultation with an experienced methodologist, biostatistician, health economist, or any other relevant team member is highly recommended when putting together the methods section and analysis plan. Include information on instruments being used (e.g., questionnaires, outcome measurements) and methods used to standardize these instruments across all participating centers.[10]

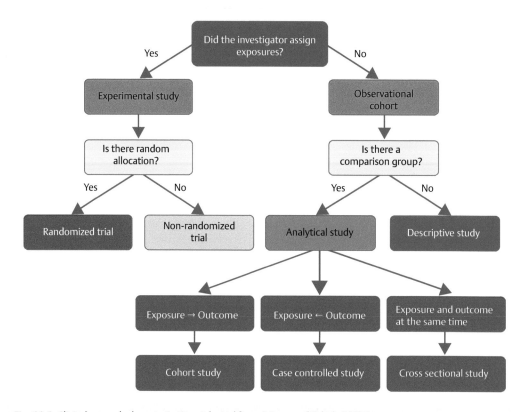

Fig. 11.1 Clinical research characterization. Adapted from Grimes and Schulz 2002.[9]

Describe how long your project will take to complete, dividing your timeline into sections: time for recruitment of subjects, follow-up, obtaining primary outcomes, analysis, and publication and dissemination of results. Plan a realistic project development and implementation timeline, allowing for unavoidable delays in each section. Some agencies ask you to consider complications that may be encountered during the course of the study and require you to propose mitigation strategies to address these. For example, how will you address problem with compliance, slower-than-expected recruitment rates, or participants lost to follow-up? Preemptively addressing potential limitations will demonstrate that you have carefully considered these and have a contingency plan in place.

Investigators/Research Team/ Environment

It is important to demonstrate that the investigator and the research team have the qualifications and expertise to complete the proposed project. Experience may be demonstrated by relevant publications, previous leadership in relevant research projects, and previous collaboration between members of the team. A curriculum vitae (CV) for investigators is required for all grant applications detailing the investigators' experience relevant to the grant application. At minimum, the CV of the principal investigator and coinvestigators is required; however, you may also require CVs for collaborators. CVs must to be formatted according to the grant agency's specific requirements, often limited to 2 to 3 pages listing prior experience directly relevant to the proposed project. Plan sufficient time to collect and reformat these documents. Describe the role of each stakeholder either in the CV or in a supporting document page, as allowed. It is a good idea to include junior investigators in the grant application so that they may gain experience for future projects. Include end users such as policy makers, industry, and patient representative groups, as appropriate. The role of patient representative groups in clinical studies has increased in recent years. They can participate in discussions about which research topics to pursue, suggest ways to minimize patient burdens, assist with developing patient-friendly consent forms, and increase awareness about real issues affecting the patient populations being investigated in the clinical study. If your research proposal involves a minority population, ensure that you have a representative of that population as a member of your research team. They can be included in the research proposal as collaborators, consultants, or as members of a steering committee, emphasizing the impact of the research on the lives of people.

Stress what makes the team of researchers the preeminent choice to tackle the research problem, and how the research will truly make a difference to the future.

Describe the resources available within the institution where the proposed study will take place, highlighting existing infrastructure, available equipment, and support from the organization's administration.

Budget

Although some granting agencies consider the budget allocation to be the least significant piece of the review process, it is certainly important to ensure that your budget accurately reflects project expenses and that it matches with the granting agencies' expense allowances. Verify the number of years of funding and the maximum amount of support per year available for the specific grant competition that you are applying for. A typical budget might include personnel (salaries), research and/or office supplies, patient-related costs (e.g., study reimbursement), animal care costs, equipment, travel costs, costs for meetings, licensing costs (e.g., for instrument use or software), and data management costs. Consider other costs usually missed such as translation services, publication costs, adjudication costs, shipping/couriers, maintenance and calibration of equipment, ethics committee fees, and archiving fees. Note any potential fees associated with laboratory, pharmacy, diagnostic imaging, or any other services required. Each item within the budget should include a justification of why it is a necessary expense. Remember to include a benefit percentage for all salaries (check with your institution as to the specific rate). If applying for multiyear funding support, be sure to include cost-of-living or merit-based yearly raises for all salaries as applicable.

When applying for more than one funding agency for the same project, be aware of overlapping budget items. Be honest about how money will be spent and do not seek funds for items that have already been funded.

Verify eligible expenses with the granting agency before including them in the budget. Some agencies prohibit expenses such as institutional overhead, equipment purchases, and support for principal investigators. Confirm that your budget does not contain any ineligible items and that the total amount falls within the total amount available in the funding announcement.

Supporting Documentation

Documentation to support your grant application may include letters of collaboration from other institutions or investigators, support letters from patient advocacy groups, justification for the proposed budget, or confirmation letters of institutional approval for the project. Including supporting documentation, if allowed in a grant application, is never a bad idea. While reviewers may not be obligated to review these documents, inclusion of appropriate supporting records provides further evidence of the thoroughness of the proposal. Written support from known and well-funded investigators will demonstrate the ability of the applicant to complete the project in the proposed time period.[11] An additional budget justification page will allow for a detailed breakdown of the proposed expenses and how they relate to the work being done. You may also include a letter from the institution where the research will take place indicating the current rates for benefits for all salaried employees to justify any benefits in addition to the base salary. As indicated earlier, some agencies will request a copy of the ethics approval or animal care committee approval letter at the time of submission. Ensure that all your documents are included and formatted according to the agency's specific submission guidelines.

Resubmissions

Success rates are often low for major granting agencies, especially on the first try, and a resubmission is usually necessary. Once you shake off your disappointment, read the reviewer comments carefully to evaluate the concerns they had with the proposal. Carefully consider all suggestions from the reviewers for improvement of the proposal. Do not take reviewer comments personally: they review dozens of competitive applications and need to narrow down numerous great proposals to determine the highest rated projects.

Often projects are rejected due to caps on funding availability.

If your grant application was declined, you can do the following:
- Revise the grant and resubmit to the same funding agency for the next available competition.
- Revise the grant and submit to a different agency.

Verify the agency's policy on grant resubmissions; some agencies have limits on how many times a proposal can be resubmitted and may require a separate letter specifically addressing the previous reviewer comments. It is strongly advised to address every critique. Be mindful of the tone in your reply; although you may disagree with the suggestions or comments, a condescending or disrespectful reply is never appropriate. Address the comment, adjust your proposal according to the suggestions or justify why a revision would not be adequate.[12]

If you decide that the initial organization is not the most appropriate funding agency to review your grant, or if the agency has limits on the number of times a grant may be resubmitted, you may choose to apply to a different agency. Adapting a previously completed grant to another agency is not as simple as copying and pasting from one application to the other. Read all the guidelines for the new grant competition thoroughly and tailor your new grant proposal to the agency's specifications.

11.3 Conclusion

Grant writing is an extensive process requiring meticulous planning and careful time management and should not be undertaken lightly. Given the highly competitive research environment, it is of utmost importance that research teams dedicate sufficient time to the grant writing process. By starting early, collaborating with experienced investigators, having a meticulously crafted research proposal, paying attention to details, and having an organized timeline for submission, the chances for successful research funding are greatly improved.

11.4 Practical Application

Grammar Tips
- Check grammar and spelling: Do not rely exclusively on word processing spellchecker as it

often fails to recognize inappropriately placed words. Have one or two other people review grammar, sentence structure, typographical errors, and punctuation.

- Be succinct and use simple language that can be easily understood. Reduce phrases to a single word whenever possible and if you can remove a word completely, remove it.
- Avoid redundancy when writing your proposal. Highlight the point you need to make and articulate it clearly, once. Avoid common redundant expressions (i.e., cooperate together, important essentials, consensus of opinion).[8]
- Use headings and subtitles for important concepts.

11.4.1 Common issues That Result in Grant Rejection

- The proposal is too ambitious and unrealistic, and cannot possibly be accomplished in the proposed timeline.
- The study design is unclear or inappropriate.
- The critical appraisal of the literature is insufficient.
- Statistical power is inadequate.
- There is a lack of preliminary data or pilot studies.
- The proposal contains too many measurements or endpoints.
- The inclusion or exclusion criteria are not justified.
- The investigator is inexperienced or lacks the necessary skills to complete the project.

Definitions

- **Angel investor:** Typically a formally educated, high net worth individual, who invests personal funds at arm's length in businesses owned and operated by unrelated individuals. For more detail, see http://www.angelinvestorsontario.ca/
- **Steering committee:** Consisting of a group of individuals that are independent from the research team, the steering committee provides oversight of the practical aspects of the study as well as ensuring that the study continues to

be run in a way that is safe for the patients. The steering committee provides recommendations about starting, continuing, and stopping the study and provides appropriate safety and efficacy data to the sponsor and investigators.

- **Data Safety Monitoring Board (DSMB):** Also known as a Data Monitoring Committee (DMC), the DSMB consists of a group of expert individuals that are independent from the research team and that review data accumulated from a clinical trial at regular intervals. The DSMB is responsible for safeguarding the interests of study participants, assessing the safety and efficacy of study procedures, monitoring study data, and the overall conduct of the study.

References

[1] Gholipour A, Lee EY, Warfield SK. The Anatomy and Art of Writing a Successful Grant Application: A Practical Step-By-Step Approach. Pediatr Radiol 2014;44(12): 1512–1517

[2] Devine EB. The Art of Obtaining Grants. Am J Health Syst Pharm 2009;66(6):580–587

[3] Wisdom JP, Riley H, Myers N. Recommendations for Writing Successful Grant Proposals: An Information Synthesis. Acad Med 2015;90(12):1720–1725

[4] National Institutes of Health. How to Apply—Application Guide. 2017 [cited July 3, 2018]. https://grants.nih.gov/grants/how-to-apply-application-guide.html

[5] CIHR. Peer Review: Policies and Procedures. 2018 [cited July 9, 2018]. http://www.cihr-irsc.gc.ca/e/193.html

[6] Haynes R, Sackett DL, Guyatt G. Forming Research Questions. Clinical Epidemiology: How to Do Clinical Practice Research. In: Haynes R, Guyatt G, ed. 3rd ed. Philadelphia, PA: Lippincott Williams & Wilkins; 2006:3–15

[7] Davidson NO. Grant Writing: Tips and Pointers from a Personal Perspective. Gastroenterology 2012;142(1):4–7

[8] Bhandari M, Joensson A. Various Research Design Classifications. In: Bhandari M, ed. Clinical Research for Surgeons. Vol. 1. New York, NY: Thieme; 2009:315

[9] Grimes DA, Schulz KF. An Overview of Clinical Research: The Lay of the Land. Lancet 2002;359(9300):57–61

[10] Chung KC, Shauver MJ. Fundamental Principles of Writing a Successful Grant Proposal. J Hand Surg Am 2008;33(4):566–572

[11] Wiseman JT, Alavi K, Milner RJ. Grant writing 101. Clin Colon Rectal Surg 2013;26(4):228–231

[12] Oster S, Cordo P. Successful Grant Proposals in Science, Technology, and Medicine: A Guide to Writing the Narrative. Vol. 1. New York, NY: Cambridge University Press; 2015

12 Dollars and "Sense": A Guide to Research Finances

Johanna Dobransky, Darren M. Roffey

Abstract

The purpose of this chapter is to show research coordinators how to plan and create a budget for a research study. Many study components require careful consideration when creating a budget—several of which are contingent on direct and indirect costs. Our aim is to outline who should prepare the budget and what it should include, when to plan and how to execute the budget, and tips for budget negotiation with sponsors and granting agencies. Monitoring, ongoing maintenance, and termination of a budget will also be discussed. Finally, we will provide a practical example with recommendations on how to create a research study budget that incorporates relevant expenses.

Keywords: budget, expenses, planning, monitoring, timeline, schedule of events, milestone, payments

12.1 Introduction

Organizing finances for the duration of a research study involving human participants requires careful planning and continuous monitoring. Preparing an accurate budget is a vital but often difficult task.[1] There are many important financial considerations to take into account, including: participant sample size, number of sites involved, institution-specific fees for non standard-of-care procedures, salaries of research personnel, and the cost of equipment.[2] It is easy to focus on tangible costs such as research staff salaries and study-specific equipment. However, if principal investigators and research coordinators do not take the time to carefully consider all possible costs, this may lead to poor study execution, troublesome monitoring, funding shortages, and an early termination of the study protocol; all of which could result in the possibility of an unfinished and underpowered study. Based on a cross-sectional, descriptive study of terminated trials posted on the ClinicalTrials.gov database, 5.5% of the 905 registered studies were terminated early due to lack of funds.[3] This not only has implications for patient safety and the ability to draw valid conclusions from available data, but is also a waste of time and valuable resources. Alas, while ample budgetary recommendations exist, there is no universal budget template readily available. Based on the current literature, the purpose of this chapter is to provide guidance to research coordinators on budgetary planning for research studies.

12.2 Planning and Creating a Research Budget

12.2.1 Preplanning Phase

Prior to agreeing to coordinate a research study or prepare and approve a budget, research coordinators must understand the strategic plan of their department (i.e., mission, vision, and values) to ensure the study aligns with the research priorities of the hospital and affiliated research institution. Additionally, it is worthwhile knowing whether a priority has been placed upon attracting clinical trial funding as a source of research-based income.[4,5] If this be the case, as it is in many research institutions, then it may provide an impetus for the principal investigator to pursue the study further. Selecting the type of budgetary management (i.e., centralized vs. decentralized) should also be configured in the preplanning phase.

12.2.2 Funding Source

Determining the source of funds for a research study is an important first step. It is the responsibility of the principal investigator and research coordinator to devise a detailed and accurate budget to meet the requirements provided by the granting agency or sponsor to which they plan to apply.[1] Ideally, the budget should be prepared after a detailed protocol has been written and prior to the submission of an application for research funding. Once funding has been successfully secured, it is important to keep in mind that industry-sponsored studies and investigator-initiated studies vary in terms of budget requirements. With industry studies, the study sponsor will generally provide a budget template. The research coordinator must ensure that any such budget template incorporates appropriate direct and indirect fees unique to institution-specific procedures, including pharmacy fees, laboratory tests, and diagnostic imaging.

12.2.3 Centralized versus Decentralized Budgetary Management

Choosing a centralized system of budgetary management means that all budgeting decisions will occur at a single location. This scenario may be convenient when conducting a randomized control trial, especially when all patient randomization is conducted at one site or via one electronic platform. Centralization ensures that budgetary tasks are performed only once, reducing duplication of efforts and facilitating a more effective method of tracking funds. Furthermore, it provides the sponsor with greater control over recruitment strategies and materials used to attract participants into the study.

Decentralization is a more traditional model, and is typically employed when the budget does not need to be managed by the study sponsor. This decentralized method is favorable when the number of participants in a study is small as it provides the principal investigators with more control over site finances. However, in recent times, a combination model is becoming increasingly popular, wherein the budget is maintained centrally, but part of the study budget is allocated to each individual site for the implementation of site-specific activities.[2] Dedicating time on budgetary management decisions in the preplanning phase will facilitate faster and more efficient budget drafting and execution.

12.2.4 Financial Lifecycle

The study budget should always be prepared in conjunction with the final version of the study protocol. Brescia[2] recommends that the amount of time spent on research finances should be allocated as: 80% at the planning stage versus 20% on monitoring and maintenance. According to Cavalieri and Rupp,[6] the financial lifecycle of a clinical trial involves many stages, including (1) feasibility evaluation of a clinical trial, (2) building or assessing a proposed budget, (3) negotiating the contract for research services, (4) tracking and reconciling revenue and site expenses, and (5) evaluating the financial outcomes. Stages 1, 2, 4, and 5 will be featured in this chapter, while stage 3 will be showcased in its own separate chapter.

12.2.5 Planning the Budget

The planning phase should help research coordinators determine whether the study is feasible. Assessing study feasibility is crucial, as spending more time upfront on whether the conduct of a research study is viable will increase the chances of successful patient recruitment, study execution, and results dissemination.[7] Anecdotal evidence suggests that the majority of studies are delayed due to inadequate staffing and low recruitment numbers, which are often downstream effects of poor planning. Major cost differentials associated with the conduct of a study largely depend on the number of sites involved and the number of participating subjects.[1]

Principal investigators are regularly offered a lump sum of funds from which they must accommodate study expenses, commonly referred to as "top-down budgeting." A better and more accountable method to calculate site expenses is through "bottom-up budgeting," which involves a thorough understanding of site resources.[6] Using this bottom-up budgeting approach, all expenses based on the study protocol are documented line by line. The research coordinator can act as a delegate of the principal investigator in this instance and plan and create the budget in minutiae accordingly, given their intimate knowledge of the study requirements and expenses. Despite the fact the sponsor is responsible for the initiation, management, and financing of a study,[8] it is the role of the principal investigator and research coordinator to finalize the study budget in direct collaboration with the sponsor.[6]

12.2.6 Key Expenses

Significant time is invested in initiating a research study, completing such task as ethics submission, development of case report forms, preparing screening and recruitment strategies, attending off-site investigator meetings, and participating in on-site initiation visits.[7] It is important that the budget account for all of these tasks, as they are often overlooked in favor of providing a detailed summary of expenses in line with the procedures that will take place at each patient visit.[9] Granted, the cost of procedures completed at every visit will form the largest contingent of the per-patient portion of the budget. As such, the protocol needs to be very specific, which in turn will assist the

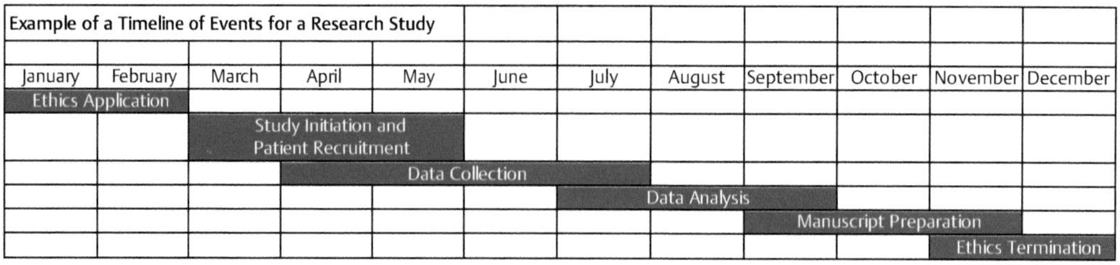

Example of a Timeline of Events for a Research Study											
January	February	March	April	May	June	July	August	September	October	November	December
Ethics Application	Ethics Application										
		Study Initiation and Patient Recruitment	Study Initiation and Patient Recruitment	Study Initiation and Patient Recruitment							
			Data Collection	Data Collection	Data Collection	Data Collection					
						Data Analysis	Data Analysis	Data Analysis			
								Manuscript Preparation	Manuscript Preparation	Manuscript Preparation	
											Ethics Termination

Fig. 12.1 Timeline of events that can be used as the basis for budgetary planning.

research coordinator in listing all of the activities that will take place and who will be facilitating its conduct. When integrating all of the personnel involved in the study into the budget, it is imperative to consider the time required to perform all of the necessary tasks.[10] Documenting the hourly rate of these personnel is therefore a must.[10,11]

▶ Fig. 12.1 displays a Gantt chart that highlights an example of a timeline of events for a research study. This chart contains the major constituents of a research study involving human participants that ideally needs to be followed in a reasonable semblance from start to finish. Research coordinators can utilize this chart as a starting point to assess what the key expenses of the study will be, in accordance with the protocol and study events. Used in combination with the Gantt chart, the detailed outlines of the common financial considerations at each stage of the time of events for a research study delineated in ▶ Table 12.1 can further assist the research coordinator in putting together a detailed budget.

It is important to note that the featured Gantt chart and sample financial considerations provided are applicable for a simple research study and budgetary plan. A more detailed schedule of events will be necessary for larger, more complex, clinical studies.

12.2.7 Direct and Indirect Costs

Direct and indirect costs of performing clinical research differ widely between institutions. Direct costs are the expenses directly related to the proposed study, including research personnel salaries, equipment and consumable supplies, equipment maintenance, publication fees, and laboratory and diagnostic imaging costs. Indirect costs are those not directly related to the project, such as human resources, finance, contracts, general administration, and building maintenance. Indirect costs can be referred to as institutional overhead fees.[12] Principal investigators and research coordinators should undertake an internal costing analysis, independent of the proposed budget, to thoroughly appreciate the direct and indirect costs that may be associated with a study. This analysis can be accomplished by assessing the protocol and considering each task and the personnel involved, and then assigning a monetary value to every specific activity. This process must be detailed, particularly surrounding research activities that are not standard or routine clinical care.[13]

12.2.8 Negotiating the Study Budget

When reviewing the protocol provided by a study sponsor, research coordinators should look for potential problems related to study feasibility. Principal investigators and other research team members with experience managing studies are encouraged to do likewise, particularly as they can provide expertise and perspective to uncover any hidden budgetary costs.[7] When negotiating with a sponsor, it is important to have standard, nonrefundable, and nonnegotiable fees for each service specific to the institution to alleviate any ambiguity in costs.

Research coordinators and principal investigators need to identify milestones when negotiating the study budget that will in turn trigger payments and help ascertain if adequate funds will be available between payments. The following are some common considerations specifically pertaining to industry-sponsored studies that need to be negotiated:
- Will the sponsor cover the initial ethics committee fees?

Table 12.1 Detailed outlines of the common financial considerations at each stage of the time of events for a research study

Study timeline	Financial consideration	Description
EC application	• Review fee • Annual renewal fee • Amendment fee	Fees charged for initial ethics review, work associated with ongoing correspondence, processing protocol changes (e.g., $5,000 initial review, $1000 annual renewal, $500 amendment)
	• Preparation of EC documentation • Ongoing EC correspondence	Preparing and submitting EC application and then addressing any concerns brought forward by the EC, plus submission of necessary updates (e.g., SAE forms)
Study initiation and patient recruitment	Budget preparation	Preparing and finalizing the budget
	• Creating source documents • Creating case report forms	Creating and amending source documents, and confirming case report forms
	Attendance at off-site meetings	Costs for transportation, accommodation, food, and time spent at the meeting
	On-site initiation visit	Time spent with investigators and sponsor representatives
	Screening patients	Screening and documenting eligible patients
	Obtaining informed consent	Corresponding with study participants to obtain informed consent
Data Collection	Conducting patient visits	Time spent with patients completing functional assessments and questionnaires and patient-reported outcome measures
	Source documentation	Completing all documents after each patient visit
	Maintaining regulatory documents	Complying with institutional and/or sponsor guidelines in the maintenance of study documents
	Communicating with sponsor or other sites	Regular correspondence with sponsor or other sites
	Monitoring visits	Preparation time to ensure files are ready for the study monitor and then being present for the monitoring visit
	Invoicing sponsor or sites	Submitting invoices on quarterly basis
	Maintenance of paper and electronic records	Organization and filing
	Data entry	Inputting data into data management systems
Analysis	Data manager	Staff needed to oversee data analysis, hourly rate, and time spent
	Data management software	Electronic data capture system (e.g., RedCap, ConEHR)
	Statistician	Statistician time for interim and final analyses
Manuscript preparation	Manuscript preparation and submission	Time to prepare knowledge dissemination via manuscript preparation and submission
EC termination	Study closeout paperwork	Paperwork completed at the end of a study
	Study audit	Time spent with auditors

(Continued)

Table 12.1 (*Continued*) Detailed outlines of the common financial considerations at each stage of the time of events for a research study

Study timeline	Financial consideration	Description
Administrative costs	Randomization software	Often necessary for conducting multicenter randomized control trials
	Computer hardware	Computers, printers, and laptops necessary to conduct the trial
	Licenses	Licenses for statistical package software, imaging analysis software
	Patient stipends	Parking and transportation should be included in per patient budget only if all patients are eligible for this
	Conference attendance	Travel to meetings, registration, accommodation, flights, food
	Printing supplies	Necessary for administering questionnaires
	Postage and courier	Necessary for mailing out questionnaires at follow-up
Overhead fees	Institutional overhead	Anywhere between 20 and 40% depending upon the institution

Abbreviations: EC, ethics committee; SAE, serious adverse events.

- Is the time required to train the principal investigator to use or insert a device reimbursed by the sponsor?
- Will the sponsor provide money to cover the costs of research staff to prepare study start-up?
- Will the sponsor pay for subjects who are screened but determined to be ineligible for enrollment?
- If pharmacy is involved, will the sponsor pay for storage and dispensing of study drugs?
- In a device trial, who will pay for the cost of the device?

While negotiating with a sponsor, it will be necessary to justify each fee allocated to every service. This can be done by creating a memo. For example, an often-overlooked element is serious adverse event reporting and the time it takes to diligently document and submit them to the sponsor and ethics committee. Such a memo would state: "$500 serious adverse event fee is for coordinator/principal investigator time needed to complete the paperwork for sponsor or ethics committee requirements."[7]

If there is any disagreement with the study sponsor, the research coordinator and principal investigator should engage in discussion to reach an alternative arrangement that is amenable to all parties. These financial decisions should be made alongside the business manager to ensure financial compliance with the institution.[14]

12.2.9 Need for a Contingency Budget

Studies often require ongoing efforts to retain patients, which may necessitate additional funding requirements to be added to the budget for the research coordinator. Alternatively, overages for other research personnel may not warrant a contingency budget, but rather the principal investigator may choose to budget more money than is necessary in the main budget and then only plan to spend a certain portion of it.[2] Both of these so-called contingency "safety nets" are acceptable, and in most instances, it comes down to preference and compliance with any study sponsor regulations. Other factors that may necessitate a contingency budget include the following: ethics committee materials that are not approved on schedule, removing or adding another site during the recruitment phase, and substantial protocol amendments.

12.2.10 Pitfalls Associated with Budgetary Planning

Time spent by the principal investigator and research coordinator on planning and executing any type of research study has a tremendous impact on the study budget, and is often vastly underestimated.[7] There may be time-consuming tasks that are not fully realized until after the study is underway. As such, there is always a degree of uncertainty when planning a budget. Patient screen failure is one such example, whereby most of the requirements for a potential study participant are completed, only to find out for one reason or another that the patient is a screen failure. Clinical research sites should be paid in full for screen failures, so as to account for all of the time research coordinators may potentially spend on this task.

Large tertiary care and academic research institutions may require a provision that research personnel be afforded an annual salary increase of approximately 2 to 3%. This percentile increase can be comprised of cost of living allowance (COLA) increments in line with inflation and consumer price index, and/or satisfactory performance reviews adjusted for the yearly COLA. For studies that last over a year, it can be difficult to adequately quantify this necessary salary incremental raise, the end result being a potential shortfall in the study budget of 1 to 2% if the estimated increase does not synchronize with the institutional requirements.

Another area of concern is the practice of mixing research events with standard-of-care procedures. This is especially problematic in the United States, where patients may start receiving bills for medical services performed under the guise of the research study that were thought to be standard-of-care. Charging a procedure to insurance, rather than it being covered by research funds, could result in a case of insurance or Medicare fraud.[14]

12.3 Ongoing Monitoring of a Research Budget

After the planning phase, tracking and reconciling revenue and site expenses and evaluating the financial outcomes of the study should be the focus.[6] Ongoing monitoring is especially important when coordinating a multicenter study, as regular payments need to be made to the additional clinical sites when data are submitted or in accordance with their payment plan. It is at this point that adhering to milestone payments based on the schedule of events is essential.

12.3.1 Invoicing and Payments

Payment plans may be arranged in installments with defined timepoints.[15] It is imperative to review the schedule of assessments included in the protocol to obtain an accurate summary of examinations, lab tests, and procedures that are required throughout the study. The research coordinator should then prepare a detailed schedule of events based on the protocol, detail all expenses separately that are necessary to run the study, and then create the milestones accordingly. During the process, it is important to ask the following questions:

- How often will site payments occur?
- What milestones must a site reach to generate a payment?

It is important to recognize that payment plans can vary in their design and complexity. Industry funders and granting agencies may insist on releasing funds by time (e.g., every quarter or every 6 months, with the total amount based on the number of agreed-upon milestones that have been reached during that time period), or it may choose to release study payments only when agreed-upon milestones are achieved by a proportion of patients or finite study-related tangibles are delivered (e.g., 50% patient study enrollment, 100% patient follow-up at 3 months, final report submitted). A checklist can be helpful to ensure that all required costs are covered in the budget, including reimbursement for often-missed fees such as phone calls, stipends, and ancillary services.[7]

Over the course of a multicenter study, regular payments are to be made to other sites involved. There are two common models used: (1) Fixed-cost model, where costs are based on the simulated scope of work; the projected costs per site and payments are made based on the direct and indirect costs of each site over the duration of the study. (2) Variable cost model, where payments are made based on successful patient enrollment and follow-up visits and case report forms submitted.[16] The variable cost model is analogous to the milestone payments that are set up in the planning phase, where sites are reimbursed by activity that takes place. Sheffet et al[16] demonstrated that changing from a fixed-cost to a variable-cost model allowed for an extension of the project that subsequently permitted other clinical sites to join and increase patient enrollment. A variable-cost model provides transparency so far as the productivity is concerned, and has been shown to promote compliance. Also referred to as performance-based budgets, the variable-cost model conserves funding and provides effective management without compromising the scientific integrity of the study.

12.3.2 Amending the Study Budget

While the study is ongoing, it is a valuable exercise to determine the amount of hours research personnel are spending on patient recruitment and study visits, and whether the total number of hours is exceeding the estimated hours that were budgeted.[14] If, on average, the number of estimated hours is within range, it is safe to assume that the approved budget was accurately estimated. However, if the total number of hours is regularly exceeding the estimated hours, research coordinators and investigators need to explore why, by posing such questions as the following:

- Are procedures taking longer to complete because of the nature of the research participants?
- Are there logistical hurdles in the clinics?
- Is it because the study called for only one research coordinator but as enrolment progressed, it was realized that two coordinators were necessary?

It is advisable at this stage to go back to the sponsor and provide thorough justification on why the study is costing the site more than anticipated and, if possible, renegotiate the study budget.[14]

12.4 Study Termination

12.4.1 Premature Study Termination

When physicians, surgeons, or clinical researchers decide to take on a study, they naturally expect that the study will be completed and some form of knowledge dissemination will occur (e.g., conference presentation, journal publication, etc.).[7] Unfortunately, studies may have to be prematurely terminated for reasons related to efficacy, safety, or feasibility.[17] Randomized control trials are generally regarded as the gold standard for evaluating interventions,[18] but due to their very nature, are prone to poor recruitment targets.[19] McDonald et al[19] found that only 31% of trials reached their recruitment target. Poor recruitment can lead to an underpowered study, which may lead to clinically important effects being missed.[20] It is not uncommon for investigators and sponsors to apply for recruitment extensions to achieve the desired patient sample size, which invariably adds to the cost of running the study.[21]

Other studies may just need to be temporarily halted, which is not as risky or complicated as completely terminating the study. According to Williams et al,[3] an estimated 39% of terminated trials on ClinicalTrials.gov are halted due to slow recruitment.[19] To avoid prematurely terminating a study, it is recommended that a Data Safety Monitoring Board be involved with any decision regarding an amendment to the existing study protocol or financial prudence. Patient representatives on the board should also play a role with regard to financial decisions, and understandably consider patient safety as the utmost priority in any such processes.

12.5 Practical Application

In this practical application example, a research coordinator is provided with a complete protocol written by an industry sponsor describing a randomized control trial comparing two minimally invasive hip approaches. Patients are required to visit the clinic preoperatively and postoperatively, with a target sample size of 50 in each

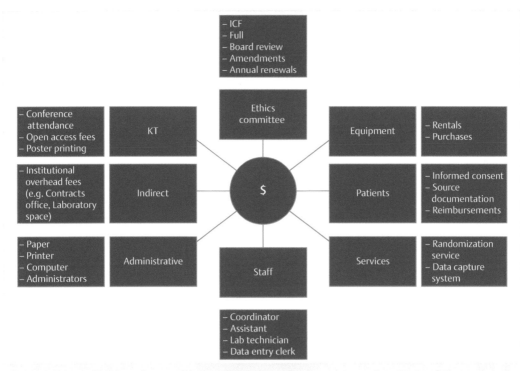

Fig. 12.2 Core considerations of a research budget. (*Abbreviations:* ICF, Informed consent form; KT, Knowledge translation.)

group. In addition, 15 patients in each group will be recruited to participate in a separate gait analysis. Each patient will be followed up at 12 months postoperatively, with the expected duration of the study being 2 years.

After thoroughly reading the provided protocol, the research coordinator should keep in mind the core considerations of a research budget to adequately plan and also visualize hidden costs (▶Fig. 12.2). The following checklist should be applied:

Ethics committee:
- How much time will be required to handle ethics-related activities, including creation of informed consent forms, attendance at ethics committee full-board reviews, addressing the letter of concerns, amendments to the protocol, and annual renewals?
- Does the ethics committee charge for annual renewals?

Equipment:
- What study-related equipment, if any, will need to be rented or purchased?

Patients:
- How much time will each study visit take?
- How many times will the coordinator need to see each patient?
- Will study participants receive reimbursement for parking?

Services:
- What are the costs of any non standard-of-care imaging, such as nontraditional X-rays?
- What are the costs of any external services being used, such as a randomization service and data capture system?

Staffing costs:
- Who are all the individuals that will need to be paid during the course of the research trial?
- Does the institution require budgetary adjustments for annual salaries in multiyear studies to reflect COLA increases and satisfactory performance reviews?

Administrative fees:
- How much paper and other office supplies will be required?
- Will any administrative support be required?

Indirect costs:
- What are the institutional overhead fees?

Knowledge translation:
- Will results be disseminated in journal that has open access fees?
- Will travel to conferences be required?

Using milestones in the form of a variable-cost model[16] as performance indicators and tying payments to these milestones is an acceptable method of securing funding for this research study. A schedule of events is created to visualize the timeline required from every studyparticipant (▶ Table 12.2). Once the research coordinator and investigator have a firm grasp of the schedule of events, the next step is to highlight all the anticipated expenses specific to the study protocol (**Toolbox A**). The final step is to then combine the schedule of events in ▶ Table 12.2 with the tasks outlined in **Toolbox A** and arrive at a proposed fee schedule (▶ Table 12.3). It is up to the principal investigator to work with the sponsor to come to a consensus as to how much monetary weight should be allocated to each study event. The costs of the anticipated expenses and proposed fee schedule should ideally align.

12.6 Conclusion

There is no current gold standard for creating a budget—only guidelines and templates are available in the literature. There are many different types of studies, all of which warrant careful planning inclusive of direct and indirect expenses. Thorough planning conducted by the principal investigator and research coordinator may enable research personnel to fully comprehend the financial requirements of the study and ensure that it is completed without financial distress. If there are potential roadblocks and unanticipated circumstances that can be envisioned during the planning phase, then having a back-up plan is critical to ensuring the budget and study are both executing correctly to ensure the success of the research study.

Definitions

- **Sponsor:** An individual, company, institution, or organization that takes responsibility for the initiation, management, and/or financing of a clinical study.
- **Investigator:** A person responsible for the conduct of the clinical study at a study site. If a study is conducted by a team of individuals at a study site, the investigator is the responsible leader of the team and may be called the (site) principal investigator.
- **Direct costs:** Costs that can be specifically attributed to a particular person or service for a research trial, for example, research staff salary and non standard-of-care.
- **Indirect costs:** Costs that cannot be attributed to one specific thing and generally encompass a mandatory service or fee at institution, for example, 30% institutional overhead that pays for administrative support, contracts office, printers, and paper within the department.
- **Schedule of events:** A table that outlines the timeframe (duration) of study and specifies all of the events that take place at each timeframe.
- **Milestones:** Selected events based on the schedule of events for which payment may be received.

Acknowledgments

We would like to acknowledge William Read, MCS, MBA, PMP, CD, Senior Research Project Manager at the Ottawa Hospital Research Institute, who provided guidance on the ***Pitfalls Associated with Budgetary Planning*** section.

Table 12.2 Schedule of events

Event	Pre-op screening (<60 d prior to surgery)	Operative	Postoperative period					
			1 d	2 wk	4 wk	6 wk	3 mo	12 mo
Informed consent	X							
Inclusion/exclusion	X							
Basic demographics	X							
Waist circumference	X				X			X
Operative information		X						
Device information		X						
WOMAC	X				X		X	X
HOOS	X				X		X	X
EQ-5D	X				X		X	X
VAS pain scores	X		X	X				
Narcotic usage	X							
Pre-post Hgb	X		X	X				
Complications						X	X	X
Readmissions						X		
TUG	X		X	X		X		X
TSC	X		X	X		X		X
IR and ER ROM at flexion and extension	X		X	X		X		X
Motion capture for gait analysis[a]	X					X		X
Gait data processing	X					X		X
Patient stipend (parking + gift certificate)	X					X		X
Dissemination of results								X

Abbreviations: EQ-5D, EuroQol-5D; ER, external rotation; Hgb, hemoglobin; HOOS, Hip disability and Osteoarthritis Outcome Score; IR, internal rotation; ROM, range of motion; TSC, timed stair climb; TUG, timed up and go; VAS, visual analogue scale; WOMAC, Western Ontario and McMaster Universities Osteoarthritis Index.
[a]Gait analysis to occur in subset of 15 patients per group

Table 12.3 Proposed fee schedule (CAD)

Event	Preoperative (<60 d prior to surgery)	Operative	Day 1	2 wk	4 wk	6 wk	3 mo	12 mo
					Postoperative period			
Informed consent	100.00							
Inclusion/exclusion	65.00							
Basic demographics	28.00							
Waist circumference	24.50				24.50			24.50
Operative information		50.00						
Device information		50.00						
WOMAC	50.00				50.00		50.00	50.00
HOOS	50.00				50.00		50.00	50.00
EQ-5D	50.00				50.00		50.00	50.00
VAS pain scores	35.00		35.00	35.00				
Narcotic Usage	45.00							
Pre-post Hb	50.00		50.00	50.00				
Complications						50.00	50.00	50.00
Readmissions							50.00	
TUG	50.00		50.00	50.00		50.00		50.00

(Continued)

Table 12.3 (*Continued*) Proposed fee schedule (CAD)

			Postoperative period						Total per patient	
TSC	50.00	50.00	50.00	50.00		50.00		50.00		
IR and ER ROM at flexion and extension	50.00	50.00	50.00	50.00		50.00		50.00		
Motion capture for gait	459.00					459.00		459.00		
Gait data processing	430.50					430.50		430.50		
Patient stipend (gift card)	50.00					50.00		50.00		
Cost per patient (n = 100)	647.50	100.00	235.00	235.00	174.50	200.00	250.00	374.50		
30% institutional overhead fee	841.75	130.00	305.50	305.50	226.85	260.00	325.00	486.85	2,881.45	Cost per 100 patients $288,145.00
Cost per patient (n = 30)[a]	939.50	0.00	0.00	0.00	0.00	939.50	0.00	939.50		
30% institutional overhead fee	1,221.35	0.00	0.00	0.00	0.00	1,221.35	0.00	1,221.35	3,664.05	Cost per 30 patients $109,921.50
Dissemination of results										$3000.00
									TOTAL	$401,067

Abbreviations: EQ-5D, EuroQol-5D; ER, external rotation; Hgb, hemoglobin; HOOS, Hip disability and Osteoarthritis Outcome Score; IR, internal rotation; ROM, range of motion; TSC, timed stair climb; TUG, timed up and go; VAS, visual analogue scale; WOMAC, Western Ontario and McMaster Universities Osteoarthritis Index.
[a]Subset of patients who will undergo gait analyses.

References

[1] Bhandari M, Joensson A. Clinical Research for Surgeons. Stuttgart: Thieme; 2011

[2] Brescia B. Budgeting and Contracting in Patient Recruitment. In: Anderson DL, ed. A Guide to Patient Recruitment. Boston, Mass: Center Watch; 2001

[3] Williams RJ, Tse T, DiPiazza K, Zarin DA. Terminated Trials in the ClinicalTrials.gov Results Database: Evaluation of Availability of Primary Outcome Data and Reasons for Termination. PLoS One 2015;10(5):e0127242

[4] Blumenthal D. Academic-Industrial Relationships in the Life Sciences. N Engl J Med 2003;349(25):2452–2459

[5] Rahman S, Majumder MAA, Shaban SF, et al. Physician Participation in Clinical Research and Trials: Issues and Approaches. Adv Med Educ Pract 2011;2:85–93

[6] Cavalieri RJ, Rupp ME. Clinical Research Manual: Practical Tools and Templates for Managing Clinical Research. Indianapolis, IN: Sigma Theta Tau International; 2013

[7] Gaa M, Baker C.. Evaluating the Protocol: Can the Clinical Research Site Really Do this Study? SOCRA 2018(96):21–25

[8] Medicines for Human Use (Clinical Trials) Regulations 2004. Bull Med Ethics 2004(196):6–11

[9] Developing an Investigator Site Budget for Clinical Trials. J Oncol Pract 2007;3(2):94–97

[10] Pitler LR, Bonomi PD. Developing an Effective and Compliant Plan for Billing Clinical Trials. J Oncol Pract 2006;2(6):265–267

[11] Pfadenhauer JB. Navigating the Clinical Trial Billing Maze. J Oncol Pract 2006;2(6):280

[12] Beal K, Dean J, Chen J, Dragaon E, Saulino A, Collard CD. Budget Negotiation for Industry-Sponsored Clinical Trials. Anesth Analg 2004;99(1):173–176

[13] Lazar EL. Budgeting for a Clinical Trial. In: Itani K, Reda D, eds. Clinical Trials Design in Operative and Non Operative Invasive Procedures. Berlin: Springer; 2017: 435–440

[14] Klein P. Evaluating a Protocol Budget. In: Gallin J, Ognibene F, Johnson LL, eds. Principles and Practice of Clinical Research. 4th ed. Amsterdam: Elsevier; 2017: 571–587

[15] Amin D. A Clinical Trials Manual from the Duke Clinical Research Institute. Lessons from a Horse Named Jim. Br J Clin Pharmacol 2011;71(5):791–792

[16] Sheffet AJ, Flaxman L, Tom M, et al. CREST Investigators. Financial Management of a Large Multisite Randomized Clinical Trial. Int J Stroke 2014;9(6):811–813

[17] Lièvre M, Ménard J, Bruckert E, et al. Premature Discontinuation of Clinical Trial for Reasons not Related to Efficacy, Safety, or Feasibility. BMJ 2001;322(7286): 603–605

[18] McDonald AM, Treweek S, Shakur H, et al. Using a Business Model Approach and Marketing Techniques for Recruitment to Clinical Trials. Trials 2011;12:74

[19] McDonald AM, Knight RC, Campbell MK, et al. What Influences Recruitment to Randomised Controlled Trials? A Review of Trials Funded by Two UK Funding Agencies. Trials 2006;7:9

[20] Warlow C. Advanced Issues in the Design and Conduct of Randomized Clinical Trials: The Bigger the Better? Stat Med 2002;21(19):2797–2805

[21] Campbell MK, Snowdon C, Francis D, et al. STEPS group. Recruitment to Randomised Trials: Strategies for Trial Enrollment and Participation Study. The STEPS Study. Health Technol Assess 2007;11(48):iii,ix-105

13 Maintaining Records and the Trial Master File

Alisha Garibaldi

Abstract

The Trial Master File is a requirement for every clinical study, but its content is dependent on a number of factors. This chapter covers the contents and requirements for a Trial Master File for both a participating clinical site and Methods Center. It explains why the Trial Master File is so important, its different components and when they may be required, and at what timepoint during the trial they should be collected.

Keywords: Trial Master File, documentation, regulatory

13.1 Introduction

A Trial Master File (TMF) is an essential part of any clinical study. Its content includes documents that detail how to conduct the study, as well as many documents that record how the study was executed. The TMF should contain all of the mandatory regulatory documents required by Good Clinical Practice (GCP) guidelines, health authorities, and the Research Ethics Board (REB)/Institutional Review Board (IRB)/Ethics Committees. For the purposes of this chapter, the TMF will encompass the full collection of documents that are important to the conduct of a clinical study, including documents that are not a requirement for GCP, health authorities, and the Ethics Committees, and those that are. Although the contents of a TMF will differ depending on the nature of the study, there are a few key documents that will appear in every TMF. The contents of a TMF will be impacted by the study design, funding agency(ies), and health authority oversight. This chapter aims to explain the contents of a TMF, as well as provide insight into assembling one as both a clinical site and a Methods Center and explain the difference between them. Also note that studies that are not randomized controlled trials should also have a TMF, but not all of the documents noted here may be required.

Throughout this chapter, the term Methods Center and study sponsor will be used often. Methods Center refers to the group responsible for study oversight and day-to-day study management. Methods Centers may be a formal Contract Research Organization or a team of researchers working with an investigator. The study sponsor may be an industry company or may be an investigator or institution that is funded by a granting organization. For some studies, the study sponsor may also be the Methods Center.

The direction provided in this chapter should be used as a guide and should not be followed in place of the requirements of updated GCP guidelines, health authority, or ethics requirements.

13.1.1 What Is a Trial Master File?

A TMF is a collection of documents that outline how a clinical study should be conducted and provide evidence to demonstrate how the processes and procedures of the study were executed. Often referred to as a regulatory binder, the contents of the TMF should tell a story of compliance and rigor in the conduct of the study to ensure a high level of data integrity at its completion. This chapter will discuss the TMF as a whole, including documents that are required as part of GCP, health authority, and the ethics committee requirements, as well as documents that are essential to the conduct of the study, such as charters, guidelines, and study-specific procedures. Although referred to as a singular file, the documents of a TMF may be contained between a few binders, or throughout several folders when stored electronically.

The collection of the documents for a TMF will begin long before the first participant is enrolled into the study and will continue to grow throughout the study; however, the contents that are required in accordance with GCP guidelines, health authority, and ethics committee requirements should be determined prior to study initiation. The study sponsor, when relevant, will determine what is required as part of the TMF, and will often provide many of the documents and templates to the clinical site directly. A single-site, nonregulated, investigator-initiated TMF will be substantially different than an international, multisite, industry-sponsored TMF. The contents of a TMF will differ substantially between a Methods Center and a participating clinical site. An overall list of documents that may appear in a TMF is outlined in ▶ Table 13.1. Please note that this table may not include all documents and forms that are necessary in a TMF.

Table 13.1 Key Trial Master File (TMF) documents

Document	Collection timeframe	Relevance (methods center or clinical site)	Requirement (GCP or study specific)	Purpose
Protocol	Prior to study initiation	Both	Both	The study sponsor will provide clinical sites with the protocol, which will be the document most referenced during the course of the study. It will contain background information regarding the purpose of the study, the study objectives, outcomes, design, methods, eligibility criteria, statistical plans, data management, and safety information. Although informative, the protocol may be supplemented with additional documents that outline the conduct of the study. The protocol may be amended throughout the course of the study, which will require approval from all local Ethics Committees.
Informed consent form	Prior to study initiation Throughout study	Both	Both	The study sponsor will often provide clinical sites with a template of an informed consent form. Each clinical site is required to have the informed consent form approved by the local ethics committee, which will often have specific requirements regarding what information the informed consent form must contain. In addition to specific statements that may be added, local investigator and research coordinator contact information should be added. The informed consent form may be amended throughout the course of the study if the study protocol is updated, or to update research coordinator contact information. Any amendment to the informed consent form will need local ethics committee approval.
Ethics committee documents	Prior to trial initiation Throughout study	Both	Both	Ethics committee documents are likely to span a few tabs or folders, including, but not limited to: • Initial application • Correspondence • Initial approval • Amendment application and approvals • Continuing review approvals • Reported serious adverse events • Reported protocol deviations It is immensely important to ensure that ethics board's approvals are up-to-date and easily accessible in case of an audit or monitoring visit. Serious adverse events must be reported to the ethics committee as per local guidelines. This will often differ from what is required to report to the study sponsor.
Delegation log	Prior to study initiation Throughout study	Both	GCP	A delegation log is exactly what it sounds like—a log that documents to whom the local principal investigator (or for the methods center the study principal investigator) delegates study responsibilities. Each individual at a clinical site who is involved in the study should be included on the delegation log, including, but not limited to, participating doctors, research coordinators, regulatory staff, pharmacists, and laboratory technicians. The delegation log should be updated in real time when an individual joins the team, or leaves. It is a reference point for auditors and monitors to know who should have up-to-date CVs and training documentation. Please see ► Fig. 13.1 for a sample delegation log.

Table 13.1 (*Continued*) Key Trial Master File (TMF) documents

Document	Collection timeframe	Relevance (methods center or clinical site)	Requirement (GCP or study specific)	Purpose
Site personnel CVs	Prior to study initiation Throughout study	Both	GCP	Signed and dated personnel CVs are often a requirement for the TMF. CVs should be signed and dated to indicate how up-to-date they are and should ideally be updated every 2 years. For clinical sites running multiple studies, it may be advantageous to keep all personnel CVs in one location to avoid duplicate copies of CVs in multiple TMFs. Keeping a tracker of the dates of CVs can be helpful to easily determine when they need to be updated. If CVs are stored in a central location, include reference to this in the TMF.
Training documentation	Prior to study initiation Throughout study	Both	GCP	Training documentation refers to both research training documentation and study-specific training documentation. Research training includes documentation that GCP training is current (often within 3 years), as well as any other certification that site personnel has obtained. Training documentation may also include medical licenses for participating doctors. This training documentation may be filed with site personnel CVs and may need to be updated throughout the course of a study if training is not current. It is also helpful to keep a tracker of this. Study-specific training documentation will indicate that site personnel have been properly trained on the conduct of the study. This will vary depending on the requirements of the study sponsor as well as local institution requirements. If the study sponsor is conducting training, they may provide a certificate of training. Alternatively, document training logs may be completed for each study document to indicate that personnel have reviewed each document. This method allows for training to be updated easily when study documents are amended, as a new training log may be completed for that specific document. Please refer to ▶ Fig. 13.2 for a sample document training log.
Investigator's brochure	Prior to study initiation Throughout study	Both	GCP	If required, an investigator's brochure will be provided by the study sponsor. An investigator's brochure will be provided when a drug or investigational product is being used in humans for the first time, or for a new indication. It should be updated at least annually, or more frequently at the discretion of the sponsor. The investigator's brochure will provide a summary of the information gathered on the drug or investigational product to date.
Financial documents	Prior to study initiation	Both	GCP	The financial documents that are required for the study will be at the discretion of the study sponsor. At a minimum, a fully executed clinical study agreement between the study sponsor and participating clinical site is required prior to initiating recruitment. Please refer to Chapter 15 for additional details on clinical study agreements. In addition to the clinical study agreement, the study sponsor may require financial conflict of interest forms or financial disclosures to be completed for the local principal investigator, or all investigators at the clinical site.

(Continued)

Table 13.1 (*Continued*) Key Trial Master File (TMF) documents

Document	Collection timeframe	Relevance (methods center or clinical site)	Requirement (GCP or study specific)	Purpose
Health authority documents	Prior to study initiation	Both	GCP	If the study is regulated by a health authority(ies), such as the U.S. Food and Drug Administration, Health Canada, or the European Medicines Agency, there will be additional forms that must be completed prior to study initiation. The study sponsor should inform the site personnel which forms are required prior to study initiation, and if any forms need to be completed on an ongoing basis.
Account-ability logs	Prior to study initiation Throughout study	Both	GCP	Accountability logs may be required if a drug or investigational product is being studied for the study. Depending on the nature of the study and the source of the drug or investigational product (e.g., provided by the sponsor or supplied by the clinical site), multiple logs may be required. The study sponsor should provide the clinical site with a template for use during the study. Accountability logs may include (but are not limited to) shipping information, lot numbers, batch numbers, storage information (e.g., temperature, humidity), expiry dates, date destroyed, and study participant ID numbers.
Monitor-ing visit reports	Throughout study	Both	Both	If the study will involve formal monitoring by the study sponsor or delegate, monitoring visit reports will be written and sent to the clinical site following the visit. These reports will summarize any findings from the visit and action items that need to be addressed, as well as who is responsible for each item. These reports should be filed in the TMF.
Data and safety monitoring Committee reports	Throughout study	Both	GCP	If a Data and Safety Monitoring Committee (or Board) is monitoring study safety, a letter of continuation will often be prepared following meetings to state that the Data and Safety Monitoring Committee confirms the study should continue, with or without modifications to the protocol. Many ethics boards require this letter to be submitted, and it is the responsibility of the site personnel to request and file these letters.
Significant correspon-dence	Throughout study	Both	Both	Significant correspondence is often part of the TMF and is exactly what it sounds like. It is a place to document significant correspondence, such as emails, from the ethics board, study sponsor, or other site personnel. It provides a location for this information to be kept so that everyone on the study team can access, rather than storing it in one individual's email.
Notes to file	Throughout study	Both	Both	A note to file is written to explain a discrepancy in the conduct or documentation of a clinical study. It should include a description of the issue, the cause of it, what corrective actions were taken, and when it was resolved. It should be signed by the author and filed in the TMF to be easily accessible to auditors or monitors.

Table 13.1 (*Continued*) Key Trial Master File (TMF) documents

Document	Collection timeframe	Relevance (methods center or clinical site)	Requirement (GCP or study specific)	Purpose
Participant documentation: • Informed consent forms • Case report forms • Source documents • Tracking documents	Throughout study	Clinical site	Both	Original participant documentation, such as informed consent forms and source documents, should be kept at the clinical site, as per GCP requirements. The clinical site should also keep a list of the participants and their corresponding participant IDs. This list should not be kept with completed case report forms. Both the Methods Center and clinical site will have access to completed case report forms in the database, the Methods Center to all sites and the clinical sites to their own. Other participant tracking documents and spreadsheets may exist at both the Methods Center and clinical site.
Randomization documents	Prior to study initiation Throughout study	Both	Both	Randomization documents may include the requirements for programming the randomization system and applicable testing (Methods Center specific), randomization processes for the clinical site (e.g., when and how to randomize a patient), and a backup randomization process in case the electronic system is unavailable.
Site feasibility questionnaire	Prior to study initiation	Methods Center	Study specific	If necessary, a site feasibility questionnaire is completed by the clinical site and returned to the Methods Center. This questionnaire will help the Methods Center determine if the clinical site is a good fit for the study (e.g., adequate infrastructure, patient population and volume, research experience). The questionnaire will be drafted prior to study initiation, but sites may continue to be recruited as participating clinical sites after the study begins.
Clinical site manual/ study guideline documents	Prior to study initiation	Both	Study specific	The clinical site manual or study guideline documents exist to add clarity to the protocol and explain study conduct in detail. Although not a requirement per GCP, this document or documents are important. They will be drafted prior to study initiation but are likely to be updated throughout the study.
Site initiation checklists	Prior to study initiation	Methods Center	Study specific	Site initiation checklists are used at the Methods Center to ensure that all initiation activities and documents have been completed and collected at a site before they begin enrollment. It is a final check before giving a clinical site the go ahead.
Data management plan	Prior to study initiation	Methods Center	Study specific	The purpose of a data management plan is to outline the procedures for managing the clinical data for the study. It is a Methods Center–specific document that will be drafted long before study initiation. It is not to be confused with requirements documents and testing plans for the database. Please refer to Chapter 19 for additional information on study databases.

(*Continued*)

Table 13.1 (*Continued*) Key Trial Master File (TMF) documents

Document	Collection timeframe	Relevance (methods center or clinical site)	Requirement (GCP or study specific)	Purpose
Clinical site monitoring plan	Prior to study initiation	Methods Center	Study specific	The clinical site monitoring plan outlines monitoring activities. Even if on-site monitoring is not being conducted as part of the study, this plan may describe remote data monitoring or data validation. It is a Methods Center document that is developed prior to study initiation.
Committee charters	Prior to study initiation	Methods Center	Study specific	Any formal committee that is established for study oversight, such as a Data and Safety Monitoring Committee, Adjudication Committee, Executive Committee, or Steering Committee, should have a charter outlining the purpose of the committee and its members' responsibilities. These charters tend to be Methods Center–specific documents, and with the exception of the Data and Safety Monitoring Committee are not a GCP requirement.
Committee agendas, meeting materials and minutes	Throughout study	Methods Center	Study specific	Further to the charters, committee meetings should be documented with drafted agendas, materials, and minutes. Any decisions made during meetings should be documented for future reference.
Study-specific procedures	Prior to study initiation	Methods Center	Study specific	Any steps that Methods Center personnel must take as part of the study that need to be consistent each time they are completed (e.g., preparing committee reports, preparing adjudication materials) should be written into a study-specific procedure. These may be very short procedures, but the formalization of the document ensures that if a team member is unexpectedly absent, another team member will be able to follow the processes.
Statistical analysis plan	Prior to study initiation	Methods Center	Study specific	A statistical analysis plan outlines exactly how the study team intends to analyze the data collected for the study. It includes templates for flow diagrams and tables that will be populated, as well as the statistical methods that will be used. It should ideally be drafted prior to study initiation, and is often a requirement when submitting a manuscript to a journal.

Abbreviation: GCP, Good clinical practice.

Task Delegation Log

PROTOCOL NUMBER : _____ PRINCIPAL INVESTIGATOR (PI) : _____ SITE NUMBER : _____

STUDY TITLE :_____ INSTITUTION :_____ SPONSOR NAME : _____

Name and title	Full signature	Initials	Authorized responsibilities	Start date	Authorized signature	End date	Authorized signature

Task delegation/responsibility list :

1 Develop study documents
2 Maintain trial master file
3 Data management
4 Clinical site oversight
5 Monitoring activities
6 Subject identification, recruitment
7 Obtain informed consent
8 Physical examination
9 Medical history
10 Affirmation of inclusion/exclusion criteria

11 Instruction on investigational product administration
12 Investigational product dispensing
13 Review AEs/SAEs
14 Review, assessment of AE/SAE criteria
15 Ethics board reporting
16 Questionnaire and survey administration
17 Data management
18 Budget management
19 Regulatory agency reporting

20 Training new personnel
21 Internal quality assurance reviews
22 Data analyses
23 Study report writing
24 Other :
25 Other :
26 Other :
27 Other :

Fig. 13.1 Sample delegation log.

13.1.2 Why All of the Documentation?

The research version of the phrase "*pictures or it didn't happen,*" is more along the lines of "*if it isn't written down it didn't happen.*" Documentation is vital to demonstrate that a study was conducted in a manner that was respectful of participants' safety and well-being and completed with rigor, so that results of the study may be considered accurate and sound. All clinical studies are susceptible to an audit, whether from a study sponsor, Ethics Committees, or health authority (e.g., Health Canada or the U.S. Food and Drug Administration). If research processes are not being properly documented throughout a study, an auditor may need to pause study activities or stop the study completely to remediate any concerns.

13.1.3 Setting up a Trial Master File at a Participating Clinical Site

If you have never set up a TMF before, the list of documents in ►Table 13.1 may look extremely daunting. How do you know what to include? Where do you start? Depending on the study, the Methods Center or study sponsor may create the site TMF (also known as an Investigator Site File or ISF) and send it to the clinical site directly. Otherwise, a sample table of contents may be sent along with a few key documents provided by the sponsor (e.g., protocol, investigator's brochure) for the clinical site personnel to set up. It is also important for clinical site personnel to be aware of what is required by their local ethics committee. What the study sponsor or Methods Center requires may not include all of the documents required by a local ethics committee.

A good place to start is always asking the Methods Center or study sponsor for the requirements. Once the content requirements are known, it is helpful to use the table of contents as a checklist for collecting the documents. Review the table of contents frequently to ensure that you are being proactive in collecting the documents and follow up with the Methods Center or study sponsor for documents that are their responsibility.

Document Training Log

Document name : _____   Version number   _____

Project : _____   Version date   _____

Name	Date completed	Signature

Fig. 13.2 Sample training log.

If an initiation visit will occur, aim to have the TMF complete prior to the visit.

Once the site TMF is set up and the study has been initiated, clinical sites also need to keep participant-specific documents. With the advancement of technology, these documents and trackers may exist almost entirely electronically. They include signed informed consent forms, participant tracking lists, completed case report forms, and source documents. The study sponsor or Methods Center will dictate which documents need to be kept as originals (most likely signed informed consent forms, source documents) and which may exist entirely electronically. Many studies now encourage direct data entry into the trial database to avoid keeping binders of completed case report forms, and some will even allow electronic consent to be established to avoid paper consent forms.

Toolbox B shows an example site TMF/ISF table of contents for a clinical site. This site TMF is separated into a main TMF and a separate binder for participant information, which is referred to at the bottom of the table of contents. This makes it apparent why no participant-specific documents appear in the site TMF. When setting up a hard copy of a site TMF in addition to an electronic version, it is helpful to set up the electronic version to be identical to the hard copy and make a numbered folder for each tab in the binder.

13.1.4 Setting up a Trial Master File at a Methods Center

Even more intimidating than setting up the TMF at a clinical site is setting it up at the Methods Center, because there isn't a Methods Center outlining what to include in the files and sending the documents or templates. However, the study sponsor may have a list of required documents that must be included as part of the TMF. Part of setting up the TMF at the Methods Center is also determining what is required at the clinical site.

To begin, it is helpful to draft a table of contents for both the Methods Center and the clinical sites and start adding to it as the protocol develops. Some documents are more cut-and-dried with respect to their requirement in the TMF, such as the informed consent form, delegation log, training documentation, personnel CVs, and ethics approvals, whereas others will depend on the study. If the protocol is examining on-label use of a surgical device, an investigator's brochure will not be required, whereas a study looking at an approved drug for a new indication will. The need for accountability logs will depend on the source of the investigational product or device. If the study sponsor is providing and shipping the study drug to clinical sites, accountability logs will be mandatory. A study looking at two different surgical techniques is unlikely to need an investigator's brochure or accountability log. Financial disclosure forms may not be required for a study if it is not investigating a branded product, but a study being sponsored by an industry company will likely require disclosure.

Another important step of study start-up and TMF development is to determine if a Medical Monitor or Data and Safety Monitoring Committee will be required for safety oversight. If so, charters and processes will need to be drafted and included in the TMF. The Food and Drug Administration has an excellent reference for determining if a Data and Safety Monitoring Committee is required, titled "The Establishment and Operation of Clinical Trial Data Monitoring Committees."

Other documents such as plans, charters, and procedures may be left up to the discretion of the study team, but it is important to remember two things: (1) documented procedures and processes allow for study success if there is turnover in team members and (2) once a procedure is drafted and versioned, it must be followed. It is never ideal to have only one individual know the ins and outs of study oversight, and having well-documented processes helps avoid extreme challenges if a team member were to unexpectedly leave. On the other side of having well-documented processes and procedures is writing documents that will be impossible to follow. If the Methods Center does not have the bandwidth to monitor every clinical site quarterly for 3 years (and it is not a requirement per the study protocol), do not write this into the Clinical Site Monitoring Plan, or you will soon find yourself to be out of compliance with your own processes. It is important to meet as a study team and work through the TMF together, while recognizing that throughout study start-up the contents of the TMF may change from what you originally thought they would be. It is the responsibility of the study sponsor along with the Methods Center to ensure that the TMF is complete.

It is important to note that the TMFs for a clinical site and the Methods Center will rarely be the same. This discrepancy comes from the fact that what is relevant to the Methods Center may not be relevant to the participating clinical site, and vice versa. A study will often have a number of committees that oversee the study such as a Steering Committee or Data and Safety Monitoring Committee. These committees will communicate with the study sponsor, or Methods Center regarding the study, and should have a charter that outlines their responsibilities. The Methods Center may also have study-specific procedures associated with these committees that go into detail to outline exactly how the committees' responsibilities should be carried out, and how their activities should be documented. These charters and procedures are not typically distributed to participating clinical sites and will be filed only with the Methods Center, as participating sites are not involved in these aspects of the study. Likewise, a participating clinical site will have an approved informed consent form, whereas the Methods Center may not if there are no participants are being recruited at the center. However, although the Methods Center may not have an approved informed consent form, it may file all of the ethics committee–approved informed consent forms for the participating clinical site. The Methods Center will also likely file an informed consent form template.

Toolbox B shows an example TMF table of contents for a Methods Center. Note that it contains many different documents from the clinical site version, including charters and plans. A Methods Center will often keep copies of documents that the clinical site has, such as their ethics approval letter, approved informed consent form, and health authority forms (e.g., FDA form 1572), but these may be filed separately rather than being included with the main TMF.

13.1.5 Document Control and the Trial Master File

Maintaining records in the TMF is a true art of document control. While drafting new documents, it is best practice to mark them as "Draft" using a watermark and in the file name, and to update the date each time changes are made. It is also helpful to include the initials of the last individual to edit the document in the file name. Save old versions of draft documents in an electronic folder titled "Draft" in case it is necessary to revisit them. When the document is finalized, ensure that all mention of "Draft" is removed throughout the document and a version number is assigned. Be sure to sign off on document training as soon as possible after the document is finalized.

If an existing document is being updated, ensure that it is marked as the draft of the next version, and follow the same tips above while it is being updated. It is helpful to include a document revision history to indicate the previous versions of the document, and what was updated in each version. When final, file the older version in an archive folder electronically and the hard copy in an archive binder, if relevant. It can be helpful to begin a draft version of a document if minor changes are needed, but a new version is not yet warranted. Minor updates can be added to a draft document over a series of months before it becomes necessary to version up the document.

13.1.6 When the Methods Center Is also a Participating Clinical Site

It is not uncommon for the Methods Center to be a participating clinical site when the study sponsor is an investigator. In this situation, it is not always clear how the TMFs should be set up, when a lot of the documents will overlap. Ideally in these situations, a TMF should be set up for the Methods Center, and a separate TMF should be set up for the clinical site. This will include having two separate delegation logs and at times two separate ethics board approvals, although some ethics boards will approve both the Methods Center and the clinical site in one application. Although it may seem redundant, the separation of the Methods Center and clinical site TMFs is the cleanest approach when it comes to audits or monitoring. If the clinical site is being audited, only their TMF will be reviewed. Similarly, if the Methods Center is undergoing an audit, the clinical site files would not be included in the review.

13.1.7 Do I Really Need a Binder?

TMFs have traditionally existed as hard copies of documents neatly organized in a binder. This method of storing files allows for easy review and access to its contents, and is especially advantageous for studies that involve on-site monitoring for compliance. However, with the advancement of technology and the trend toward reducing paper use, electronic TMFs are becoming increasingly more common.

The use of an electronic TMF will tend to be at the discretion of the study sponsor. If an electronic TMF is acceptable and on-site monitoring is a requirement of the study, it should be noted that clinical site personnel will need to give monitors access to these files to review, similar to how a monitor would review a hard copy of a binder or file. However, there may be some documents, such as original informed consent forms and the delegation log for which original copies and wet ink signatures will need to be kept in a binder. Whether being stored as a hard copy or electronically, the contents of the TMF should be organized, clearly identifiable, and found easily. This is also applied if an audit is necessary; if documents are being stored electronically, clinical site personnel must be prepared to give an auditor access.

13.1.8 Spotlight: The Clinical Site Manual

From a regulatory perspective, the mandatory documents of the TMF often do not include all of the necessary information that a clinical site will need to execute a study. It is the responsibility of the Methods Center or study sponsor to develop additional documents that provide more detailed instructions on study execution. These documents will exist in harmony with the study protocol and should provide clarification on study procedures that are not fully detailed or covered in the protocol. These documents may include but are not limited to the following:

- Investigational product storage and handling guidelines.
- Eligibility guidelines.
- Randomization guidelines.
- Case report form completion guidelines.
- Follow-up guidelines.
- Study event and serious adverse event reporting guidelines.
- Database manual.
- Training presentations.

These documents may be written separately or may exist in one large clinical site manual. They should be filed at both the Methods Center and the participating clinical sites, and training on them should be formally documented in the TMF.

13.1.9 Internal audits

Internal audits of the TMF should be conducted at a minimum on an annual basis. These audits do not necessarily need to be formal within the institution but should be conducted informally to ensure that the TMF is complete and up-to-date. When reviewing the TMF, here are some key items to look at:

- Have new personnel signed off on all training?
- Are CVs current within the last 2 years?
- Are GCP certificates still valid?
- Are ethics approvals up-to-date?
- Have end dates been documented for individuals who are no longer working on the study?
- Do any documents need to be updated?

If there are findings from internal audits, take all necessary measures to correct them, or if necessary, write a note to file explaining the gap in documentation. Internal audits help ensure you are prepared in case of an external audit.

13.1.10 Practical Application

The author was recently involved in the study start-up for a large cluster-randomized crossover trial. This was new to the author for two reasons: (1) she was more accustomed to data cleaning and study close-out and (2) she had never been involved in a cluster trial before. For this particular study, the author was acting as the project manager at the Methods Center, and the study sponsor was another university that received the funding award; the Methods Center was subcontracted because of existing infrastructure.

The process of protocol development took about 3 months to finalize from the time of the funding award. Although the grant proposal described the planned study, there were major decisions to be made and input needed from stakeholders. The Methods Center began setting up the TMF as the protocol was being developed. The study team researched to determine the requirement for a Medical Monitor or Data and Safety Monitoring Committee, drafted charters for the established committees, developed case report forms, initiation checklists, data management, and monitoring plans, and wrote study-specific procedures relevant to us as the Methods Center. During this time, a draft table of contents for the TMF was kept. This table of contents changed almost weekly as new documents were added or removed documents that seemed redundant, but it was vital to keeping study start-up on track. Two additional columns in the table of contents indicated the status of each document, who was responsible for it and the deadline for completion. The Methods Center team met weekly to review the status of the TMF with one of the Principal Investigators to ensure that study start-up was moving forward. When the day came to finalize the protocol, a number of other key documents were also ready to be finalized, and our ethics application was prepared and ready to be submitted.

The clinical site manual was also being written during this time. It is a document that was developed for all the previous studies of the study team and had worked well in the past. However, it was realized that this cluster study did not fit the neat template used previously for other randomized controlled studies. They went back to the drawing board and began developing a study resource binder. This binder became a road map that explained exactly how to conduct the study. It included study team contact information, case report forms, a series of smaller guidelines for study procedures, presentations, posters, outcome definition documents, and even pulled the protocol and informed consent form from their typical home in the TMF. The series of smaller documents has allowed us to update one or two procedures without updating a 100+ page document. The smaller documents are also far more manageable for reading and training.

Setting up a TMF from a Methods Center perspective is a big job. It takes an enormous amount of time, thought, and care to get it just right, and one can never assume that what worked for a previous study will work for the next one. For this study, our diligence in preparing the TMF alongside protocol development allowed for a smooth and efficient study launch.

13.2 Conclusion

A clinical study cannot be conducted without a TMF in place. From a regulatory perspective, it provides evidence that the study was conducted safely and rigorously. From a methodological perspective, it provides a road map for how to get from a funded study to a published paper. Its contents are drafted prior to study initiation and updated throughout the course of the study, and should be neatly organized and accessible the entire time. Following study completion, TMF documents should be stored per the appropriate regulations (e.g., 25 years for Health Canada–regulated studies). The TMF as a whole should be reviewed internally for quality control on a regular basis to ensure that all documents and signatures are up-to-date and present. A complete and organized TMF is one of the key steps to a successful clinical study!

Definitions/Acronyms

- **Methods Center:** A group of individuals who oversee and facilitate the conduct of a multisite clinical study. The Methods Center has responsibilities such as day-to-day clinical site management, data management, monitoring, document development, and data analyses. The Methods Center may share responsibilities with the investigator and the sponsor.
- **Investigator:** The individual who is in charge of a clinical study. A study may have multiple investigators, in which case the ultimately responsible investigator is the Principal Investigator(s). In some cases, the investigator is also the sponsor, or affiliated with the sponsor institution.
- **Sponsor:** An individual, company, institution, or organization that takes responsibility for the study initiation, management, and/or financing.
- **GCP:** Good clinical practice
- **IRB:** Institutional review board
- **REB:** Research ethics board
- **TMF:** Trial master file

Further Readings

FDA Guidance for Clinical Trial Sponsors: Establishment and Operation of Clinical Trial Data Monitoring Committees. https://www.fda.gov/media/75398/download

FDA Guidance for Industry: Investigator Responsibilities—Protecting the Rights, Safety, and Welfare of Study Subjects. https://www.fda.gov/regulatory-information/search-fda-guidance-documents/investigator-responsibilities-protecting-rights-safety-and-welfare-study-subjects

Health Canada Guidance Document: Master Files (MFs)—Procedures and Administrative Requirements. https://www.canada.ca/en/health-canada/services/drugs-health-products/drug-products/applications-submissions/guidance-documents/guidance-document-master-files-procedures-administrative-requirements.html

International Council for Harmonisation of Technical Requirements for Registration of Pharmaceuticals for Human Use (ICH). ICH Harmonised Guideline. http://www.ich.org/fileadmin/Public_Web_Site/ABOUT_ICH/Articles_Procedures/ICH_EWG_IWG_SOP_v3.0_final_22Jun2017-.pdf

14 Ethics Submissions

Bregje J.W. Thomassen, Michel Sourour, Kesh Reddy

Abstract

This chapter endeavors to provide an outline of the steps and processes of approval of research projects by Research Ethics Boards or Research Ethics Committees (RECs). We provide guidelines as to whether REC approval is required, and when it is required, we try to address how this may be best achieved. We focus on research ethics guidelines recommended by the World Health Organization (WHO) and address the differences in the process in different parts of the world.

Keywords: submission, research ethics committee, Research Ethics Board approval, research file

14.1 Introduction

Once an appropriate research question is generated, depending on the nature of the question, most jurisdictions require that a formal protocol be generated and a submission be made to a Research Ethics Board (REB) or Research Ethics Committee (REC). In some jurisdictions, such as the United States, the term Institutional Review Board (IRB) is used. In this chapter, we will use the term REC except when discussing specific jurisdictions. The World Health Organization (WHO)[1] defines research with human subjects as:

"...any social, biomedical, behavioural, or epidemiological activity that entails systemic collection or analysis of data with the intent to generate new knowledge, in which human subjects: (1) are either exposed to manipulation, intervention, observation, or other interaction with investigators either directly or through alteration of their environment, or (2) become individually identifiable through investigator's collection, preparation, or use of biological material or medical or other records."

In practice, it may not be immediately evident if a specific project requires ethics board approval or not. We recommend looking up guidelines in your own institution on what types of projects require ethics board review. If the guidelines are unclear, we suggest calling the chair of your institution's REC.

14.1.1 Research Ethics Committee

The REC is the board responsible for review and approval of various studies that involve human subjects. Although the members that constitute this committee vary slightly by country/institution, there are some consistent themes. In general terms, there is a chair for the committee and the members are balanced in terms of gender, age, discipline, and sociocultural diversity.

The following are some useful generalizations that relate to the composition of RECs:

- The REC panel should include individuals with different scientific backgrounds and experience. This would include expertise in health care, behavioral, and social sciences, as well as expertise in legal and ethical matters pertaining to the region.
- The panel should also include lay members from the communities from which the research participants are likely to come from. These members provide insight about the community and will provide a research subject's perspective to the panel.
- There should ideally be a mix of members both affiliated and nonaffiliated with the institution to which the REC belongs.
- The committee should be large enough to allow different voices and perspectives to be heard and to ensure that there is a quorum for the meetings.

North America

Canada requires at least five members to be part of the review committee[2]:

- At least two members are experts in the field being studied.
- At least one member is an ethics professional.
- A member who is knowledgeable in law (but not the institution's legal counsel).
- One community member not affiliated with the institution.

In the United States,[3] the requirement of membership is slightly different and broader than in Canada. The minimum number of members required is similar, but the specifics of recommended composition of the panel are as follows:

- Membership should be diverse in terms of gender, race, and cultural background.
- At least one scientist and one nonscientist should be members of the panel.
- There should be at least one member who is not affiliated with the institution.

Interestingly the United States also has private ethics committees that have differing memberships and requirements. The major difference is accountability. In the ethics committee associated with specific institutions, the committee is accountable to the institution. With private RECs, they are self-governing with oversight by the Office of Human Research Protection (OHRP). This office is tasked with licensing and regulating private RECs. Often the private RECs are composed of individuals with experience in the institutional RECs.

Europe

In Europe,[4] typically there are institutional and noninstitutional RECs. They are independent research review bodies that operate in accordance with the laws of the area. The panel should generally include both experts and lay people. The ethics review boards are empowered to give opinions and in particular take into account the views of patients and patient communities/organizations. The composition of the committees seems to be similar to that in North America though there is significant variability in different countries.

Asia

In Asia, the Forum for Ethical Review Committees in the Asian and Western Pacific Region (FERCAP; http://www.fercap-sidcer.org/whatsfercap.php) was formed in 2000 in Thailand. Although not strictly recognized as a governing body, there are currently seven member states including China and India with over 100 ethics boards that participate in this collaboration. In order to be recognized by FERCAP, the following standards should be met in terms of membership in the REC:
- At least five members.
- Gender balanced.
- Experience and knowledge are balanced in terms of ethics, science, and social science.
- Lay person.
- Nonaffiliated person.
- Terms and conditions of appointment should be clear.

▶Table 14.1 summarizes the differences and similarities between the different areas and the requirements for ethics committees.

Among the FERCAP member countries, Australia[5] has strict rules and guidelines for their RECs. This is all outlined in their National Statement on Ethical Conduct in Human Research (NSECHR). The minimum number of people required for the REC is eight (four men and four women). Furthermore, one-third of the individuals have to have no affiliation with the institution from which the research would be conducted. There should be at least two lay persons (one man and one woman), one health care professional, one ethical/religious leader, one lawyer, and two researchers.

Africa

Africa has a complicated history with ethics review and there have been several historical

Table 14.1 Summary of Research Ethics Committee member requirements

	North America		Europe[a]	Asia	Australia
	Canada	United States			
Number of members	5+	N/A	5+	5+	8
Scientific members	2+	1+	1+	1+	2
Nonscientist	N/A	1+	1+	1+	2
Ethicist	Yes	N/A	N/A	N/A	1
Legal expert	Yes	N/A	N/A	N/A	1
Community member	1+	1+	1+	1+	2

[a]In Europe, this is highly variable by country; however, we have provided a general guideline that seems to apply to most countries in Europe.

trials that have caused significant harm to both patients and the reputation of the scientific community among many communities in Africa. An example of this was an experimental drug (Trovan) used to treat meningitis and was used in studies comparing it to ceftriaxone in Nigeria. Unfortunately, the dosage of ceftriaxone used in this study was inadequate and there was no ethics committee review done at that time resulting in significant adverse outcomes in many children including the death of 11 children.[6]

As a consequence of all this, there has been a specific drive through various foundations to strengthen the ethics review process in Africa. Many countries now have well-structured and well-developed ethics review committees and there have been continued efforts by the WHO to increase research oversight in Africa. This has been established based on the WHO principles.

14.1.2 Research Ethics Committee Submission

The research file that must be submitted varies by country. Applications are normally accompanied by supporting documents. The package of supporting documents you will need to provide will depend on the type of research activity and the country where the reviewing process will be done.

The typical research application to the REC includes the following documents:
- Application letter with basic information of the study and relevant information regarding the submission.
- Research protocol.
- Participant information and informed consent form (ICF).
- Contracts and study agreements.
- Participation agreements of each center, in case of multicenter study.
- Budget.
- Approval from regulatory bodies, if required.

14.1.3 Review Process

Ethics review is where the REC examines the proposed research to consider the various aspects as outlined below. Usually research ethics review is required in the following situations:
- Research involving human subjects.

- Research involving human biological materials, as well as human embryos, fetuses, fetal tissue, reproductive materials, and stem cells. This applies to materials derived from living and deceased individuals.

Typically, no less than two reviewers review each protocol and the protocols are discussed by the REC panel before a communication goes out to the investigator. In some jurisdictions, the REC members are expected to be certified in GCP (Good Clinical Practice).

There are many country- and institution-specific guidelines used by the various RECs to decide whether a study should be approved or whether it requires further modifications. In general, the following domains are evaluated during the approval process:
- Scientific design, importance of the research question, feasibility, and conduct.
- Risk and benefits.
- Study population selection and recruitment.
- Financial benefits, costs, and any conflicts of interest.
- Safety and privacy of participants/personal health information.
- Informed consent process.
- Research team—all research personnel must be qualified and appropriately trained (e.g., GCP certified).

We will examine each of the above issues in sequence based on the Canadian experience and point out any differences in other parts of the world when possible.

Scientific Design

The REC needs to consider the appropriateness of the research question, the feasibility of the study as presented, and should ensure that the study can be completed within the temporal, financial, and other constraints in the study protocol.

Risk and Benefits

When a review board approaches the research proposal, one of the key factors they need consider is the risk-to-benefit ratio. The balance is clearly between minimizing harm to the research subjects and maximizing possible benefits to the research subject and the general population.

Study Population Selection and Recruitment

The REC needs to ensure that there is no inherent bias in the case selection that would prejudice the results of a study. Specifically, if age, ethnicity, and gender restrictions are in the study design, they need to be reviewed carefully to ensure that the results do not compromise the generalizability of the study results.

Financial Benefits, Cost, and Any Conflicts of Interest

The REC also needs to ensure that the study is adequately funded so it can be completed satisfactorily. The REC should also be alert to any financial inducements to the investigators. In Canada, RECs do not allow any monetary payment to investigators that may be perceived as an inducement. Typically, the allowable payment is no more than the standard provincial payment. Also, the investigator is not allowed to "double dip," (i.e., collect from the provincial health plan and the study). The study budget needs to be reasonably balanced.

Safety and Privacy of Participants/ Personal Health Information

All personal health information is protected by law in Canada[2] and in most countries. The REC needs to ensure that all personal health data are anonymized as soon as possible and kept under lock and key. If the data are transmitted to other center(s) (as in a multicenter study), it must be encrypted and the encryption protocol specified in the REC application.

Informed Consent Process

The ICF is a document that is very thoroughly reviewed by the REC. The ICF guidelines are usually posted on the REC website, but in general, the ICF should identify at the outset the names of the investigators and any sponsors on the appropriate institutional letterhead. The ICF font size should be large enough for most people to be able to read it and the reading level should be appropriate for the population. All risks for the subjects should be clearly spelled out with quantification of the risks where available—ideally in an easily readable

format such as a table. Any consent to store biological material is especially vital as the material may be stored for a long time and used for research that the subject did not consent to in the first place. Strict guidelines exist for the use of genetic material in most jurisdictions. In particular, if subsequent studies are conducted on genetic material for profit, this should be clearly outlined in the ICF.

North America

In the United States, as of January 1, 2018, the National Institutes of Health sponsored studies are required to have a central IRB approve all their studies.[3] This has proven to be problematic as the institutional IRBs see this as a threat to their autonomy. On the other hand, a centralized review process does intuitively streamline the process considerably. The implications of this decision will become obvious in the near future.

Europe

In 2014, the European Union (EU) released a document guideline for all member states of the EU regarding clinical studies.[4] The guidelines state that a clinical study should only be conducted if "the rights, safety, dignity and well-being of the subjects are protected and prevail over all other interests" and "it is designed to generate robust and reliable data." When reviewing submissions, the ethics committees look at the degree of intervention proposed (low vs. high intervention), the risks to subjects, anticipated benefits to individuals involved, and compliance with various laws regarding medicinal products. Furthermore, in the EU, research involving more than one member state would require three additional steps:

- The primary investigator sends the submission to a central portal where one committee reviews the submission.
- Other member states have 14 days to conduct a coordinated review.
- The primary member state consolidates all the information.

Australia

In Australia,[6] REC review is required for all human research except in research where there is "negligible risk," which is defined as "research where there is no foreseeable risk of harm of discomfort; and any foreseeable risk is no more than inconvenience. Where the risk, even if unlikely, is more than inconvenience, the research is not negligible risk."

The following things are discussed by the REC when deciding upon giving REC approval for a research study:
- Research merit and integrity.
- Justice—recruitment of participants and benefits are fairly distributed.
- Beneficence.
- Respect.
- Risks.
- Consent.

Asia

The FERCAP recommends the following for all member RECs for their review process:
- Should focus on value or research, design, and conduct.
- Ethics of the study including risk, harm, confidentiality, and informed consent are just some elements mentioned.
- The boards should be involved in monitoring and ensuring safety of the patients by reviewing Data Safety Monitoring Board progress reports.

Africa

When reviewing research ethics in Africa, several resources are available through the WHO for the use of the RECs. Generally, the following recommendations are made for the review process:
- Study design with focus on scientific validity and the rights and welfare of participants.
- Risk and benefits of the study to both the patients and the community.
- Equitable selection of research participants especially if the population selected is a vulnerable population. The ethics committee should review with the investigator the necessity of selecting this particular population of participants.
- Confidentiality of participants.
- Informed consent, with special focus on cultural issues surrounding consent.
- Qualifications of the primary investigator conducting the study.

"Experts" in this context will usually include views from relevant clinicians, allied health professionals, and other professional groups, methodologists, patients, and members of the public. In most countries, the majority of RECs are linked to an institution, for example, a university medical center or hospital. A number of RECs are not linked to an institution. Some studies must be reviewed by a REC that is "flagged" for the type of research, which is to take place. This information can be found on the websites of the government regulations of the specific country you have to submit your research proposal. The REC is entitled to charge an amount for costs related to the review.

The review process requires that a complete research file be submitted. Some files are necessary during the primary submission and some will be requested during the review before a final decision is made. Based on your submission, a decision would be made to do either of the following:
- Accept research proposal and given a REC number to proceed with research.
- Modify and resubmit.
- Reject research proposal.

Before submitting a research application, it is advisable to contact the reviewing REC for specific information regarding their process. Applicants are strongly encouraged to attend meetings in person in most countries. To prevent delay of a research project, checking the timelines (deadlines) and required documentation, etc., and submitting early would likely be rewarded with a smooth process. A single review process normally takes 6 to 8 weeks. It is also important to note that any changes to the initial REC proposal will require an amendment to be submitted and reviewed by the REC. In some places, this also includes any new members that will be performing the research (e.g., coinvestigators) that need to be added to the proposal.

14.1.4 Multicenter Human Studies and International Studies

For multicenter research, the process is more complicated. Generally, separate REC reviews may be required by each institution involved, although this sometimes may vary by the type of research and the country/countries where the research is to take place. In a typical procedure, there is a primary REC (where the primary principal investigator is conducting their research) and this is the first site of approval. After that, each separate institution will have to complete an REC review before the study can go on. In some jurisdictions, a central REC for a geographical area can approve studies at multiple sites in that area (e.g., cancer studies in Ontario, Canada). If submissions are required by each institution separately, then a Site Principal Investigator will be required to help with submission.

In some jurisdictions, in addition to REC approval, hospital board approval is also required. Only after all applicable approvals are obtained can a study commence in the center concerned.

14.2 Conclusion

Ethics submission is an essential administrative task. It is important to contact the reviewing committee about the submission. They can provide you with specific information about the submission. Each REC has its own standards, documents, and requirements. Not all RECs are authorized to review all research types.

Acknowledgment

Dr. Thomassen and Dr. Sourour contributed equally to the authorship of this chapter as first authors.

References

[1] WHO. Standards and Operational Guidance for Ethics Review of Health-Related Research with Human Participants. Geneva: WHO; 2011

[2] Ethical Conduct for Research Involving Humans. CIHR. (2014)

[3] Hemminki E. Research Ethics Committees in the Regulation of Clinical Research: Comparison of Finland to England, Canada, and the United States. Health Res Policy Syst 2016;14(5):5

[4] Regulation (EU) No 536/2014 of the European Parliament and of the Council of 16 April 2014 on Clinical Trials on Medicinal Products for Human Use, and Repealing Directive 2001/20/EC. (2014). Official Journal of the European Union

[5] National Health and Medical Research Council. National Statement on Ethical Conduct in Human Research. Canberra: NHMRC, Australian Government; 2018

[6] Smith D. Pfizer Pays out to Nigerian Families of Meningitis Drug Trial Victims. The Guardian. August 12, 2011

15 The Basics of Research Contracts

Caroline Woods

Abstract

A key part of clinical research coordination is managing the relationships between the many parties involved in a study including study funders, study sponsors, and study sites. Once everyone has agreed to a plan for the conduct of the study, a formal agreement clearly laying out this understanding between parties can be a useful guide for the ongoing relationships and prevent many issues as the study moves forward.

Keywords: grant, investigator-initiated study, industry-initiated study, sites, contracts

15.1 Introduction

This chapter will provide an overview of the key aspects of standard research contracts for clinical research. Every clinical research contract contains standard clauses that are important for the overall conduct and administration of a clinical study. However, the type of study, source of funding support, and jurisdiction where the study is being conducted can also require the use of specific clauses for that situation and different agreement formats.

No matter the type of study or the role of the parties to the agreement under negotiation, a key aspect is to ensure that not only does the agreement cover the basics of applicable laws and regulations for the study, but also each agreement in the study is consistent with the others and there is no conflict in the terms between the agreements for the different parties involved. The agreement terms should reflect the needs of the study itself with respect to funding, roles of the parties, and timelines. Specific clauses would be used to address agreed-upon payments, the management of intellectual property, and the terms under which the results would be published.

There are two main types of clinical studies as determined by who initiates the research. The first is the investigator-initiated study where the protocol is written by an investigator affiliated with a hospital or university. The second is the industry-initiated study where the protocol is written or prepared on behalf of a company usually looking to evaluate their products in a clinical trial to support regulatory approvals. Investigator-initiated research is usually funded through a grant either from a granting agency or from an industry partner; therefore, the study sponsor and study funder are not the same. Industry-initiated studies are usually funded by the company themselves and so the study funder and the study sponsor are the same.

15.2 Different Types of the Agreements

There are several different types of agreements that may be used in a study. They are determined by and the clauses included are based on the following:

- Who wrote the protocol (whose idea is it)?
- Who is providing the funds?
- Who is recruiting the patients?

15.2.1 Grant Funding

Grant funding agreements are common for investigator-initiated academic study where the idea for the study comes from a lead investigator and the funding support comes from another source such as a not-for-profit grant agency. The study sponsor would normally be the institution where the lead investigator holds a faculty or clinical position. These agreements will cover the provision of the funding and will ask for reporting in the form of a financial report on the use of the funds. They may also require a final report on the results of study and for the results to be published within a certain period. The funding provider will have no input into the overall conduct of the study, will assume no responsibility for the study itself, and will usually have no rights to the results and intellectual property generated by the study.

15.2.2 Collaboration

Collaboration agreements are becoming more common in clinical research with the development of research institutes globally and the increasing ease of global communications. These agreements come into play where there are multiple investigators at different institutions who prepare a protocol for a clinical study together and who may or may not also be contributing grant funding sourced at their institution. There could be investigators acting as study sponsors in each jurisdictions and a study committee would provide the oversight of the whole study. These agreements will address which party is responsible for each aspect of the study. It could be providing funding support or oversight of the conduct of the study jurisdictions. A key component of the agreement will be the need for each party to assume equivalent responsibility for the study and to have rights to the study results and intellectual property.

15.2.3 Sites

Site agreements are entered into between the study sponsor, the investigators conducting the study, and the institutions where the clinical activities of the study are being carried out.

These agreements detail the step-by-step conduct of the study from patient recruitment and treatment to the transfer of the results to the sponsor. They will include a payment structure, which is normally a cost reimbursement based on a per patient amount for recruitment and treatment milestones. Also addressed will be publication rights and licensing of any intellectual property.

15.2.4 Industry Involved in Investigator Initiated Study

Industry partners can be involved in investigator-initiated studies in several ways. The industry partner can provide funding for the study in the form of a grant or they may be providing the study drug or device as an in-kind (for free) support for the study or at a discount. These types of agreements will resemble a grant funding agreement but will likely include clauses addressing ownerships and licensing of the study results and intellectual property to the industry partner in return for their support of the study. Should the agreement involve the provision of a study drug or device, the agreement will include clauses around product liability and warranties on quality and manufacturing standards being met.

15.2.5 Industry-Initiated Study Agreement

Studies can also be initiated by a company itself. The protocol would be prepared by the company and they would also be providing the funding. They are therefore both the sponsor and the funder for the study. Normally only site agreements are used for this type of study and they would be directly between the company and the sites recruiting the patients. In this case, the intellectual property and results would normally be owned by the company themselves. The sites would likely negotiate a license to use the results and intellectual property for academic purposes along with a right to publish. Sites would also request indemnification from the company. In this case, agreements tend toward a service type of relationship between the sites and the company and have less collaborative clauses than those in an academic investigator–initiated study.

15.3 The Parts of an Agreement

No matter the type of the agreement used in a study, there are standard parts and clauses that will appear. Each clause has a purpose to provide the terms for an aspect of the arrangement between parties.

15.3.1 The Parties

The first section on any agreement will lay out the parties to the agreement. Parties are who is involved in the relationship that the agreement is about and who is assuming the legal responsibility for the conduct of the study.

Normally for clinical study agreements, the sponsor is a party to all of the agreements as they are coordinating all the activities of the study with all the other groups involved. For example, a grant agreement would be between the sponsor and the granting agency, while a site agreement would be between the sponsor and the site.

A common question is whether the investigators themselves should be a party to the agreement. The answer is "that depends." A party to an agreement should be a legal entity with appropriate policies, practices, and insurance in place to ensure that they can assume the responsibilities laid out in the agreement. Most investigators have an affiliation with an institution that supports them in their research. Where the investigator is an employee of that institution, normally the institution as the legal entity would enter into the agreement on behalf of their employee and not require the investigator to be a party. Other institutions consider clinicians to be independent contractors and would require the investigator they represent to also be a party to the agreement.

15.3.2 The Preamble

This section leads into the clauses of the agreement and is intended to provide background and context for the agreement. It may include the title of the study, indicate where the funding is coming from, and if there are multiple groups leading the study.

15.3.3 The Clauses

Clause Content Determined by the Study

- *The scope of work:* This clause will address the protocol itself and requirements for the conduct of the study including obtaining consent, expected recruitment targets, and timelines to study completion. It will also include requirements regarding compliance with applicable laws, regulatory requirements, and registration of the study in a clinical study listing. These will vary with the type of study and the jurisdiction where the study is being conducted.
- *Budget and payment:* This should be established between the parties before the agreement is drafted, so this section will normally just lay out that understanding and include any financial restrictions or requirements needed based on the arrangement under which the study funding is initially obtained. For funding agreements, this clause would include the terms under which the funds are received to the lead institution. This is normally installment-based advance set to a timeline. For site agreements, the most common format is a set per patient amount paid out as a cost reimbursement per patient when certain study milestones are met.
- *Intellectual property and publication:* Much like the budget, this should be established between the parties before the agreement is drafted. Its

important for this clause to keep in mind that the rights provided between the parties here must be compatible with the rights granted between parties in all the other agreements in the study. For example, should the study involve an industry partner they would likely have requested some control of the intellectual property, which would have to be addressed in each site agreement. Freedom to publish is also important in academic studies, but it is important to ensure that each site and the lead institution have the same rights.

Standard Clauses

- *Assurances:* This clause would cover the need for the parties to comply with any laws applicable to the study in the jurisdiction where it is being conducted as well as require ethical compliance.
- *Privacy:* Privacy laws are specific to each jurisdiction in a study. The data obtained from patients often must be handled in compliance with the law in the jurisdiction where the data are gathered, so this clause will provide the direction and balance between those laws for the study. It should be noted that this applies to identifiable data and requirements will vary depending on the type of data being shared and the definition of de-identified or anonymized data in the jurisdictions involved.
- *Confidentiality:* Confidentiality language is standard to most agreements and will lay out what is considered confidential and how to mark things confidential. Most important is the conditions under which information would not be considered confidential including being required to be disclosed under law or if it is obtained legally from a source outside of the agreement. Confidentiality requirements should not be perpetual (forever) and normally include a term of 5 to 10 years.
- *Liability and indemnification:* This clause can be a deal breaker in agreements. The terms lay out who is going to be held responsible for what should something go horribly wrong during the study. Most academic studies use their own liability language, which holds each party responsible for its own actions and the claims against them. The next step from that is reciprocal indemnification where each

party assumes responsibility not only for their own actions, but also for claims against the other party because of first party's actions, should there be any. The clauses will lay out under what conditions each party will assume responsibility for claims against the other. In an industry-initiated study, normally sites would ask for the company to assume complete responsibility for any claims arising from the study and provide what is called full indemnification.

- *Record retention:* Varying from jurisdiction to jurisdiction, this clause simply states that time for which each party will keep records on file. The time is usually determined by regulatory requirements. In Canada, for clinical trials, the requirement is 25 years.
- *Relationship of parties:* This clause clarifies normally that the parties while working together are separate entities and do not represent each other.
- *Representations and warranties:* This clause is a statement that the parties are what they are stating they are in the agreement and a surety of the quality of what they are providing for the study as well as the limits of that surety.
- *Termination:* This clause addresses under what conditions other than simply the end of the term of the agreement can the parties end the agreement early. It would also include statements on the process of the early termination.
- *Incorporation by reference:* Frequently, agreements include attached documents referenced in the clause as schedules or appendices. As these documents can frequently be large files themselves, and would not be considered part of the legal terms themselves unless they are physically included in the agreement, an incorporation by reference clause allows those documents to be added to the agreement without being physically attached. The clause would also contain a priority statement that would indicate which document would be considered the correct one should there be any conflict between the parts of the agreement.
- *Governing law and jurisdiction:* This is one of the most commonly negotiated clauses for studies that work in multiple jurisdictions. It designates which jurisdiction laws should a court use to interpret the clauses in the agreement. Most sponsor agreements utilize the jurisdiction the study sponsor is located in.

Sites typically prefer their home jurisdiction. Commonly, parties can agree on silence, which means the jurisdiction would be determined at the time a legal action is initiated between the parties. Parties can also agree on "jurisdiction of the defendant," which means should a legal action be initiated between the parties the laws and courts of the defending party's jurisdiction will be used.

- *Insurance:* Again, this is a frequently negotiated clause. Insurance is a key requirement of clinical studies. Institutions that conduct clinical research frequently and act as sponsor in academic studies often have their own program of insurance or self-insurance to cover their clinical research actively. However, smaller institutions and particularly those in smaller or less developed countries would not have their own insurance. For industry-initiated studies, along with providing indemnification, the company may also purchase insurance for the sites in their studies. Academic investigator–initiated studies frequently do not have sufficient funding to purchase additional insurance for sites and must require the sites to have their own insurance. In some jurisdictions, sufficient insurance is a regulatory requirement and special arrangements must be made between the sponsor and the site.
- *Entire agreement, amendment, and assignment:* These clauses would state that the agreement laid out is complete and there is no other relevant document other than what is already contained in the agreement. It would also state that amendments or changes to the agreement must be made in writing and signed by all the parties. Assignment, which is a party handing its responsibilities under an agreement to another third party, is normally only allowed with approval of the other parties in writing.
- *Notices:* The notice section is a list of who should be contacted for any communications regarding the agreement and should include a statement on when a notice should be considered received. For example, an email would be received the next business day, whereas for couriered documents it could be 5 business days.
- *Use of name:* Public disclosure of a study and the parties involved is a common requirement for academic purposes and regulatory requirements. A use of name clause lays out

the condition, methods, and amount of information a party can disclose to the public about the agreement and the other parties involved.

- *Conflict of interest and misconduct:* These clauses can be presented separately as well as together. Parties that fund clinical studies often require that institutions have policies in place regarding the definition, tracking, and reporting of incidents when the investigators participating in the clinical may be in a conflict of interest or have committed scientific misconduct.
- *Severability:* This clause is standard in most agreements and simply states that if a court deems a clause in the agreement to be invalid, unenforceable, or illegal, the clause will be changed either by the parties or by a court to a clause that is valid.
- *No adverse construction:* This clause simply states that regardless of who wrote the initial agreement there would be no bias in the interpretation of the clauses.
- *No waiver:* Sometimes it becomes necessary for parties to negotiate a one-off exception to the "rules" of an agreement. A waiver clause describes the process should a party decide to waive a provision of a clause in an agreement for the other party.
- *Survival:* Agreements have a "term," which is a start date and end date under which all the clauses of an agreement are in effect. However, some clauses such as publication, intellectual property, governing law, and indemnification do need to remain in effect beyond the agreement itself. This clause would list those.
- *Provision of product:* This clause would be specific to the situation where a company is involved in the study either as the sponsor of an industry-initiated study or where they are providing their study drug or device in support of an investigator-initiated study. The clause would appear in the agreement between the study sponsor and the company as well as in all the site agreements related to the study. The key components of the clause would be the continued provision of the product sufficient to conduct the study, a warranty or guarantee that the product is manufactured appropriately in compliance with applicable laws, and an indemnification for the sponsor and the sites should there be any defect in the product or adverse effects on the patients specific to the product.

15.3.4 Signatories

This section is where the formal acceptance of the terms of the agreement is indicated by the parties. Each party will have their own policy on who is authorized to sign on their behalf. For most large institutions, it would be someone in a senior management position. Investigators who are employees of the institution are not normally authorized to sign for their institutions alone, but often are listed as "read and acknowledged." This means they are not a formal party to the agreement, but they are aware and understand the terms of the agreement if they are the individual carrying out those terms.

15.4 Practical Application

15.4.1 Examples of Clauses

The most common areas for negotiation in a clinical study agreement are study budgets, intellectual property, publication, indemnification, and governing law and jurisdiction.

Indemnification/liability and governing law and jurisdiction clauses can be complex to negotiate and are best handled by your institution's legal representative.

In the following sections, we list sample clauses for study budgets, intellectual property, and publication as the content of these clauses are usually determined by the nature of the study itself. The clauses represent typical language in academic or collaborative agreements. It is important when negotiating changes in these particular clauses to keep in mind the need to maintain consistency with the agreements with other collaborators in the study as well as fair terms for all the parties involved.

15.5 Study Budget

15.5.1 Overview

The key components of a study budget clause are the following:

- To set a fixed maximum amount for the cost of the study to the site (Article 1.2). Normally, this is tied to a set recruitment target for the site that is part of the study performance clause.
- To set terms under which payments can be controlled or withdrawn (Articles 1. 4 and 1.6).

- To establish the right to audit the financial documents (Article 1.7).
- To set the currency, and provide guidance as to the process of requesting and receiving payment.

15.5.2 The Terms

1.1 Payments made to the Investigator and the Institution will be made by XXXXX on behalf of itself and the Principal Investigator. The Institution and the Investigator shall be responsible for all tax payments (if any) owing on the amounts paid.

All payments shall be made payable to Institution and sent to:

Attention: (Enter Name)

(Enter Address)

1.2 The total payments that XXXXX shall be obligated to make or cause to be made to the Institution to complete the Study is a maximum of XXXXX Canadian dollar per participant as detailed below:

(i) XXXXX Canadian dollars on recruitment.

(ii) XXXX Canadian dollars on treatment.

(iii) XXXX Canadian dollars on follow up visit.

(iv) XXXXX Canadian dollars on final receipt of Study Data by XXXXXXX.

1.3 Funds release is dependent on the receipt of documentation verifying research ethics board's approval from the ethics review board within the Institution and a fully executed original agreement.

1.4 XXXXXX shall issue payments quarterly based on enrollment, submission of case report forms, and adjudication materials as per the Study Protocol, and completion of required data clarification forms subject to receipt of invoice.

Invoices shall be submitted to:

Insert name and address

1.5 All funds shall be paid in Canadian dollars (CAD). Payments will be conditional upon continued support of the Grantor to XXXXXX in accordance with the terms of the support awarded.

1.6 The Principal Investigator and XXXXX reserve the right to withhold payment or request to return of funds to the extent that Participants were not properly enrolled under the terms of the Study Protocol and/or the Study was not conducted under the conditions set out in the Study Protocol.

1.7 Institution shall maintain appropriate accounting records according to generally accepted accounting practices for costs claimed as incurred in the performance of this Agreement and shall keep these records for a minimum of seven (7) years.

Institution shall also make such records available, upon request, to authorized XXXXXX representatives for audit purposes.

15.6 Intellectual Property

15.6.1 Overview

The key components of an intellectual property clause are the following:

- To establish the ownership of the raw data set obtained from the work on the study under the protocol (Article 1.1). This is normally a set of de-identified data that are gathered by the multiple sites in the study and combined into the study database. It is important to have the ownership of the data set clearly established and preferably solely owned by the study sponsor or lead institution who initiated the study. This is important for the overall administration and any potential future use of the data. If the data were to remain owned by each individual site in the study, then the study database would have multiple owners, which can create an administrative burden and confusion should there be any secondary analysis or use desired or should the data become key to any intellectual property. Sites are normally given a license to use for specific purposes (Article 1.2). Sites also frequently ask Article 1.1 to clearly state that the Study Data does not include medical records.
- To set the ownership and licensing of any other intellectual property that may be created from the study separately from the data (Article 1.3).

15.6.2 The Terms

1.1 All rights, title, and interest in and to any and all data arising out of the Study "(Study Data")" shall be the sole and exclusive property of XXXXXX.

1.2 Without limiting the foregoing, the Investigator and Institution shall have a nonexclusive, royalty-free, irrevocable, perpetual right to use the Study Data generated at the Institution for the purpose of the Study and internal and academic research purposes.

1.3 Investigator and the Institution shall promptly and reasonably disclose to the Principal Investigator and XXXXXX any patentable or unpatentable inventions or improvements made or conceived by the Investigator in the course of or as a result of the work done hereunder in relation to the Study (hereinafter "Inventions"). Inventorship will be determined in accordance to Canadian patent law and ownership will follow inventorship. Where a joint Invention is made by naming at least one entity as inventor from each party, Institution and Investigator agree to enter into an agreement with XXXXX to administrate such joint Inventions. Each Party agrees to grant to the other Party a royalty-free, nonexclusive license to use Inventions for internal and academic research purposes.

15.7 Publication Clause

15.7.1 Overview

The key components of a publication clause are the following:

- To establish a fair process for publication that does not infringe on the rights of any of the parties involved and prevents the disclosure of confidential information and "scooping" of the publication.

15.7.2 The Terms

1.1 All Parties agree that there will be a strict moratorium on any release of preliminary or final Study findings (including any correspondence, meetings, media releases, presentations, posting on web sites, reports, or publications whatsoever) until the dissemination plan has been approved by the Principal Investigator. All Parties further agree that the first publication of the Study should be made as a joint, multicenter publication involving all participating Investigators and Institutions. Authorship of the multicenter publication shall be in accordance with academic standards for authorship. If such a multicenter publication has not been submitted to an academic journal within eighteen (18) months after conclusion, abandonment or termination of the Study at all participating Sites, or if the Principal Investigator confirms in writing that there will be no multicenter Study publication, the Investigator may publish the information and/or results from the Institution in accordance with Article 1.2. The Investigator will have the right to disclose information resulting from this Study or any background information provided by Principal Investigator and XXXXX that is necessary for inclusion to allow other scholars to verify research results.

1.2 Subject to Article 1.1, Institution and Investigator will have the right to publish and/or disclose publicly information and/or data arising from the Study and the Study Protocol provided, however, that the text of any such publication and/or public disclosure (collectively referred to as the "Publication") shall be submitted to the Principal Investigator to review for confidential or proprietary information and for comment at least thirty (30) days prior to the Publication's submission for disclosure. Further, any information identified by the Principal Investigator or XXXXX as being Confidential Information shall be deleted from the Publication, provided, however, that XXXXX shall not request the deletion of, and the Investigator shall not be required to delete, data or information related to research methods used in the Study. At the request of Principal Investigator or XXXXX such submission shall be delayed for a further period not exceeding sixty (60) days to enable XXXXX to protect its rights in such confidential or proprietary information. If the Investigator does not wish to delay the Publication, then the Institution and Investigator shall delete the confidential or proprietary information identified by the Principal Investigator or XXXXX from the Publication prior to its disclosure.

15.8 Conclusion

As the drafting and negotiation of clinical research agreements is complex and involves knowledge of the conduct of clinical studies, regulatory requirements, legal clauses, and institutional policies, most companies and institutions involved in clinical research have their own contracts department or legal counsel that handles the drafting, review, and negotiation of research contracts for clinical research studies.

Before starting negotiations for study agreements, you should contact your contracts department to discuss how the process for drafting, negotiating, and finalizing your agreements is done at your institution. Most institutions have a standard template agreement that they prefer to use that contains most of the clauses listed above drafted to be specific to their institution and needs. The study-specific information would then be inserted into the template and the draft agreement provided to the parties to begin the negotiation of the details. In most cases, someone in the contracts office would be assigned to assist with the negotiation of the clauses to ensure that the final agreement is compliant with legal, regulatory, and institutional requirements to clinical research.

Definitions

- **Investigator-initiated study:** A study where the protocol is written by an investigator alone or in collaboration with other investigators who are not associated with the company that owns the product being tested.
- **Sponsor:** The legal entity assuming responsibility for the content of the protocol and any reporting needed to regulatory authorities.
- **Industry-initiated study:** A study where the protocol is written by or on behalf of the company that owns the product being tested.
- **Clinical study:** A clinical study is medical research conducted on human volunteers.
- **Clinical trials:** Studies to evaluate the effectiveness and safety of devices, drugs, and procedures by investigating their effects on groups of people.
- **Observational studies:** Investigators observe and evaluate the effect of interventions on groups of participants receiving an already established intervention as part of their routine medical care, which can include medical products such as drugs or devices or procedures.
- **Grant:** An agreement to provide funding to support a study with no control and oversight of the study from the funder.
- **Contract:** An agreement to perform a clinical study as a service for a sponsor or funder where they retain oversight and ownership of the results.
- **Coordinating Center:** An institution or group overseeing the conduct of the study at all the institutions involved. Contracts and agreements with the sites are normally initiated by this group.
- **Site:** An institution performing the clinical protocol on participants.

Further Readings

Agreement Clauses

http://www.ccmo.nl/en/legal-framework—agency providing guidelines and practices for clinical studies conducted in the Netherlands

https://www.cancer.gov/about-nci/organization/ccct/resources/start-clauses-info.pdf—document on standard clauses that can be used in clinical study agreements

https://www.lawinsider.com/clauses—online archive of standard legal clauses

Government Sites and Regulations

https://ec.europa.eu/health/human-use/clinical-trials/directive_en—European Union

https://www.australianclinicaltrials.gov.au/—Australia

https://www.canada.ca/en/health-canada.html—Canada

https://www.clinicaltrials.gov/—U.S. Registry Site

https://www.nih.gov/—United States

16 How to Start-Up a Study

Ellie B.M. Landman

Abstract

Large multicenter clinical studies are essential contributions to the knowledge base that supports the practice of evidence-based medicine. The overall success of clinical studies depends on the contribution in time and effort of local investigators. The recruitment of suitable sites and the careful preparation of participating sites are crucial to ensure the study is completed according to predefined timelines and within budget, and ultimately resulting in reliable and qualitative data. With thorough preparation during study start-up, problems resulting in delays or additional costs can be avoided, or at least minimized. However, the start-up of a clinical study can be challenging in itself, and is prone to cause delays when not carefully planned out. Generally, preparation and careful consideration of how to realistically reach goals is as important for providing the evidence aimed for as the scientific basis for the study. The aim of this chapter is to outline the steps involved in the study start-up phase and the challenges that can be faced. A guide on how to successfully go through study start-up is provided, to enhance the chances of successful completion of the study.

Keywords: study start-up, feasibility, regulatory approval, site activation

16.1 Introduction

Large randomized controlled trials (RCTs) are considered the highest level of evidence to support evidence-based clinical practice. As it is often impossible for a single center to conduct a large RCT, multicenter trials are needed. By having multiple sites (in different countries) participate in a study, it becomes possible to recruit large numbers of patients to provide sufficient power to reliably answer a research question. Also, participation of different sites provides a heterogeneous study population, enhancing the generalizability of study results. However, to ensure successful conduct of such large study at multiple sites requires careful planning and a solid study set-up. Large investments of financial resources and time and effort invested by research personnel are required to successfully conduct these large trials. Although

a lot of effort is spent on protocol development and application to funding agencies, this is not enough to guarantee successful conduct of the trial. An important first step toward success can be made during the start-up phase of the study. Proper planning and preparation during study start-up can ensure a smooth start and provide the grounds for an efficient study.

The aim of any clinical study is to provide a reliable answer to its research question. Collecting reliable data is crucial in this respect. Also, meeting recruitment goals within time and budget targets not only plays a key role in the overall success of a clinical study but also provides the main challenges in conducting the study. As proper preparation can set off the study to success, the aim of this chapter is to outline the steps to take during the start-up phase of a clinical study.

16.2 Study Start-Up Phase

After protocol development and obtaining regulatory approval, the study start-up phase is a costly and time-consuming but an inevitable and important step. However, investing in this step can prevent problems and delays later on and proves to be worthwhile in the long run. A successful start-up phase of a clinical study can provide a solid basis for successful completion of the study. ▶ Fig. 16.1 shows a schematic overview of the steps involved in the study start-up phase. During the start-up phase, recruitment of appropriate sites, and training of site study personnel aims to ensure recruitment goals are met and reliable data are collected. Proper preparation plays a key role in the overall success of a clinical study. Therefore, time and effort should be spent during the start-up phase of the study to ensure a smooth takeoff and set the correct course for the study.

During the study start-up phase, all preparations needed to secure successful conduct of the study are completed. One of the main tasks to take care of during study start-up (for a multicenter study) is to select investigator sites that have the capacity and ability to successfully conduct the study. Also, appropriate training of participating sites is provided during study start-up to ensure protocol adherence and proper data collection. As many

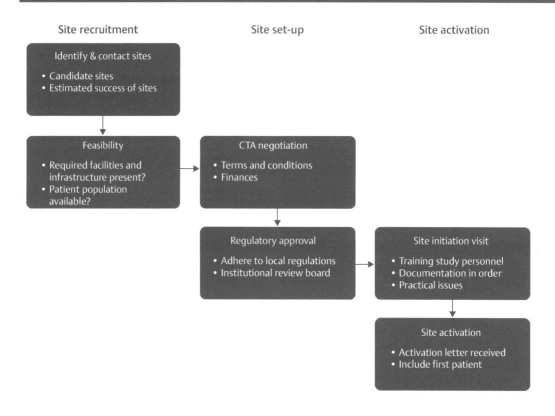

Fig. 16.1 Schematic overview of study start-up.

clinical studies fail to meet the recruitment target within the predefined time, efforts should be aimed at optimizing conditions to ensure successful patient recruitment. A recruitment plan based on the study protocol and the available budget and time can provide a basis for planning study start-up. The number of sites needed to meet recruitment goals within time and the practical necessities for conducting the study determine which sites might be suitable to participate in the study and which sites are most likely to be successful in participating. It is important to set realistic goals, to avoid deviation from the initial plan. Selecting suitable sites and streamlining processes of agreement negotiation and the application for regulatory approval can contribute to meeting recruitment targets and deadlines in a timely manner within budget. In order to go through study start-up efficiently, each step (▶ Fig. 16.1) needs to be carefully considered and planned for in advance.

16.2.1 Identify and Contact Sites

The success of large multicenter RCTs depends on the participation of clinical sites that can quickly go through the process of regulatory approval, make necessary arrangements before site activation, and eventually enroll a large number of patients in the study.[1] Therefore, critical selection of participating sites plays an important role in the final success of a clinical study.

The first question to be asked when identifying potential sites to participate in a study is whether the facilities and requirements to conduct the study according to the protocol are in place. The success of a large multicenter clinical study is largely dependent on meeting recruitment goals and adhering to the study timelines. The critical selection of study sites plays a crucial role in meeting targets. When sites are selected that have a high capability of meeting recruitment goals within the set timeframe, delays can be avoided, preventing additional costs.

The identification of suitable sites can be a time-consuming first step, but when done carefully, it can prevent disappointing recruitment rates and thus study delay. Evaluating past performance in clinical studies and the availability of suitable patients to participate in the study are main factors to consider when identifying participating sites. Sites that have proven successful in previous studies are more likely to be successful in a new study as well. A risk lies in recruiting sites that are new to conducting clinical studies, as there is no comparison of past performance.

The intended local lead investigator has the responsibility to consult with the involved colleagues whether there is an interest in participating in the study. Often, collaboration between different specialties is needed to conduct a study. When there is no agreed interest in the study, it will be impossible for a local investigator to make the study a success. It has been shown that a committed investigator and study team are important contributors to a high recruitment rate.[2]

16.2.2 Feasibility

Once the initial contact with sites is set up and the interest in participating in the study is expressed, feasibility assessment is the next step in site recruitment. The aim of feasibility assessment is to evaluate whether the required facilities and staff are available to guarantee a successful conduct of the study. This evaluation can be performed by filling out a feasibility questionnaire. The feasibility questionnaire can include questions about the intended study population and the availability of involved departments, as well as the presence and capabilities of dedicated study personnel.

First, identification of the specific patient population is required to enable sites to review the availability of eligible patients. A (preliminary) patient recruitment plan can assist in evaluating the ability of sites to meet recruitment goals.[3] Setting specific, detailed goals for recruitment enables sites to realistically estimate whether these goals can be met. Reviewing the anticipated study population at site provides a first indication of the possibility to adhere to the intended recruitment plan. This includes the number of patients per unit of time that meets the inclusion criteria, as well as the estimated number of patients that can actually be included. One needs to take into account not only the number of patients eligible

to participate, but also the likelihood of patients to consent to participation in the study.

In addition, it is important to evaluate whether all facilities needed to conduct the study are available. All necessary facilities and practical requirements for adhering to the study protocol need to be assessed. When laboratory assessment or imaging, for instance, are required, agreements with the relevant departments need to be set up. For studies concerning medicinal products, the hospital's pharmacy plays a key role. It is important to seek collaboration and come to an agreement with required facilities in an early stage, as time and effort spend would be wasted when it turns out later on that there is no support for participation in the study.

In addition to the feasibility questionnaire, a site visit can be part of the feasibility assessment. During a site visit, the capabilities of study personnel and the availability of required equipment and infrastructure can be verified. The hospital's pharmacy, if applicable, should be involved during the site visit as well. It is important to verify the capacity regarding storage and handling of the investigational products when selecting participating sites. Especially when recruiting new sites, a site visit can be informative. Also, in-person contact with investigators and other members of the study team makes it easier to communicate later on.

Often, detailed information from the study protocol is required to determine whether participation of a particular site is feasible. When sensitive information is shared during the initial recruitment of sites, setting up a confidentiality agreement can be part of the process. Since signing such, or any, agreement is a likely cause for delay in this initial step, it is important to handle this as efficiently as possible, by strictly holding on to set deadlines.

16.2.3 Clinical Trial Agreement Negotiation

Once the feasibility of successful conduction of the study at a particular site is confirmed, the terms and conditions of participating in the study can be discussed. The clinical trial agreement (CTA) comprises an agreement of legal, financial, and intellectual property issues. In particular, financial reimbursement and ownership of intellectual property can be subjects of negotiation. As participation in the study can be dependent on financial compensation, CTA negotiation can be part of the early phase of study start-up. It is important for participating sites to carefully review all costs involved in participating in the study to make sure no financial setback is encountered along the way. Ownership of intellectual property and authorship on publications derived from the study can be issues to negotiate as well. To adhere to authorship regulations, but to compensate clinicians for their efforts to recruit patients, group authorship for those involved can be an option. Also, the availability of the collected data at site for substudies can be issues to negotiate.

As careful consideration of all issues included in the CTA is necessary, CTA negotiation can evolve into a lengthy process.[4] Eventually, the goal of CTA negotiation should be satisfactory to all parties involved. Negotiating terms and conditions of participation in a clinical study and obtaining signatures of those involved can be a major delaying factor. Keeping track of communication and the sites' status along the process can facilitate smooth completion of this important step.

16.2.4 Regulatory and Ethics Approval

Some studies of experimental or not-yet-approved drugs and devices need to be approved by a national or regional regulatory agency (e.g., Health Canada, U.S. FDA, European Medicines Agency). In addition to central regulatory approval, participation of each site in the study needs to be approved. Moreover, each site needs to obtain local ethical approval for conducting the study. For detailed discussion of obtaining ethical approval, see Chapter 14. In the case of multinational studies, participating sites in different countries can be subjected to different regulations. Although many documents that are required for obtaining central approval will be applicable for local ethical approval as well, certain documents need to be specifically adjusted to each particular site. For instance, patient information and consent forms, insurance, and investigators' qualifications need to be adapted to each specific site. Some sites may need documents in their own local language, which can be challenging. Documents need to be applicable to the local situation, yet comparable to the original versions. Both collecting and adjusting

all required documents for regulatory approval, as well as responding to potential questions from the regulatory board, can take a lot of time and are a notorious cause for delays.[4]

16.2.5 Site Initiation Visit

After obtaining central and local regulatory approval, but before the first patient can be enrolled, the site initiation visit is the last step before site activation. During the initiation visit, which can be done either in person or by telephone or video conference, site staff will be trained. It is important to ensure detailed understanding of the protocol and all study procedures by all members of the study team. Training of site personnel needs to be documented on a staff training log, signed by the responsible person giving the training.

Even though the local principal investigator is responsible for proper execution of all study-related tasks according to the study protocol, specific tasks can be delegated to members of the study team. All members involved in conducting study-related tasks should be listed on a specific study task delegation log, signed off by the local principal investigator.

Going through all practical issues involved in the study during the initiation visit ensures adherence to the protocol and, ultimately, good data quality. Standard operating procedures (SOPs) are used to outline all study-related tasks. SOPs can provide detailed instructions for all day-to-day tasks involved in conducting the study and the responsible members of the study team. It includes directions for enrolling patients and follow-up visits, data collection and management, and keeping track of study progress. Adhering to the execution of study tasks according to SOPs guarantees the standardized execution of tasks and transparency to all members of the study team.

An initiation visit at the hospital's pharmacy is required when medicinal products are involved in the study. During the pharmacy visit, training for proper storage and handling of the medicinal products as well as registration of stored and dispensing of medication should be arranged.

Finally, the initiation visit can be utilized to ensure all required documents are in place. An Investigator Site File (ISF), also known as a site Trial Master File (site TMF) should be kept on site with all regulatory documents, such as study protocol, regulatory approval letters, and signed informed

Table 16.1 Required documents for site initiation

Document	Required information
Site training log	Name and role of study personnel Training date Lead investigators signature
Study staff delegation log	Name and role of study personnel Delegated study tasks Start and end date of participation in the study Lead investigator signature
Screening and enrolment log	Screening date Included/excluded/missed Reason for exclusion
Patient identification log	Patient name, age, gender Study ID
Standard operating procedure	Study-related tasks Responsible member of the study team
Drug accountability log	Details of study medication Temperature of storage location Details of issued medication

consent forms, and also the site training log, delegation log, and SOPs. In addition, the screening and enrolment log and patient identification log are essential documents in the ISF. For studies involving drugs, a drug accountability log and a temperature log should be maintained by the pharmacy. All medication in storage as well as the details of all dispensed medication should be registered. All documents needed for proper documentation of all study-related actions are listed in ▶ Table 16.1.

16.2.6 Site Activation

Much effort has been spent once sites are activated and recruitment of patients can be initiated. However, continued efforts are needed to ensure successful conduct of the study. Although the study start-up phase can provide all positive input to support a good start, guidance and encouragement along the way is inevitable. It is important to stay in touch with local investigators and continuously review patient enrolment to identify pitfalls as they occur. Updating investigators about study progress keeps investigators aware of the continuous effort needed to reach the study goals. A positive report on patient recruitment rates can support a positive flow and encourage local investigators to keep an ongoing interest in the study.

16.3 Challenges Encountered During Start-Up

Although study start-up can be a time-consuming and costly process, it can prevent problems and save time and money in the end. That is, when it is done right. As is true for each phase of conducting a clinical study, many challenges can be encountered during study start-up.

16.3.1 Protocol Adherence

The first challenge in conducting a large clinical study is protocol adherence. For results to be meaningful, it is of the utmost importance that all patients are treated the same way and data are collected in a standardized manner. Providing a reliable answer to the research question is dependent on the reliability of data collected. Having a clear view on the exact data required, and the analyses to be performed, one can ensure that the specific data needed are collected in the appropriate way. Deviations in execution of study procedures or data collection should be avoided. Occasional interim data safety monitoring can be employed to detect errors at an early stage in order to be able to correct them and avoid similar mistakes later on. This will aid in facilitating data clearance at the final stages of the study.

16.3.2 Meeting Recruitment Goals

For a clinical study to be considered successful, it needs to not only provide the reliable data to answer the research question but also meet the recruitment goals within the set time and budget. In practice, 45% of trials reach only 80% of their targeted sample size eventually. Many studies fail to meet their recruitment targets within the set timeframe, resulting in the need for an extension in time and money to meet the recruitment goal.[5] Only when the predefined recruitment target is met can a clinical study provide a reliable answer to its research question. As this seems quite straightforward, meeting recruitment goals within time and budget can be a major difficulty faced in many clinical studies. Therefore, effort should be made before initiation of the study to ensure patient recruitment will be efficient.

16.3.3 Delaying Factors

Generally, each step of study start-up is prone to cause delays. Awaiting responses of local investigators, signing of the confidentiality agreement or CTA, and going through ethics and/or regulatory approval can take a lot of time and are likely to be stretched due to delayed replies. Therefore, it is important to keep track of each step of the process in all sites, and to set out specific timelines to remind people of their actions when deadlines are not met. In order to streamline the process of identifying participating sites and go through it as efficiently as possible, keeping track of the status of different sites is needed. Keeping track of each sites' status along the way enhances the process of recruiting and setting up participating sites.

16.3.4 Guidelines for Good Clinical Practice

The guidelines of good clinical practice (GCP) aim to set a standard for ethical and scientific quality for the design, conduct, and reporting of clinical studies involving humans. These guidelines are founded on the principles of protecting participants, improving the quality of research, and the possibility to check afterward. GCP guidelines aim to result in better use of human (and animal) materials, decrease unnecessary delays in development, and faster availability of new medication. In short, taking into account the GCP guidelines helps ensure the safety and rights of participants and provide reliable and qualitative data. A major aspect in GCP is proper documentation of everything involved in a clinical study. During the start-up phase of a clinical study, one needs to take into account the GCP guidelines, to guarantee adherence to the guidelines during the active study phase. Also, working according to GCP guidelines provides a uniformity in conducting clinical studies across countries.

16.3.5 Drug, Device, or Procedure

Clinical studies involving medicinal products require elaborate attention during all phases of the study, including the start-up phase. However, when medical devices or surgical procedures are the subject of study, different rules apply. For studies involving medicinal products, strict rules apply; they need to be tested in randomized clinical studies in the particular patient population, for the particular indication it is aimed to be used in practice, before it can be actually used. In contrast, for medical devices, clinical data from literature and judging safety and performance in a particular situation on available data can be sufficient. Medical devices are classified into class I, II, or III, and regulatory control is required accordingly. Class I devices require no notification, class II devices require premarket notification, and class III devices require premarket approval. Although surgical procedures have a large share in medical treatments provided to patients, no specific regulations apply to the introduction of new surgical techniques in medical practice. Techniques might vary between countries or regions, but it is not known whether different approaches in surgery result in different outcomes.[6]

16.4 Practical Application

The key to a smooth and efficient study start-up is a detailed plan outlining required actions and deadlines. In order to set up a solid plan for study start-up, it is crucial to have an overview of all tasks to go through in this phase and making a realistic estimation of the time needed to complete each task. Next, adhering to the timeline aids in an efficient study start-up, thus providing a basis for successful conduction of the study. This often requires making sure that local investigators and study staff keep to their deadlines as well.

When planning study start-up, upfront identification of all tasks that need to be completed along each step facilitates overview of the process. Generally, most tasks will be independent of the size, objective, or duration of a study, but adjustment to a particular situation might be required (a sample checklist for study start-up tasks is provided in **Toolbox D**).

16.5 Keys to Success

- Set up a realistic and practical recruitment plan.
- Clearly define necessary facilities and required characteristic of study sites.

- Set and adhere to strict deadlines.
- Keep track of status of all (potentially) participating sites from initial contact until study close-out.
- Stay in contact with local study team, during start-up (and active recruitment).

16.6 Conclusion

The overall success of a study depends not only on providing a reliable answer to the research question, but also on the timely completion of the study within budget. Much effort is spent on writing the research protocol and obtaining ethical approval and funding, but the study start-up phase is of crucial importance for a successful conduct of the study. Time and effort spent in the preparation phase pays off in success during the execution phase of a clinical study.

A successful clinical study initially relies on selecting appropriate sites and proper assessment of the feasibility of sites. CTA negotiation and obtaining regulatory approval can be time-consuming but are inevitable in reaching agreement regarding finances and ownership of intellectual property, and adhering to (local) regulations. Before recruitment of the first patient, site initiation is aimed at providing necessary training as well as arranging required documents. Going through study start-up provides all support needed for successful conduct of the study, but continuous support and effort is needed to ensure successful completion of the study.

Definitions

- **Clinical trial agreement:** Signed agreement between sponsor and local investigator concerning legal, financial, and intellectual property issues.

- **Confidentiality agreement:** Signed agreement between sponsor and local investigator to keep confidentiality of shared protocol and study-related information and documents.
- **Feasibility questionnaire:** Questionnaire aimed to evaluate the required facilities and staff available at candidate sites.
- **Investigator Site File:** File to document all required regulatory documents at site.
- **Regulatory approval:** Authorization by regulatory board to allow conduction of the study at site.
- **Site initiation visit:** Visit during which training is provided and protocol and study procedures are reviewed.

References

[1] Demaerschalk BM, Brown RD Jr, Roubin GS, et al. CREST-2 Investigators. Factors Associated with Time to Site Activation, Randomization, and Enrollment Performance in a Stroke Prevention Trial. Stroke 2017;48(9): 2511–2518

[2] Abraham A, Jones J, Vikram S. How to Minimize Low Enrolling Sites: A Case Study in Diabetes. Perspect Clin Res 2010;1(1):25–28

[3] Huang GD, Bull J, Johnston McKee K, Mahon E, Harper B, Roberts JN; CTTI Recruitment Project Team. Clinical Trials Recruitment Planning: A Proposed Framework from the Clinical Trials Transformation Initiative. Contemp Clin Trials 2018;66:74–79

[4] Duley L, Gillman A, Duggan M, et al. What are the Main Inefficiencies in Trial Conduct: A Survey of UKCRC Registered Clinical Trials Units in the UK. Trials 2018;19(1): 15–017

[5] Farrell B, Kenyon S, Shakur H. Managing Clinical Trials. Trials 2010;11:78–6215

[6] Darrow JJ. Explaining the Absence of Surgical Procedure Regulation. Cornell J Law Public Policy 2017;27(1): 189–206

Further Readings

ICH-GCP guideline, accessible through: https://www.ich.org/fileadmin/Public_Web_Site/ICH_Products/Guidelines/Efficacy/E6/E6_R1_Guideline.pdf

Regulations regarding trials involving medicinal products or devices: https://www.fda.gov/ and https://ec.europa.eu/health/human-use/legal-framework_en

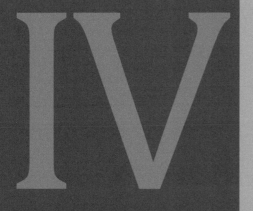

Part IV

Study Execution and Close-Out

17 Screening and Recruiting
    Participants   *178*

18 Obtaining Informed
    Consent   *187*

19 Collecting Data: Paper
    and Electronic Data
    Capture Systems   *193*

20 Follow-Up: Why It Is
    Important and How to
    Minimize Loss to
    Follow-Up   *203*

21 How to Close Out a Study   *214*

22 Knowledge Dissemination:
    Getting the Word Out!   *222*

IV

17 Screening and Recruiting Participants

Nienke Wolterbeek

Abstract

Recruiting and screening participants is often one of the most challenging aspects in the execution of a clinical study. Recruitment problems could lead to study delays, increased costs, selection bias, reduced statistical power, and eventually also early termination of the study. As each study is different and varies in screening complexity, each study needs its own approach. It is important to create not only an effective recruitment and screening setting but also an ethical one that complies with all the applicable regulations. This chapter will help investigators to address recruitment and screening issues in advance. The aspects that are discussed are definitions of recruitment, prescreening and study screening, barriers for inclusion, ethical considerations, how to improve recruitment and screening, and practical applications. Also, a number of practical tips about the target population, a recruitment plan, different contact methods, screening mechanisms, automatic screening alerts, different study designs, and a checklist are presented.

Keywords: recruitment, prescreening, study screening, participants, inclusion

17.1 Introduction

Performing clinical studies is impossible without the help of willing participants. At the same time, recruiting these participants is often one of the most challenging aspects in the execution of a clinical study. Recruitment problems could lead to study delays, increased costs, selection bias, reduced statistical power, and eventually also early termination of the study.[1]

Study recruitment is often not discussed; however, it is worthwhile to think of a strategy in advance and evaluate it regularly throughout the study to secure enrollment timelines. As each study is different and varies in screening complexity, each study needs its own approach taking into account the potential participants, participating study sites, study design, provision of information, and different investigators.[1,2] This chapter will help investigators to address recruitment and screening issues before a study begins. Points to consider

and some practical tips and tricks, including a checklist, are presented to serve as a resource to improve recruiting and screening strategies when planning a clinical research study. The aspects that are discussed in this chapter are definitions of recruitment, prescreening and study screening, barriers for inclusion, ethical considerations, how to improve recruitment and screening, and practical applications.

17.2 Recruitment, Prescreening, and Study Screening

It is important to distinguish and acknowledge the differences between recruitment, prescreening, and study screening procedures. Recruitment is the process of finding potential participants by providing information and obtaining information on their interest and eligibility. Subsequently, prescreening includes any screening activity to determine eligibility before approaching the patient. During prescreening, available patient data from the patient chart are checked relative to the prescreening inclusion and exclusion criteria. Prescreening criteria consist of, for example, demographic or medical characteristics such as gender, age, diagnosis, radiological findings, and other medical or surgical history. To protect the privacy of (potential) participants, it is mandatory to only record a minimal amount of patient-identifying information necessary for determining eligibility. Finally, study screening is where there is interaction or an intervention with the patient to determine eligibility that would not have been performed if not for the study. Examples are laboratory tests to see if the results are within the required range and written or oral screening questionnaires for accessing private (medical) information. Study screening can only be performed with ethics approval and with the consent of the participant.[3] As studies vary in screening complexity, for some studies it is possible to determine full eligibility based on merely prescreening criteria prior to informed consent. For these studies, study screening is not applicable. However, other studies require a multistep screening process with prescreening and study screening steps to determine final eligibility. The required complexity needs to be determined separately for each clinical study and should be clearly outlined in the study protocol.

17.3 Barriers for Inclusion

There are several reasons why there may be a delay with the inclusion of patients. They can be roughly divided into three categories: clinician, patient, and system barriers.[4]

Possible clinician barriers that lead to low inclusion rates are lack of time (informing the patient and informed consent procedure), lack of motivation, limited resources, and limited awareness of the clinical study. Furthermore, clinicians may have concerns or feel reluctant about the time requirements, especially when recruitment has to take place during practice hours. Also, clinicians may not be convinced of the scientific value of the study.[4] Also, clinicians can presume that the patient does not want to participate because of, for example, old age, without informing them. Most of these barriers can be resolved by providing adequate guidance to the study staff.

Patient or individual barriers are mainly caused by experiencing a loss of control over decision-making and the experimental aspect of clinical studies.[4,5] Patients might feel uncomfortable participating in an experiment and feel uncertain about risks or side effects and the provided information. Furthermore, patients might not want to change their current medical treatment or physicians if necessary for the study. In the case of randomized controlled trials, patients might question whether a decision based on chance is as good as the decision of their treating physician. Adequate patient information, sufficient time, and attention for the individual patient might help solve these barriers.

System or organization barriers are, for example, the location or distance to the center, transportation costs, lack of medical or research staff, and availability of resources necessary for the research protocol. The follow-up frequency, time requirement, restrictive inclusion or exclusion criteria, complexity of the study, or impractical or inconvenient protocol requirements are protocol-related issues that influence the decision for participation.[3,4,5] During the designing and initiation of the study, these barriers can be contemplated and minimized as much as possible. Furthermore, a pilot or feasibility study prior to full-scale study implementation could help overcome possible system or organization barriers.

17.4 Ethical Considerations

There are several ethical considerations that need to be considered when planning and executing a clinical study. This also applies to the recruiting and screening phase. It is important to create not only an effective recruitment and screening setting but also an ethical one that complies with all the applicable regulations. There may be local differences, but generally the following points need to be considered:

- Ensure that selection of participants is equitable and appropriate for the study.
- Respect the privacy of participants; ask questions in a private setting and do not use speakerphone.
- Give an unbiased presentation of the study without misleading emphasis that makes the study more attractive.
- Avoid therapeutic misconception where patients conflate the clinical study with clinical treatment. Ensure patients understand the clinical study and that they might not benefit.
- When there is a doctor–patient relationship, be very clear why certain tests are being conducted and which tests are solely performed for the clinical study and are therefore not required for their medical care.
- Minimize the pressure on patients to participate. Allow patients sufficient time to consider participation without imposing time limits.
- Avoid conflicting concerns. Patients might find it hard to say "no" to their treating physician. Treating physicians might experience conflicting concerns between their clinical judgment and the pressure to enroll patients.

First contact with patients must be initiated by a member of the health care team directly involved in their medical care. The health care team can refer or hand off a patient to the study team with the permission of the patient. It is recommended to document this permission in the study and medical record of the patient. The person explaining the study should be thoroughly knowledgeable about the study, regulations, able to answer questions, and trained in the voluntary nature of research participation.

17.5 How to Improve Recruitment and Screening

There are several topics that can be taken into consideration when designing a new clinical study to improve the recruitment and screening of patients. In the following sections, a number of practical tips about the target population, a recruitment plan, different contact methods, screening mechanisms, automatic screening alerts, and different study designs are presented.

17.5.1 Target Population

Based upon the inclusion and exclusion criteria, you should identify the target population of the study. Ask yourself if there are specific characteristics attributable to this specific patient group and if you can use these characteristics for the benefit of the study. Patients are more likely to participate when there is a personal benefit, such as extended medical expertise, promising therapies, or personalized medical care. Other motivations for patients might be boredom, altruism, and confidence in their physician.[4] Therefore, try to identify what will be the most appealing for the target population and emphasize this in the information material.

17.5.2 Recruitment Plan and Contact Methods

When you know your target population, you can start developing a recruitment plan. First, determine how many patients you need to approach in order to be able to enroll the desired number of patients. Especially for longitudinal studies, also take into account a certain percentage of lost to follow-up, death, and voluntary withdrawal during the study. Determine the number of potential participants that the recruiting clinic typically sees in a certain period of time to determine if your goal is achievable. Conclude if you are able to perform a single-center study or if you need to set up a multicenter study. Then establish the recruitment timelines (▶ Table 17.1).

Second, establish how you can reach your target population, which sources can you use, and what their preferred method of receiving information is. Examples of recruitment methods are direct recruitment in the clinic, referrals from colleagues, advertisements, paper brochures, flyers, information letters, patient support groups, internet, and social media (▶ Fig. 17.1). Match the recruitment method to the target population. A good, attractive, and clear information package can help convince people to participate in your clinical study. Bear in mind that if the clinical study requires reviewing of an ethics committee, the information package also needs to be approved by this committee. After approval, you are not allowed to make changes to the information package without informing the reviewing ethics committee.

When sending an information package to a potentially eligible patient, use a good-quality envelope with corporate identity (logo), personal addressing, preferably not handwritten, and clear sender's details. This will increase the chance that the patient will open the envelope.

Table 17.1 Depending on the design of the study, recruitment timelines can be established

	Total study	Per month	Per site
Expected number of patients to be identified/prescreened	X	x	x
Expected number of patients to be randomized/enrolled	x	x	x
Anticipated end of enrollment date	dd-mmm-yyyy		
First patient enrolled date	dd-mmm-yyyy		
Actual last patient enrolled date	dd-mmm-yyyy		
Target goal for the site	X		
Expected conversion ratio (number identified to number enrolled)	x to x		
Number of months remaining to enroll	x		

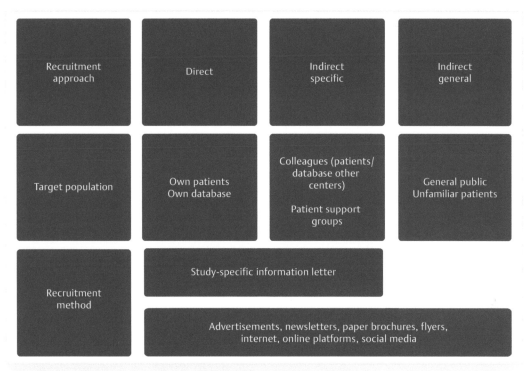

Fig. 17.1 Overview of recruitment approaches, methods, and target population.

In the envelope should be an attractive and clear information letter that encourages people to read. Writing a professional information letter is very difficult but well worth the effort to spend time on. The AIDA (attention, interest, desire, action) formula and BALD (baker able leaflet design) criteria are examples of available tools to help you write a good-quality information letter.[6,9] Also, most ethics committees or institutions have their own templates you can use. A few things to keep in mind are the following: (1) keep it short; additional information can be provided in a folder. (2) Make it easy for the patient to answer by providing a prepaid return envelope or reply card with the response address preprinted. (3) Create boxes that the recipient can tick instead of open questions. (4) Layout, color scheme, and content should be well thought through. Use the house style of the institute when available. (5) Specify when you will contact the potential participant again, for example, by telephone. By piloting the information letter on friends and family, certain pitfalls can be addressed before submission to an ethics committee.

When contacting patients by telephone for initial contact, prescreening questions, or conducting research (questionnaires), use a phone script approved by an ethics committee and adhere to the script as closely as possible. It is essential to speak clearly in a professional and polite manner and respecting the rights of the potential participant. Introduce yourself in a proper way and include the name of the center and department. Double check that you are speaking with the potential participant or designated representative and not with a family member or other person. Address the patient appropriately and never address an unfamiliar patient by their first name. You can also ask the patient how they would prefer to be addressed. Do not provide further information about the reason for your call to anyone but the potential participant. Always refer the patient to their treating physician when they ask for medical results or advice unrelated to the study. For privacy reasons, do not use speakerphone. Avoid leaving voicemail messages as you cannot confirm the identity of the person who will listen to the message. If you do want to leave a voicemail message, do not leave private or medical information such as diagnosis, treatment, or the nature of research. Additionally, do not use your private phone or protect your personal telephone number when calling patients. Because anonymous calls are often not answered, use a phone that displays the general number of the hospital, the number of the department, or a specific research number when calling. Another advantage of having the appropriate phone number displayed is that when patients call back after having received a missed call, they immediately reach the right person.

If using email to communicate with patients, the same rules apply as when contacting patients by phone; however, privacy issues are even more present. Use secure email and never include private or medical information that might identify the participant's medical condition or disease. Keep in mind that patients might use shared email accounts with a spouse or family member and that email accounts are easily accessible by third parties on the patient's phone or tablet as automatic logoff is not often used on such devices.

17.5.3 Screening Mechanism

It is advisable to develop a screening mechanism for what happens once potential participants are identified. Include a process to ensure rapid appointment scheduling for additional testing or enrollment in the study if required by the protocol. Each center is different, so determine the best way to include patients for that specific study site. How is the workflow, who is involved, who identifies eligible patients, who needs to be trained for screening? Ensure that all persons involved know the study protocol, the inclusion and exclusion criteria, and what they have to do with a potential participant. Do not inform only the treating physicians; inform the residents, physician assistants, skilled nurses, nurse practitioners, physiotherapists, research assistants, back office, and other health care professionals as well. Develop a training protocol including the instructions that need to be provided, who is responsible for conducting the training, and whether the training is given several times during the clinical study. Keep a training and delegation of responsibilities log that provides an overview of the training levels and tasks of the involved study staff. Posters with the flowchart of the study or pocket cards for the study staff might

be useful tools during the recruitment and screening phase.

Automatic prescreening with e-mail notifications improves screening efficiency and seems to be an effective tool to support clinical research coordinators.[2] Ideally, a screening module is built into the hospital information system. Based on inclusion and exclusion criteria, the study physician or research coordinator will then receive a notification about potential study patients after which they can verify eligibility.[2,7]

17.5.4 Study Design

The decision whether or not to participate, and thus the enrollment rate, is influenced by the methods and complexity of the study design.[3,4,5] The more complex the study, the fewer patients willing to participate. When a complex design is needed to answer the research question, it is advised to perform a pilot study to give an indication about a realistic recruitment plan. A different study design, deviating from the standard randomized controlled trial, could also be considered. Willingness to enroll in a clinical study appears to be higher for studies where both arms of the study have an active treatment compared to placebo-controlled studies.[1,8] Furthermore, it appears that patients are more willing to participate if they know which treatment they are receiving before giving informed consent, even if the treatment was randomly predetermined.[1] Therefore, consider alternative designs wherein patients, for example, are randomized before they are approached and inform them about the assigned treatment arm before obtaining informed consent or a randomized controlled study nested in a longitudinal cohort study. Although there may be other disadvantages, alternative designs might result in higher enrollment rates.[1]

17.6 Practical Application

Participants in clinical studies go through different stages of recruitment, prescreening, and screening.[2] The different stages are described below with reference to ▶ Fig. 17.2. To keep track of each point of contact with potential participants, maintain a screening log. In ▶ Fig. 17.3, an example of a (pre) screening and enrollment log is given, which contains basic demographic information, (pre)

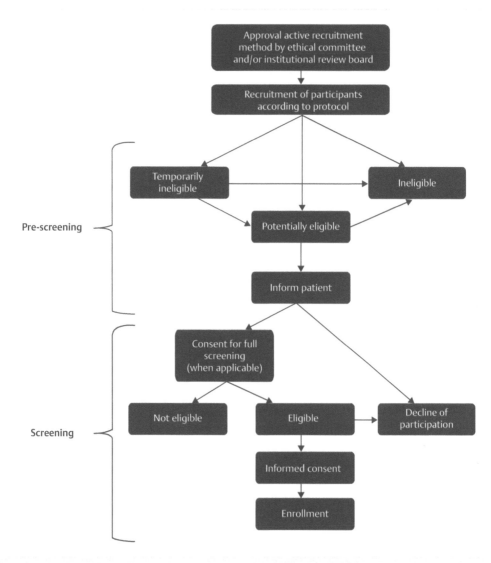

Fig. 17.2 Recruitment flowchart including the different stages of prescreening and screening.

screening date, eligibility, enrollment, and the reason if not enrolled. This log can be adjusted so that it is in accordance with your study. The log, when properly filled in, will give an indication of possible selection bias of participants and will demonstrate the investigator's attempt to enroll a representative sample. Selection bias is present when results of subjects in the study differ from what you would have gotten if you had enrolled the entire target population. Selection bias is often unavoidable, all the more reason to examine and

acknowledge possible selection bias. Consult with your privacy officer, ethics committee, and/or Institutional Review Board about which patient-identifying information may be collected for patients who refused participation or were ineligible. These logs must be archived in the investigator site file. Besides the study logs, there may be opportunities to record the points of contact into the hospital information system. Provide standard sentences for the different points of contact (e.g., identified, informed, and waiting for consent, sending

Site number		Study name	
Site name		Protocol number (EC / IRB)	
Principal investigator		Sponsor	

Subject number	Date of birth (ddmmyyyy)	Gender	Date of (pre) screening	Eligible (yes / no)	Reason if not eligible	Enrolled (yes / no)	Reason if not enrolled

Fig. 17.3 Example of a (pre)screening and enrollment log, which contains basic demographic information, (pre) screening date, eligibility, and enrollment. (*Abbreviations:* EC, ethics committee; IRB, Institutional Review Board.)

information package) and instruct study staff to always record their name and date when they add a comment.

17.6.1 Recruitment

Develop a recruitment plan and information package and include this in the submission to the ethics committee. After approval of the active recruitment method by the ethics committee and/or Institutional Review Board, you can start recruiting according to the protocol. Evaluate the effectiveness of the recruitment plan on a regular basis and keep the involved study staff informed about the progress of enrollment. When there are delays or enrollment issues, identify alternative strategies and implement these after informing the ethics committee and/or Institutional Review Board.

17.6.2 Prescreening Phase

In the screening phase, available patient data such as gender, age, and diagnosis are checked relative to the prescreening inclusion and exclusion criteria to identify eligible patients. It is convenient to have a research-specific checklist including these criteria. Only medical data already available in the patient file can be assessed without first obtaining consent. In some jurisdictions, it may be possible to add a "reminder" to the medical chart of a potential patient so that the physician can discuss participation during the next visit. If it turns out that a patient is not eligible for the study during prescreening, the study procedures stop (ineligible). If a patient is temporarily ineligible but there is a possibility that this might change, add a reminder to the medical chart or patient list and check this patient again at a later moment. If a candidate in prescreening is potentially eligible for participation in the study, the patient needs to be informed about the study by the investigator (or their designated representative). Inform the patient about the purpose of the study, study duration, follow-up schedule, all foreseeable risks and potential benefits, the patient information letter, when applicable randomization, and the inform consent procedure. Determine the patient's interest in participation and discuss that the patient is free to refuse study participation or to withdraw from the study at any time without compromising future medical care and that the confidentiality of the patient will be maintained at all times.

Always handle patients with care and approach the patients with generally accepted courtesy and respect.

17.6.3 Screening Phase

After being informed, the patient can decline participation, which means you have to stop all research procedures. When applicable for the study, patients can agree to full screening to determine relevant inclusion or exclusion criteria. It is advised to schedule a screening visit as quickly as possible. During this visit, the patient can be more fully informed about the study, the informed consent for full screening or informed consent for the entire study can be obtained, and screening data can be collected. Research procedures may not take place unless informed consent has been signed or a waiver of consent has been issued by the ethics committee. The process of obtaining informed consent and enrollment will be discussed in Chapter 18. With the results of the screening data, patients can be again divided into eligible or ineligible. If there are no additional screening tests, this step can be skipped and the informed consent procedure can be conducted for the eligible patients. After signing informed consent, a patient is considered enrolled. Informed consent forms that have been signed by patients need to be kept in a secure place in the study center. Also, informed consent forms of patients that are considered ineligible after full screening must be carefully kept. **Toolbox E** shows an example of a screening form used in a randomized controlled trial of two fracture care interventions.

17.7 Conclusion

Take the time to develop a proper recruitment plan and information package for your clinical study. Spending this time in an early phase is well worth the effort and will make a difference later on. Evaluate the effectiveness of the recruitment plan on a regular basis and keep the involved study staff informed about the progress of enrollment. Involve not only the treating physicians but also all health care professionals that can contribute to recruitment and screening to increase the success rate of the enrollment. Make sure that all involved study staff are properly trained and provide flowcharts or pocket cards describing the clinical study and study processes. Always handle patients with care and approach the patients with generally accepted

courtesy and respect. Ensure that study participants receive all necessary information before and throughout the research.

Definitions

- **Clinical study:** Any research study that prospectively assigns human participants one or more health-related intervention, such as drugs, biological products, surgical procedures, radiological procedures, devices, or behavioral treatments to evaluate the effects on health outcomes.
- **Recruitment:** The process of finding potential participants and obtaining information on their interest and eligibility. Recruitment does not require the consent of the potential participant.
- **Prescreening:** Identification of potential participants for a clinical study before approaching them based on available demographic or medical data in the patient chart. For prescreening, no signed informed consent is required.
- **Study screening:** Apply relevant inclusion or exclusion criteria specifically for the study in question to determine final eligibility. Study screening can only be performed with the consent of the participant.
- **Investigator Site File:** File that contains all essential documentation generated before, during, and after undertaking the clinical study.

References

[1] Caldwell PHY, Hamilton S, Tan A, Craig JC. Strategies for Increasing Recruitment to Randomised Controlled Trials: Systematic Review. PLoS Med 2010;7(11):e1000368
[2] Weng C, Batres C, Borda T, et al. A Real-Time Screening Alert Improves Patient Recruitment Efficiency. AMIA Annu Symp Proc 2011;2011:1489–1498
[3] Campillo-Gimenez B, Buscail C, Zekri O, et al. Improving the Pre-Screening of Eligible Patients in Order to Increase Enrollment in Cancer Clinical Trials. Trials 2015;16:15
[4] Grand MM, O'Brien PC. Obstacles to Participation in Randomised Cancer Clinical Trials: A Systematic Review of the Literature. J Med Imaging Radiat Oncol 2012;56(1):31–39
[5] Mills EJ, Seely D, Rachlis B, et al. Barriers to Participation in Clinical Trials of Cancer: A Meta-Analysis and Systematic Review of Patient-Reported Factors. Lancet Oncol 2006;7(2):141–148
[6] St. Elmo Lewis E. Financial Advertising. New York, NY: Garland Pub.; 1908
[7] Dugas M, Lange M, Müller-Tidow C, Kirchhof P, Prokosch HU. Routine Data from Hospital Information Systems

can Support Patient Recruitment for Clinical Studies. Clin Trials 2010;7(2):183–189

[8] Welton AJ, Vickers MR, Cooper JA, Meade TW, Marteau TM. Is Recruitment More Difficult with a Placebo Arm in Randomised Controlled Trials? A Quasirandomised, Interview Based Study. BMJ 1999;318(7191):1114–1117

[9] Baker J. Who Can Read Consumer Product Information? Aust J Hosp Pharm 1997;27:126–131

Checklist: Study Recruitment and Screening Plan

1. Design of the clinical study.
    - ☐ Determine complexity of the study: single-step or multistep screening process.
    - ☐ Identify the target population of the study.
    - ☐ Minimize barriers for participation.
    - ☐ Perform a pilot study to give an indication about a realistic recruitment plan.
    - ☐ Consult with privacy officer, ethics committee, and/or Institutional Review Board which patient-identifying information may be collected.

2. Developing a recruitment plan.
    - ☐ Determine how many patients you need to recruit in order to be able to enroll the desired number of patients.
    - ☐ Compare the sample size with the typical number of potential participants in a certain period of time to determine if your goal is achievable.
    - ☐ Conclude if you are going to perform a single-center or multicenter study.
    - ☐ Establish the recruitment timelines.
    - ☐ Evaluate the effectiveness of the recruitment plan on a regular basis.
    - ☐ Ensure an ethical recruitment and screening setting.
    - ☐ Define the sources of patients (e.g., database, clinical patients, referrals from other health care professionals).
    - ☐ Determine the recruitment tactics (e.g., database, chart review, contacting referring colleagues, support groups, advertising, social media).
    - ☐ Establish the preferred method for patients to receive information.
    - ☐ Create an information package.
    - ☐ Ensure participants receive all necessary information before and throughout the research study.
    - ☐ Create a recruitment log.
    - ☐ Obtain approval of ethics committee for the recruitment plan and information package.

3. Developing a screening plan.
    - ☐ Take into account center-specific issues or processes in multicenter studies.
    - ☐ Ensure rapid appointment scheduling for additional testing or enrollment, if required.
    - ☐ Develop a training protocol.
    - ☐ Create a training and delegation of responsibilities log.
    - ☐ Create posters with the flowchart or pocket cards for the study staff.
    - ☐ Create a research-specific checklist including (pre)screening inclusion and exclusion criteria.
    - ☐ Explore the possibilities of the hospital information system such as automatic prescreening.
    - ☐ Create a screening log.
    - ☐ Evaluate the effectiveness of the screening procedure and identify alternative strategies.
    - ☐ Inform study staff regularly about the progress of enrollment.

18 Obtaining Informed Consent

Chandni Patel, Nazanin Barkhordari

Abstract

Obtaining informed consent is a process that involves providing the potential participant with appropriate information required to make an informed decision about participating in the clinical investigation. The potential participant should be well informed regarding the research being conducted and voluntarily agree or be free to decline to participate in research without any undue influence or coercion. Furthermore, researchers should be aware of all the legal and regulatory requirements with regard to decision-making capacity. Finally, the language used during the informed consent process or consent documents must be written in a simple, easy-to-read, and understandable language.

Keywords: informed consent, informed consent process, informed consent in clinical research, exculpatory language

18.1 Introduction: What Is Informed Consent?

This chapter is intended to provide information regarding requirements for consent in clinical research that involves human participants.

Informed consent is a process in which a potential study participant is informed about the study and voluntarily agrees or declines to participate in research. It is crucial that individuals who decide to participate in research do so willingly after understanding all aspects of the research, particularly its risks and potential benefits and what is expected of them, as fully as possible.[1] This is known as Respect for Persons according to The Belmont Report.[1,2] The Belmont Report was developed by the National Commission for the Protection of Human Subjects of Biomedical and Behavioural Research. It includes information regarding ethical principles and guidelines for research involving human subjects.[2] One of the fundamental ethical principles of research is the idea that researchers respect individuals' autonomy.[1] Obtaining informed consent can result in either agreement or refusal to participate. As a result, consent must be obtained from the potential participant prior to conducting the research.[1] Researchers should respect the autonomy of individuals who decline participation and their decision not to participate should not negatively affect their care. Informed consent is required for all research that involve human participants, including but not limited to diagnostic, therapeutic, interventional, bioequivalence, social and behavioral studies and for research conducted domestically or abroad.[3]

Furthermore, extra care and thought should be given to potential participants who are not considered competent to consent (i.e., lack decision-making capacity) such as children, people with cognitive disabilities, people with dementia or delirium, unconscious persons, etc.[1] The ethical principle of Respect for Persons also includes that individuals who lack decision-making capacity should not consent to participate in research on their own.[1] Legally authorized representatives, persons who have the authority to make decisions on behalf of individuals who lack the capacity to make informed decisions, may decide whether it is appropriate for the participant to participate or not.[1] It should also be noted that persons who are not capable of consenting should give assent to participate, where possible. Assent means that the person is willing to participate, even though they are unable to provide formal informed consent. For example, many studies involving children require the child to sign an assent form stating that they are willing to participate, and their parent/guardian also provides formal informed consent.

The goal of the informed consent process is to ensure that the participant understands the purpose of the research and the risks involved in order to make an informed decision. As a result, the informed consent form (ICF) should be written out in language that is easily understood by the participant and also to avoid the possibility of coercion or undue influence.[4] Therefore, this chapter will also discuss the use of appropriate language for informed consent.

18.2 The Informed Consent Process

The informed consent process is not exclusive to obtaining a signature on a legal document. In fact, it is a process that involves providing the potential participant with appropriate information required to make an informed decision about participating in the clinical investigation.[1] The consent process begins with screening eligible participants. After a participant is screened, a research professional knowledgeable about the research project and capable of answering potential questions and concerns addressed by the prospective participant should conduct the consent process.

The location to obtain consent should be private and appropriate for the participant's emotional, physical, and psychological well-being. Additional tools such as brochures, videos, presentations, and decision aids may be used during this process to ensure participants are well informed regarding the research.

18.3 Voluntary Consent

The condition in which informed consent is obtained can influence voluntary consent. It is reflective of how, when, and where prospective participants are recruited, but most importantly, who approaches the participants has a larger impact on the voluntariness of consent.[1] Undue influence, coercion, or offering incentives to participants may affect the voluntariness of consent.[1,2]

The relationship between the prospective participant and person obtaining consent can have undue influence. A conflict of interest can arise if the person obtaining consent is in a position of authority.[1] For example, in the case of a physician–patient relationship, when the principal investigator is also the prospective participant's physician, the physician can influence the participant to agree to participate in the research project.[1] Thus, the physician should be careful when recruiting their patients for research. Particularly, the physician should place emphasis on voluntary participation ensuring the participant understands enrollment is completely voluntary and a decision to not participate in the clinical study will not adversely affect the patient's quality of care.[1] Additionally, other power relationships such as employers and employees, teachers and students, or correctional officers and prisoners can have similar undue influence.[1] Some jurisdictions and ethics committees require someone outside the patient's circle of care to obtain informed consent.

Coercive conditions involve a threat of harm or punishment by the recruiter in order to obtain compliance.[1,2] This is an extreme form of undue influence as the willingness to participate is completely neglected. Thus, the consent process should emphasize that participation is voluntary, especially if it is obtained by someone who can heavily influence the decision to participate in a study.

Recruitment incentives are another form of influence that can pose a challenge in determining the reason for participation. Incentives are vital in assessing voluntariness because they are often used to encourage participation in a research project. Incentives that are used to compensate for inconveniences and expenses related to the research project are distinct from incentives used to attract and encourage participation.[1] This is often the case for early phases of clinical study where healthy volunteers are recruited by offering a large monetary incentive.[1] As a result, information should be delivered in a way that allows the participant to voluntarily decide whether or not to participate in the clinical trial.

18.4 Consent Should Be Informed

Informed consent involves providing adequate information to the participant to allow them to make an informed decision regarding participation in the clinical study. This should involve an in-depth discussion between the research personnel and the participant and should address the study's purpose, duration, experimental procedures, risks, benefits, and alternatives.[1] The list provided in the following section includes the most basic elements that are required for informed consent. If a study does not include some of the listed basic elements, the researcher is responsible for explaining to the ethics committee the reasons why it is not applicable to that particular study.[1] Some additional elements are also listed that might be useful for research under specific circumstances.

18.5 Basic Elements of Informed Consent

The ICF must contain the following elements[1]:
- A statement stating the study involves research.

- Information of the researcher and funder or sponsor.
- An explanation of the background and purpose of the research, an expected duration of participation, and procedures involved along with subject's responsibilities as a participant.
- A description of all known and/or anticipated benefits to the participant from being a part of the research; a statement should be included if no benefits are anticipated.
- A description of all foreseeable risks, harms, discomforts, and inconveniences to the participant from being a part of the research.
- Information regarding voluntary participation that refusal to participate will be subjected to no penalty or loss of benefits.
- A statement regarding the participant's right to withdraw agreement to participate in research at any time without any legal obligations and details on the right to request to withdraw data or biological materials, including any limitations on the feasibility of that withdrawal.
- Details on the potential opportunity of the research findings to be commercialized, including the possible conflicts of interest that may arise on the part of the researchers, their institutions, or study sponsors.
- Procedures to be used to disseminate research findings and the possibility of the participants to be identified directly or indirectly.
- The name and contact information of designated research team who can provide answers to pertinent questions about the research.
- The name and contact information of the Research Ethics Board to address any concerns regarding ethical issues the participants may have.
- A description ensuring confidentiality of data, limitations to confidentiality, and anticipate use of data.
- Details of, if any, compensation or remuneration involved with participation as well as reimbursement for cost related to participation and compensation for injury.
- A statement indicating that by signing the consent form the participant does not waive any legal rights in the event that the participant experiences any research-related harm.

The informed consent elements from the "Tri-Council Policy Statement: Ethical Conduct for Research Involving Humans" have been used to generate the list above.

Additional Elements to Consider for Informed Consent:
- An explanation indicating potential risks from the treatment or procedure to the participant or the embryo or fetus if the participant is expected to or becomes pregnant.
- The foreseeable circumstances where participant may be excluded or participation may be terminated by the investigator without obtaining participant's permission.
- The possible outcomes of decision to terminate from the research and procedures by the participant.
- A statement indicating that the participant will be informed of new findings that may become available that may be relevant to the participant's willingness to continue participation in the research.
- The number of participants that will be included in the research.

In order to ensure the consent is informed, the potential participant should be given sufficient time and opportunity to process information, ask questions, and have those questions answered.[1] The research personnel and potential participant should exchange information and discuss whether the participant will participate in the research. This process can be time-consuming as it is dependent on the complexity of the information conveyed, risks involved, and where this conversation takes place.[1] The ultimate goal of this process is to ensure that the participant is well informed and comprehends the information presented to them.

18.6 Participants Must Be Free to Withdraw

The general principle of the informed consent process is that the consent should be voluntary, participants should be able to withdraw from the research study at any given time, and if the participant withdraws consent, they are entitled to request to withdraw the data or biological materials as well.[1] However, for some research projects, withdrawal without completing the study can be hazardous as it can compromise the safety of the participant.[1] In such instances, the consent process should lay out all circumstances in which participants cannot withdraw participation, data, or human biological materials.[1]

18.7 Consent Is an Ongoing Process

The informed consent process may require additional steps to be taken even after the consent document is signed by the participants. Depending on the nature of the study, the participant may require additional information and opportunities to ask questions and receive answers throughout the period of participation.[1,2]

18.8 Decision-Making Capacity

The ability of prospective participants to understand information regarding a research project as well as the consequences of their decision to participate or not to participate is referred to as decision-making capacity.[1] This is dependent on the complexity of the choice being made, the consequences of the decision, or when the consent is obtained.[1] The decision-making capacity can change over time depending on the participant's condition. It is determined based on the prospective participant's ability to understand the nature of the research, its risks, consequences, and potential benefits.

In order to follow the principle of justice, individuals who are not capable of making decisions on their own should neither be excluded without proper reasoning nor be improperly enrolled in a research study.[1] Researchers should be aware of all legal and regulatory requirements with regard to decision-making capacity.

In addition, a potential participant may be unable to make decisions in some respects but still be able to understand the importance of research and decide whether to participate in certain types of research.[1] Thus, the researcher should accept the wishes of that individual with regard to participation.[1] Some of the individuals that are partially capable of making a decision for themselves are the following:

- Individuals whose decision-making capacity has not been completely developed, for example, children whose capacity for judgment and self-direction is still maturing.

- Individuals with disappearing or fluctuating decision-making capacity in comparison to when they were once able to make independent decisions regarding informed consent.
- Individuals with partially developed decision-making capacity, for example, those living with permanent cognitive impairment.

18.9 Language Understandable to the Participant and the Legally Authorized Representative

The language used during the informed consent process and in the consent documents must be written in simple, easy-to-read, and understandable language. The language should be nontechnical, similar to language used in newspaper or general circulation magazine.[4] It should be written using second person and in professional but conventional language. Any scientific, technical, or medical terms used should be defined in the consent document or explained in simple terms.[4] For example, words like "placebo" should be explained to the participant prior to randomizing the patient in a trial. It is suggested that language used for informed consent should be consistent with grade 5 to 8 reading level. However, the language should reflect the reading level of the individuals being recruited (e.g., minors).

The consent process should not use exculpatory language, which is language that appears to waive participant's legal rights, or releases or appears to release the investigator, the sponsor, the institution, or its agents from liability of negligence.[5] Exculpatory language is considered to be a language that clears an individual or an entity from malpractice, negligence, blame, fault, and/or guilt.[4,5]

The following examples are considered exculpatory language and cannot be used for informed consent:

- "By agreeing to this use, you should understand that you will give up all claims to personal benefit from commercial or other use of these substances."[5]
- "I voluntarily and freely donate any and all blood, urine, and tissue samples to the U.S. Government and hereby relinquish all right, title, and interest to said items."[5]

- "By consenting to participate in this research, I give up any property rights I may have in bodily fluids or tissue samples obtained in the course of the research"[5]
- "I waive any possibility of compensation for injuries that I may receive as a result of participation in this research"[5]

The following examples are considered acceptable language and can be used for informed consent:

- "Tissue obtained from you in this research may be used to establish a cell line that could be patented and licensed. There are no plans to provide financial compensation to you should this occur."[5]
- "By consenting to participate, you authorize the use of your bodily fluids and tissue samples for the research described above."[5]
- "This hospital is not able to offer financial compensation nor to absorb the costs of medical treatment should you be injured as a result of participating in this research."[5]
- "This hospital makes no commitment to provide free medical care or payment for any unfavourable outcomes resulting from participation in this research. Medical services will be offered at the usual charge."[5]

The communication process can vary from one patient to another when obtaining informed consent. Extra consideration must be taken when communicating with individuals who lack decision-making capacity.[1] The informed consent process can be challenging when dealing with this group of people as they might have a problem understanding the purpose of the research and their role as a research participant. For this type of population, the consent process should specifically address the needs of the individual providing the consent. The research personnel responsible for the consent process should be careful and consider all aspects of the patient's life and approach the participant with the best way to communicate with them.

18.10 Practical Application

Please refer to Toolbox E for "Informed Consent Form Template."

When obtaining consent from a study patient, it is important to have a clear understanding of the cognitive ability of the individual. The following example describes the challenges and proper way of obtaining consent from a patient with a history of Alzheimer's disease, a type of dementia that causes problems with memory, cognition, speech, and behavior.

A study coordinator was informed by the study principal investigator of a patient who wanted to know more about a new trial on a new drug for patients with early- to middle-stage Alzheimer's disease. The patient is 73 years old, female, divorced, lives by herself, and has a 38-year-old daughter who drives her to and from appointments. While reviewing her medical history, the coordinator realized that the patient had been recently diagnosed with middle-stage Alzheimer's disease, with low scores on her cognitive tests administered on her last visit. She was also taking a few medications for memory loss, blood pressure, and type II diabetes.

The coordinator met with the patient in the consenting room. After confirming her information, the coordinator asked the patient why she was interested in participating in the study. The patient's response was that she wanted to benefit from the new medication as she knew her cognitive behavior including her memory was rapidly declining. She mentioned she had difficulty remembering which floor her doctor's office was every time she had an appointment. Her daughter would have to drop her off at the doctor's office to ensure attendance. The patient seemed to be aware of her surroundings and could communicate relatively clearly. At this point, the coordinator believed it was best to consult with the treating physician and confirm the patient's cognitive ability in order to evaluate her decision-making abilities in order to participate in the study. The physician/principal investigator confirmed that in order to recruit the patient, there was a need for a study partner to be involved during the consenting process to protect the patient's safety and to ensure informed consent was obtained. The coordinator asked the patient whether her daughter could join them to go over the study together. She explained clearly, in order to protect the patient's safety and rights, a study partner, someone the patient has close interactions with, was best to be present while reviewing and signing the consent form.

The patient refused and insisted to continue with the consenting process without her daughter present as she completely understood what the study was about and was willing to participate voluntarily. The coordinator understood the patient's frustration and reminded her calmly that the only reason they were asking for a study partner was to protect the patient and everyone involved.

Even though the patient was not happy, she agreed to have her daughter involved as a study partner. When the daughter was back, the coordinator asked whether she would be involved in the study as a study partner. The coordinator explained the study thoroughly to the patient and her study partner and answered all of their questions. The coordinator also reminded the daughter to attend the study visits with her mother, as the consenting process was ongoing throughout the study.

18.11 Conclusion

The informed consent process is an ongoing process that involves providing the potential participants with sufficient information to allow for an informed decision about participation in a research study. This generally includes the research purpose, procedures involved, anticipated risks, alternative procedures, and potential benefits.[2] The participant should be given adequate time to review and comprehend information and be given the opportunity to ask questions. In addition, consent is considered valid only if given voluntarily; therefore, undue influence and coercion should be avoided in every aspect of the informed consent process. Participants who lack decision-making capacity should have a legally authorized representative provide informed consent instead.

Definitions

- **Coercion:** An extreme form of undue influence that involves threat of harm or punishment by the recruiter to obtain compliance.
- **Decision-making capacity:** The ability of prospective participants to understand information regarding a research project as well as the consequences of their decision to participate or not to participate.
- **Informed consent:** A process in which a participant is informed and voluntarily agrees to participate in research.
- **Undue influence:** This arises when the person obtaining consent is in a position of authority and may manipulate the participant to agree or disagree to participate in a clinical investigation.

References

[1] The Consent Process [Internet]. Government of Canada. 2018. Available from: http://www.pre.ethics.gc.ca/eng/policy-politique/initiatives/tcps2-eptc2/chapter3-chapitre3/#toc03-1d

[2] Office of the Secretary Ethical Principles and Guidelines for the Protection of Human Subjects of Research - The National Commission for the Protection of Human Subjects of Biomedical and Behavioral Research. The Belmont Report [Internet]. 1979. Available from: https://www.hhs.gov/ohrp/regulations-and-policy/belmont-report/index.html

[3] Nijhawan LP, Janodia MD, Musmade PB. Informed Consent: Issues and Challenges. J Adv Pharm Technol Res 2013;4(3):134–140

[4] Informed Consent in Human Subjects Research. 2014

[5] Exculpatory Language in Informed Consent. [Internet]. 1996 [cited July 30, 2018]. Available from: https://www.hhs.gov/ohrp/regulations-and-policy/guidance/exculpatory-language-in-informed-consent-documents/index.html

19 Collecting Data: Paper and Electronic Data Capture Systems

Esther M.M. Van Lieshout, Stephanie M. Zielinski

Abstract

A critical part of designing and preparing for a clinical study is making a list of all data to be collected. The official data collection sheets are called the case report forms or case record forms (CRF). Developing CRFs should not be done by a single research coordinator, but should be a multidisciplinary effort with input from at least the principal investigator, the research coordinator or investigator who collects the data, a monitor, and the statistician. A properly designed CRF allows for efficient and complete data entry, processing, analysis, and reporting. This chapter provides an overview of different options for data collection (from paper to fully digital) and gives guidance for CRF design. It also shows a list of electronic data capture systems available. The toolbox at the end of the book shows CRF examples that may be used for inspiration when designing a new study.

Keywords: case record form, case report form, electronic data capture system, database

19.1 Introduction

When conducting a clinical study, quality of the collected data is paramount. A perfect database is a key to efficient conduct of data collection, data export, and data analysis. In order to achieve that, one should collect all data needed for answering the research questions, supplemented with a number of items required that describe the population or intervention studied. Generating the list of data to be collected should therefore receive a high level of attention. Also, it requires a close collaboration with the principal investigator, a research assistant or research nurse, and the statistician. This chapter aims to provide an overview of different types of data capture systems. It also aims to provide guides for choosing the best system for your study and to outline the essentials to be considered when developing case report forms or case record forms (CRF) for a clinical study.

19.2 The Aim of Data Collection in a Clinical Study

The aim of data collection is to gather accurate data to answer the study question(s). Data should be collected in a specific format in accordance with the protocol and in compliance with regulatory requirements. Data to be collected should be mentioned in the protocol. For each research aim or question, the proper data should be collected, and each item collected should have a meaning for and be used in the data analysis. Do not collect data "just for fun" or "just in case you may decide later that you wanted to have it."

19.3 What Data Should Be Collected

The type of data collected differs between studies and strongly depends on the research questions. In general, there are only a few specific reasons why data are collected:
- The item is necessary for answering a research question.
- The item is necessary for describing the population or the intervention studied.
- The item is necessary for evaluating the quality of the intervention or compliance to it.
- The item may confound the association of the intervention with the outcome; knowledge of those items may be relevant for multivariable analysis or subgroup analysis.

Any items that do not fall into these categories and that will not be analyzed and are not necessary for safety or regulatory reporting should not be collected.

In a clinical study, patient outcome (either functional outcome or quality of life) will often be a parameter of interest. It may be the primary outcome measurement or a secondary outcome measurement. Patient outcome is often measured by using patient-reported outcome measures (PROMs).

These are standardized, validated question-naires (also called instruments) completed by patients to measure their perception of their functional well-being and health status. They can be generic, limb-specific, or disease-specific. Some generic PROMs (such as the EQ-5D) provide an index score, which can be used to calculate quality-adjusted life years (QALYs) that are commonly used in cost-effectiveness analyses. When designing a study and data capture system, it is important to carefully deliberate on the (dis)advantages of the PROMs that will be used, depending on the aim of the study. In general, it is recommended to use PROMs that are validated for the injury studied as well as for the language that they will be used in. This is especially important when performing an international study in countries with different native languages.

19.4 Source Data

An often underestimated issue is source data. The protocol should contain a clear description of what is to be considered as source data. Clinical data will be used as mentioned in the patients' medical files maintained at the participating site. In many cases, it will be necessary to obtain other data as well, such as other use of additional medical resources. Examples are physical therapy, general practitioner visits, medication use, or other health care facilities outside the hospital. If these are not available from the medical files, patients can be asked for the information. The official data-recording document or tool for a clinical study is called a CRF. The data can be collected on a (e)CRF directly, similar to what is done with all questionnaires. For monitoring and auditing purposes, it is crucial to mention in the protocol that these specific CRFs are also considered as source data. If there are inconsistencies between data in multiple places, it should be clear which source is "the truth."

19.5 Multidisciplinary Approach

Although a research coordinator will typically be in charge of CRF design, the CRFs are best designed using a multidisciplinary approach. At least three persons should be involved at some stages. The principal investigator should be involved throughout the process, and a statistician should be consulted in order to ensure that they can efficiently analyze the data after completion of the study. Should an electronic system be used, the software programmer should also be consulted to rule out any technical issues in the CRF. Depending on the type and complexity of the study, a monitor or other data entry personnel (e.g., a research assistant or research nurse) should also review that CRF before it is finalized. The latter is important, for instance, to assure that the data sequence is in line with the sequence in the source data where data are collected from. Often that is the patient file. Should the study be a multicenter study, other site coordinators or site (principal) investigators could be asked to confirm if the CRFs will work efficiently for them too.

19.6 Case Report Forms, Remote Data Entry, and Electronic Data Capture

Traditionally, CRFs were designed to be completed on paper, but currently the majority of studies use a digital system for data entry.

The first electronic systems became available in the 1980s and were called remote data entry (RDE) systems. These computerized systems were designed for the collection of data in electronic format. They typically provide (1) a graphical user interface component for data entry; (2) a validation component to check user data; and (3) a reporting tool for analysis of the collected data. RDE systems are installed locally on (portable) computers with a modem.

With the availability of internet, new generations of software have been developed. The currently used systems are called electronic data capture (EDC) systems. They provide the same type of functionality as the RDEs, but data trafficking takes place via the Internet using web pages. The use of electronic data capture is increasing. In general, the concepts for the design of electronic CRFs (eCRFs)/EDC screens are the same as those discussed for paper forms. Differences are that EDCs require screen review instead of paper review, and there is no need to print and distribute paper when using an EDC system. EDC allows for inclusion of validation checks, which research coordinators can use to monitor progress of data collection.

19.7 Datasheets on Paper versus eCRF

The choice for a paper or eCRF depends on the study population and setting of the study. Questionnaires in elderly may be better on paper, whereas younger patients may prefer an eCRF that they can complete on their computer, tablet, or even on their smartphone. It is a good idea to check this with the targeted population while the study is under design.

For a paper CRF, the font size, layout, and appearance are very important. Should participants receive printed questionnaires by regular mail, it is advisable to include a preaddressed and prestamped return envelope. A disadvantage of printed and postal questionnaires is that you will need additional administration to check if the patient returned the questionnaires in a timely fashion. Another disadvantage is that there is a risk that questionnaires get lost in the mail.

Data collected on paper require storage in a locked and fireproof cabinet. Both for paper and eCRF, access needs to be restricted to a limited group of persons who are entitled to access them. These persons should be mentioned in the protocol. They should also be mentioned in the informed consent form, so that patients will know that. International legislation such as Good Clinical Practice (GCP) regulates who is entitled to access study data. In multinational studies, it may vary across countries.

Although printed questionnaires and CRFs have clear advantages in specific situations, their drawback is that they require subsequent entry into an electronic database. This is often done manually, with all risks of data entry errors associated with it. As an alternative, DataFax and iDataFax systems are also available. DataFax is an EDC system with a hybrid approach that allows users the flexibility of designing a study by EDC, paper, or both. In the case of paper CRFs, the scanned document can be uploaded or faxed; the data are than read and entered into a database automatically. Most systems work with a barcode that identifies the CRF

section. In order to be without error, the answers need to be exactly where the software requires them to be, and any text answer should be written in a readable way. Although a DataFax is essentially much more efficient than manual data entry, some manual checks and corrections will always be necessary.

19.8 Examples of Available EDCs

Regardless of whether or not data are first collected on paper, in the end they will need to be entered into an electronic database (EDC). The choice of the software depends on the study design. Not every system has incorporated options for randomization or provides easy options for programming identical databases per hospital in the case of a multicenter study. Also, the more basic systems may not allow questionnaire completion by study participants directly. More advanced systems may allow connection to the electronic patient files; that allows automated data import from the medical file into the database (e.g., for data like laboratory test values or specific data like gender, age, or diagnosis codes), which saves time and makes the data collection less prone to errors. ▶ Table 19.1 shows properties of the most commonly used EDCs.

The ultimate aim of the database is to enable efficient data analysis. After the data in the database have been locked, the data are exported in a format that your statistician will work with. Most EDCs allow data export to SPSS, SAS, Access, Excel, etc. It is a good idea to check with your statistician if the export options are agreeable.

Multiple EDCs are available and the number keeps increasing. They vary largely in complexity of programming, user friendliness, and costs. When choosing the EDC for your study, make it a point to check if the functionalities match with the requirements of your study. Also check where the data are stored. GCP demands to store the data for 15 years (or 20 years in case of pharmaceutical studies), so you should need to have access to the data during that entire period. Ethics committees or hospital boards may have specific requests for this (and ideally provide in-house storage options). There may be costs involved in external storage of data.

Table 19.1 Ten commonly used electronic data capture (EDC) systems

EDC (website)	Website	Deployment					Electronic data capture features									
		Installed: Windows	Installed: Mac	Cloud, SaaS, web	Mobile: Android native	Mobile: iOS native	Audit trail	CRF tracking	Data entry	Data verification	Distributed capture	Document imaging	Document indexing	Forms management	Remote capture	Study management
CareRecord	(www.cleardinica.com)	+	–	+	+	–	+	+	+	+	–	+	+	+	+	–
Castor EDC	(www.castoredc.com)	–	–	+	–	–	+	+	+	+	+	–	–	+	+	+
Clear Clinica	(www.cleardinica.com)	–	–	+	–	–	+	+	+	+	+	+	+	+	+	+
Clinical Studio	(www.clinicalstudio.com/edc_software/)	–	–	+	+	+	+	+	+	+	+	+	+	+	+	+
(i)DataFax	(www.datafax.com)	+	+	+	–	–	+	+	+	+	+	+	+	+	+	+
Data Management	(www.deresearchmanager.nl)	–	–	+	–	–	+	+	+	+	+	–	–	–	+	+
DDI-mEDC	(www.makrocare.com)	–	–	+	–	–	+	+	+	+	–	–	+	–	+	+
Digitalis Clinical Data Collection	(www.digitalis-cdc.com)	–	–	+	–	–	+	+	+	+	+	–	–	+	+	–
LimeSurvey	(www.limesurvey.org)	–	–	+	–	–	+	+	+	+	+	–	–	–	+	–
Medrio	(www.medrio.com)	–	–	+	–	–	+	+	+	+	+	+	+	+	+	+
Mobile Data Capture App	(www.fluix.io)	–	–	+	+	+	+	+	+	+	+	+	+	+	+	+
OpenClinica	(www.openclinica.com)	–	–	+	–	–	+	+	+	+	+	–	–	+	+	+
QureClinical	(www.cleardinica.com)	–	–	+	–	–	+	+	+	+	+	+	–	–	+	+
REDCap	(www.project-redcap.org)	–	–	+	+	+	+	+	+	+	–	+	+	+	+	+
SecuTrial	(www.secutrial.com)	–	–	+	–	–	+	+	+	+	+	–	–	+	+	+
Simple Forms	(www.biopharm.com)	–	–	+	–	–	+	+	+	+	+	+	+	+	+	+
Square 9 GlobalCapture	(www.square-9.com/)	–	–	+	–	–	+	–	+	+	+	+	+	+	+	–
Viedoc	(www.viedoc.com)	–	–	+	–	–	+	+	+	+	+	+	+	+	+	+

Abbreviation: SaaS, Software as a Service.

Whichever system you plan to use, beware that in any case the system needs to adhere to guidelines as set out in the GCP guidelines (i.e., 21 CFR Part 11 Compliance), and at least have an obligatory audit trail that tracks in real time who has entered, modified, and accessed the data.

19.9 Case Report Form Design Guidelines

The concepts for the design of paper or eCRF/EDC screen are the same. A properly designed CRF allows for efficient and complete data entry, processing, analysis, and reporting. This section outlines basic guidelines that will help inexperienced research coordinators to design high-quality CRFs.

CRFs consist of multiple sections; the different sections are best organized and named in a logical and clear way. The following sections apply to most studies:

1. Patient characteristics/demographic data, such as age (or year of birth), gender, and race.
2. Medical history and medication use prior to injury.
3. Details of the cause of the studied condition (or injury), such as trauma mechanism.
4. Injury details (such as fracture type and specific items determined from radiographs) or disease details (such as severity, stage, and duration of complaints).
5. Vital signs like blood pressure, Glasgow Coma Scale, respiratory rate.
6. Details of the therapy or intervention studied.
7. General follow-up data collected at every follow-up visit, such as range of motion, grip strength, radiographic outcome, or number of physical therapy sessions.
8. Questionnaires completed by patients.
9. Adverse events.
10. Secondary (surgical) interventions.
11. Early withdrawal.

Sections 1 to 5 are often very similar across studies. Multiple options are available on the Internet, but you may also ask a colleague if you could use their generic forms. Depending on the study, some modification may be necessary. The sections 6 to 9 may be more unique to a particular study, although range of motion, grip strength, radiographic healing, general adverse event lists, and many more outcome parameters can be re-used across studies as well. When using a part of a CRF from another study, it is important to be critical as to whether it is complete and has enough details for the study you want to use it for. If necessary, adoptions should be made.

Designing your first CRF may be challenging. Below are some basic rules that will help you organize your CRF in a structured way. ▶ Fig. 19.1 and ▶ Fig. 19.2 show a selection of design examples. Sample CRFs that may be used for inspiration when developing your own CRF are shown in **Toolbox F**.

1. CRFs should have a unique header and footer that identify the study, the patient, and the date of collection. The header should contain, at minimum, the following information:
   a. Study or protocol ID.
   b. Site ID (optional).
   c. Subject ID.
   d. Name of form (e.g., baseline, vitals, comorbidities, questionnaire).
   e. Date of completion.

The footer should contain at least the following information:
   a. Name of study.
   b. Version number.
   c. Version date.
   d. Page number.

a

Patient study ID: OTC - _____

Study site ID : _____

Date of completion (dd-mm-yyyy) : ___-___-20__

b OTC study; version 1.0, date june 30.2018 Page 1 of 1

Fig. 19.1 Example of case report form (CRF) header **(a)** and footer **(b)**.

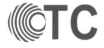

1. Height   ☐☐☐.☐   ☐ inches
                             ☐ centimeters

2. Weight   ☐☐☐.☐   ☐ pounds
                             ☐ kilograms

3. Temperature   ☐☐☐.☐   ☐ °C
                             ☐ °F

4. Blood pressure   Systolic :   ☐☐☐ (mmHg)
    (mean of 3 readings;
    patient in sitting Diastolic : ☐☐☐ (mmHg)
    position for 5 minutes)

5. Date and time of   ☐☐   ☐☐☐   ☐☐☐☐   ☐☐:☐☐
    hospital admission   dd   mmm   yyyy   hh   mm

6. Medication use   ☐ NASIDs
    before trauma   ☐ Analgesic opioid
    (check all the apply) ☐ Anti-hypertension medications
                        ☐ General cardiac medications
                        ☐ Pulmonary (respiratory system) medications
                        ☐ Osteoporosis medications
                        ☐ None; patient did not take any of these medications

7. Patient's living   ☐ Home
    status at follow-up ☐ Elderly care facility
                        ☐ Skilled nursing facility
                        ☐ Rehabilitation facility
                        ☐ Hospitalized
                        ☐ Other, specify _____

8. Was fracture healed ☐ Yes
    radiographically?   ☐ No
                        ☐ Unknown (no X-rays were made)

9. Comments (optional) _____
                        _____
                        _____

Fig. 19.2 Mixture of example of questions. Examples showing the relevance of **(1)** using a fixed format with(out) decimals (Q1–Q3); **(2)** including units of measurements (Q1–Q4); **(3)** defining measurements (Q4); **(4)** specifying date and time notation (Q5); **(5)** including the option "none' (Q6); **(6)** mentioning when multiple options may apply (Q6); **(7)** including the option "other" with specification in case the list of options provided may not be complete (Q7); **(8)** including the option "unknown" if a result is dependent on diagnostics that may be absent (Q8); and **(9)** including space for any comment that may be not be captured in the case report form.

2. Collect only data mentioned in the protocol.
3. Be clear with your data questions.
4. When designing a CRF, keep all users in mind:
   a. Provide important definitions to facilitate data entry personnel.
   b. Provide units of measurement where needed. Units of measurements may differ across sites or countries. This can be the case for laboratory tests (mmol/L vs. µg/L), height (centimeter vs. inch), distance (meters vs. blocks vs. yard), weight (kilograms vs. pounds), temperature (°C vs. °F), and many more. One solution could be to restrict data entry to one specific notation and ask data entry personnel to convert their units where necessary. A more user-friendly alternative (which is also less prone to error) is to allow all measurement units and to add a tick box for the unit used.
   c. Use as few abbreviations as possible, as they may have multiple meanings. Provide an explanation if applicable.
   d. Specify measurement guidelines if needed. An example is measurement of blood pressure, which may differ with the patient sitting or in supine position. Other examples are listing the requested minimum time between repeated measurements and the number of measurements that need to be averaged. This provides clarity to users and improves data quality.
   e. Specify the notation of dates and time as these vary across countries (dd-mm-yy vs. mm-dd-yy and 24-hour vs. 12-hour notation). A notation using three characters for the month (MMM, e.g., JAN for January) will prevent mistakes. Use the same notation throughout the CRF.
5. General data that apply to multiple studies can be collected in sheets that can be copied to other studies. Items like age, gender, comorbidities, other essentials of the patient's medical history, and medication use are collected in most studies. Ask your colleagues if they have a CRF section that you may use or modify for your study.
6. If data collected have decimals, space should be provided in the CRF. This prevents entry of data in too little or too much detail. Some software packages require programming of the number of decimals and characters allowed.
7. Provide fixed choices for each question, as that facilitates data analysis.
8. Make sure that every question has an answer option. For a list of comorbidities, for instance, always add the option "none." In other cases, "not applicable," "not done," or "unknown" may apply. If such options are not provided, it remains unclear if the question was forgotten or if none of the answer options applied.
9. Avoid free text responses as much as possible. Beware that they are more difficult to analyze or require processing by a statistician. Providing a list with fixed options and a supplemental free text option allows entering answers that you had not thought of during the CRF design.
10. Avoid duplication and ask every question only once.

19.9.1 Response Types and Coding

From the start of CRF design, the response type and coding should receive attention. Both determine how the CRF will look, what type of data can be entered, and how the content will be exported to the statistical file after completion of the study.

When using an electronic CRF or EDC system, there are multiple data types to choose from. Although names and appearance may differ between software programs, the most common options are given in ▶ Table 19.2. Some examples of how this is seen in an online database are shown in ▶ Fig. 19.3.

19.10 Conclusion

CRF design is a critical step during preparation of a clinical study. A poorly designed CRF will result in incomplete data or in too much data collected unnecessarily. A database that is based on a poorly designed CRF requires much work afterward, which is a waste of time and resources. A properly designed CRF is correctly and completely structured according to the patient workup and contains all necessary items in proper detail. It contains high-quality data that allow efficient analysis by a statistician. Answering the research questions based on a properly designed CRF is much easier than working from a CRF that requires a substantial amount of processing after the study is completed. Although it takes time to develop a proper CRF, it saves time (and thus money) at the end of the study and is certainly worth the initial effort.

Table 19.2 Overview of fields in an electronic data capture (EDC) systems

Field	Field description
CRF name	Defines the name of the CRF as it will be displayed in the user interface. A user performing data entry will identify the form by this name. It is best to include a short study identifier as part of your CRF name and specify the CRF after an underscore (e.g., TestStudy_Comorbidity).
Version	Version of the CRF; it is important for assuring you are using the latest version.
Section label[a]	Name of section in the CRF. When the CRF is accessed for data entry, each section will be a page.
Section title	The value in this field will be displayed at the top of each page when a user is performing data entry, as well as in the tabs and drop down list used to navigate between sections in a CRF. An example would be "Inclusion Criteria."
Item name[a]	The unique label or variable name for the data element. The first five characters should be unique within your study. Exporting data to SAS for statistical analysis often truncates item name to eight characters.
Left item text	Descriptive text that appears to the left of the input on the CRF; often phrased in the form of a question, or descriptive label for the form field input.
Right item text	Explanation for data entry personnel, e.g., measurement in supine position. Descriptive text that appears to the right of the form input on the CRF; often shows unit of measurement or supporting instructions for the form field input.
Header	Contains text used as a header for a particular item, e.g., Demographics or Injury Characteristics.
Subheader	This field can contain text that will be used underneath the Header, e.g., Comorbidities, Drug Use.
Column number	Data entry screens are set up by columns. By default, a blank value will put the Item in column 1. To have Items show up on a horizontal plane next to each other, specify column numbers 2, 3, etc.
Page number	To be used when CRFs are also printed for manual completion (optional).
Question number	Questions may be numbered consecutively. This is especially useful if parts of the CRF may be skipped after a specific answer (e.g., continue at Q5 if patient has no comorbidities).
Response type[a]	The type of input display you would like to use for a given Item on the CRF. It is different from Data type. Response type reflects the display on screen, while Data type defines how it is stored in the database. The following options are commonly used: • *Radio*. Round bullets showing the full list of answer options, of which only one option can be chosen for an item. Radio buttons cannot be deselected in the user interface once an option has been chosen. • *Single select*. Drop-down field showing all answer options, of which only one can be selected. This may be preferred if the list of answers is very long, but be aware that you will need to scroll down to the bottom to see all options. • *Multiselect*. Drop-down field listing all answer options, which allows multiple options to be selected at once. Always check with your statistician if this option can be used, as it requires conversion into options that can be analyzed. • *Checkbox*. Square bullets listing all answer options, which allow multiple options to be selected at once. Always check with your statistician if this option can be used, as it requires conversion into options that can be analyzed. • *Text*. A rectangular box to enter information on a single line that generally allows up to 39,999 characters of free text to be entered. • *Text area*. A multiline box for entering information over several lines that generally allows up to 39,999 characters of free text to be entered. • *File*. Allows a file to be uploaded and attached to the CRF by the data entry person. Often, there is a 10 MB size limit, but any file type is acceptable.
Response label	Create a custom label associated with a response set. This label must be defined once and may be reused by other Items with the same responses (e.g., Yes, No) and values.

Table 19.2 (*Continued*) Overview of fields in an electronic data capture (EDC) systems

Field	Field description
Response options text	List of all options to be chosen by a data entry person when they are entering data in a CRF
Response values	List of values that will be used as the values saved to the database for the corresponding options mentioned in Response options text. Lists of options are typically numbered consecutively as 1, 2, 3, etc. Commonly used standard options are 1 for yes, 0 for no, and 999 for unknown.
Response layout	The layout of the options for radio and checkbox fields. Options may be displayed in a horizontal or vertical plane.
Default value	Default text for Response options text. Commonly used for response type single select to provide additional instructions for data entry. For example, select one.
Data type[a]	This is the format in which the value is stored in the database. The following options are commonly used: • *ST (string)*. Allows any character. • *INT (integer)*. Allows only numbers with no decimal places. • *REAL*. Numbers with decimal places. • *DATE*. Allows only full dates. The default date format is DD-MMM-YYYY. • *PDATE*. Also allows partial dates. The default date format is DD-MMM-YYYY, so users can provide either MMM-YYYY or YYYY values. • *FILE*. Allows files to be attached to the item.
Width decimal	Specifies the width (the length of the field) and the number of decimal places to use for the field.
Validation	Specify a validation expression to run an edit check on this Item at the point of data entry.
Validation error message	Defines the error message provided on the data entry screen when a user enters data that do not meet the Validation, e.g., age should be >65 y.
Required	Indicates whether a value must be entered in order to save the data entered in that Section.

Abbreviation: CRF, case report form or case record form.
Note: This list shows the most commonly used items in an EDC system, but systems may have additional options. The exact naming of the items may differ between EDC systems.
[a]Completion of these items will be obligatory in most EDC systems.

Definitions

- **Case report form or case record form:** The official data-recording document or tool for a clinical study.
- **Good Clinical Practice:** Regulations and guidelines that describe the responsibilities of sponsors, investigators, and ethics committees involved in clinical studies. Their purpose is to protect the safety, rights, and welfare of participants and ensure accuracy of data collected during the study.
- **Remote data entry system:** Computerized system designed for collecting data in electronic format. It has a user interface for data entry, a validation component to check data, and a reporting tool for analysis of the collected data. These systems are installed locally on computers with a modem.
- **Electronic data capture system:** Computerized system designed for collecting data in electronic format. It is essentially similar to an RDE system, but data trafficking takes place via the Internet.
- **Patient-reported outcome measure:** Questionnaires that patients can be requested to complete. It is available for quality of life and also for specific anatomic locations like the wrist or knee, or for specific diseases like osteoarthritis.
- **Query:** A request for clarification on a data item collected for a study to resolve an error or inconsistency discovered during data review.
- **Source documents:** Original documents, data, and records. Source documents are the documents where the data are first recorded. These are often the patient's medical files, but questionnaires can also be source documents.

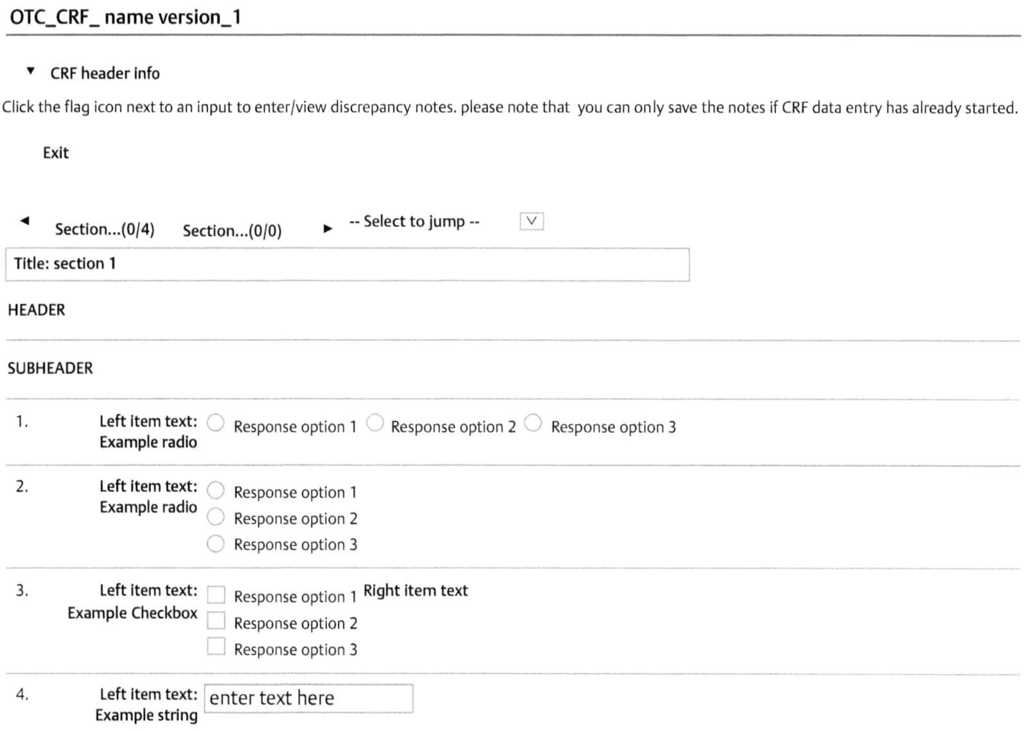

OTC_CRF_ name version_1

▼ CRF header info

Click the flag icon next to an input to enter/view discrepancy notes. please note that you can only save the notes if CRF data entry has already started.

Exit

◄ Section...(0/4) Section...(0/0) ► -- Select to jump -- ☐∨

Title: section 1

HEADER

SUBHEADER

1. Left item text: ○ Response option 1 ○ Response option 2 ○ Response option 3
    Example radio

2. Left item text: ○ Response option 1
    Example radio ○ Response option 2
                   ○ Response option 3

3. Left item text: ☐ Response option 1 Right item text
    Example Checkbox ☐ Response option 2
                     ☐ Response option 3

4. Left item text: [enter text here   ]
    Example string

Fig. 19.3 Example of where design elements appear in an electronic data capture screen.

Further Readings

https://en.wikipedia.org/wiki/Electronic_data_capture
ICH. ICH E6(R2) Good Clinical Practice (GCP) Guideline. http://www.ich.org/products/guidelines/efficacy/article/efficacy guidelines.html. Accessed June 29, 2018

20 Follow-Up: Why It Is Important and How to Minimize Loss to Follow-Up

Stephanie L. Tanner

Abstract

Adequate follow-up in clinical studies is necessary for the internal and external validity of the study results. Understanding the common reasons for loss to follow-up can help investigators properly design their study. There are a number of strategies that can be taken to help reduce the rates of loss to follow-up in a research study. Different strategies should be used by study investigators during the design phase, by methods center staff during study management, and at the individual study sites to minimize loss to follow-up.

Keywords: clinical trial retention, loss to follow-up, retention strategies, attrition

20.1 Introduction

Almost all clinical studies involve follow-up beyond study enrollment. It is at these follow-up times that the majority of the primary outcomes will be met. Therefore, for a successful completion of a clinical study, it becomes imperative to have adequate follow-up. Some loss to follow-up is unavoidable; however, there are many strategies that can be taken to minimize loss to follow-up as well as to minimize the effects of participant dropout.

This chapter will describe the importance of study follow-up on the overall conclusions of a clinical study. It will also examine potential reasons for participant dropout or loss to follow-up. Finally, it will discuss in detail strategies that can be employed to reduce loss to follow-up. Strategies will be described that should be applied at the time of study design, by the methods center during study management, and by the study sites during the conduct of the study.

20.2 Why Is Follow-Up Important?

Almost all clinical studies that include longitudinal follow-up of participants will have some missing data. This can be due to a number of factors such as participant death, the participant is "too busy" to return to the clinic or complete the questionnaire,

they no longer want to participate in the study, or they have moved and are unable to be reached by study staff. These are generally considered "loss to follow-up," "attrition," or "dropout" by researchers. While loss to follow-up is often unavoidable, it can significantly impact the results, conclusions, and validity of a clinical study. Both the internal and external validity of a study can be affected by loss to follow-up. It has been suggested that a 20% loss to follow-up can threaten study validity, while a 5% loss may lead to minimum bias.[1]

Loss to follow-up can reduce the clinical impact of a study and lead to incorrect conclusions. The overall study validity is based on the assumption that similar groups are being compared. However, if there are substantial differences between participants who are lost to follow-up and those who complete the study, bias is introduced. For example, a subgroup of participants may have more severe symptoms. This subgroup may be too sick to attend all of the study visits and thus become lost to follow-up, or the subgroup may follow-up more often than participants with less severe symptoms. Either situation may lead to systematic bias because the individuals who complete follow-up may be healthier, or sicker than those who do not complete follow-up. Depending on the type of study, adoption or rejection of the investigational product is a very important outcome. If a participant is not compliant with the use of a product or decides that the product is too difficult to use, the participant may withdraw from the study. This in turn provides a threat to the validity of a study due to systematic differences between those who withdraw and those who are retained in the study.

Attrition may also lead to a dataset being insufficient, leading to decreased statistical power in addition to the introduction of bias. In clinical studies of new drugs or devices, high rates of attrition can lead to, at minimum, a delay in reaching the required sample size. This in turn delays the time for the product to get to market and significantly increases the overall cost of the study. Attrition rates are also evaluated by the U.S. Food and Drug Administration (FDA) during regulatory review to determine what possible effects the attrition could have on the overall study outcomes. Therefore, if attrition rates are too high, submission to regulatory authorities may not be possible.

Finally, loss to follow-up can produce time delays. If the appropriate sample size is not retained, the study may need to be lengthened in order to enroll and retain enough follow-up to meet sample size calculations. This not only increases the overall burden of the study to the investigators but also causes a significant increase in the study costs. This extended study time thus leads to delays with the dissemination of data that are necessary to guide practice.

The problems arising from study attrition have led many investigators to evaluate both why participants are lost to follow-up and what strategies may be employed to counteract this.

20.3 Why Are Participants Lost to Follow-Up (Why Do Patients Leave a Study)?

It is a crucial principle in clinical research ethics that a participant has the right to withdraw from research. This must be respected to allow for patient autonomy and respect for persons. Researchers must actively plan to prevent dropouts and reduce the effects of the unpreventable loss to follow-up. To do this, researchers must have an idea of why patients withdraw or become lost to follow-up.

There are many reasons why a participant may withdraw or become lost to follow-up in a clinical study. Some of these reasons are completely independent from the clinical study and are unpreventable, such as non–study related participant death.

However, participants frequently leave a study based on the nature of the study design. Studies that require frequent or long in-person follow-up visits routinely have some missed follow-up and attrition. Studies that have cited reasons for participant withdrawal or loss to follow-up have most frequently reported excessive burden/demands of the study, competing life demands including (including time away from work or family), time required to travel to study follow-ups and procedures, cumbersome record-keeping, and lack of motivation or commitment.[2,3,4] Studies requiring additional visits or extended visits outside of the standard care may impede on the participant's work or family schedule. Visits during standard working hours often require the participant to take time off work to attend the study visits, which may lead to a reduction in wages. Additionally, participants may struggle with transportation to and from visits if private or public transportation is not easily available or if the research site is not near the participant's home.

One possibility for study dropout is a patient's perception of a lack of treatment efficacy or success of treatment efficacy.[2] If perceived lack/success of efficacy is the reason for attrition, this represents selective attrition. Attrition may also be related to ease of use of the study product or adverse effects of the product.[5]

Predictors for dropout vary based on the population being studied. It is important to understand your target population. In a study of patients with open fractures, factors associated with higher odds of study dropout included male sex, age younger than 30 years, smoking, high alcohol consumption, and fracture treatment in the United States,[6] while injury severity was associated with decreased odds of dropout. A recent review of loss to follow-up in the National Spinal Cord Injury Database showed that people who had less education, were non-whites, victims of violence, unemployed, and with no health insurance were all more likely to be lost to follow-up, while people with higher levels of education or who were more seriously injured were more likely to return for follow-up.[7] A large tuberculosis treatment study conducted in the United States and Canada showed that a history of homelessness, birth outside of the United States or Canada, and enrollment at a health department were factors associated with loss to follow-up.[8]

In general, researchers should ask participants who actively withdraw from a study for their reasons for withdrawal in a nonjudgmental and noncoercive way. Actively identifying reasons for withdrawal may allow investigators to amend their protocol to reduce burden, add additional exclusion criteria, or amend to allow innovative ways to collect study data. In the ICH (International Council for Harmonisation of Technical Requirements for Pharmaceuticals for Human Use) E-6 Good Clinical Practice: Consolidated Guidance, Section 4.3.4 addresses identification of reasons for withdrawal, by stating, "Although a subject is not obliged to give his/her reason(s) for withdrawing prematurely from a trial, the investigator should make a reasonable effort to ascertain the reason(s), while fully respecting the subject's rights."[9]

20.4 Strategies to Minimize Loss to Follow-Up

There are many strategies that can be put in place to minimize loss to follow-up in clinical research. Reducing loss to follow-up should be a concern for researchers from the beginning of study design and continue until data analysis. There have been some studies that have examined strategies to maintain study follow-up. However, most strategies are untested. Also, it is important to note that while some methods will be successful in specific populations, they may not maintain their effectiveness in other populations.

20.4.1 Study Design Strategies

There are a number of strategies that should be considered during the design of the study to help ensure a successful completion of a study and to minimize loss to follow-up. Many of these strategies are directed at improving participant selection and retention. Other strategies help account for unpreventable attrition, so as not to be detrimental to the overall impact of the study. ▶ Table 20.1 demonstrates strategies that can be incorporated into the study design to prevent or reduce the impact of loss to follow-up.

Identifying the Primary Outcome Early

The primary outcomes of the study should be identified early in the design phase and the study should be designed to meet the goal of answering the primary outcome. For most studies, participant retention is defined as meeting the primary outcome at the time point of interest.

Therefore, successfully obtaining the data required to evaluate the primary outcome of the study is directly related to the rate of attrition. Primary outcomes that involve extensive in person evaluations at extended follow-up times are more susceptible to dropout. By identifying a clinical outcome that can be easily assessed with a reduced burden to the participant, this may allow for the retention of study participants who would have otherwise been lost to follow-up. Incorporating follow-up alternatives and partial withdrawal options into the study design can also help address this. One example would be to define the primary outcome as a simple outcome that could be reliably reported by the participant via phone, mail, e-mail, or text message. An outcome such as incidence of hospitalization, reoperation, or hypoglycemia requiring treatment can reliably be collected from most study participant populations.

Inclusion/Exclusion Criteria

During the design phase of any clinical study, extensive thought should be given to the inclusion and exclusion criteria. The inclusion and exclusion criteria are very important to both the internal and external validity of a study by properly defining the study population. For the study results to be generalizable, it is important

Table 20.1 Study design strategies for reducing loss to follow-up

- Exclude individuals who are likely to be loss to follow-up:
  - Individuals who plan to move out of the area during the study follow-up time period.
  - individuals who are homeless or without a fixed address.
  - individuals who are uncertain about their willingness to complete follow-up.
  - individuals who are likely to become incarcerated (if your local regulatory approval does not allow for prisoners to be research participants).
- Study follow-ups should be scheduled to coincide with standard-of-care visit schedules as much as possible.
- If possible, select a primary outcome that can easily be obtained from medical records or by brief telephone conversations.
- Design the study to have as little of a burden as possible on both participants and study staff. Weigh the effort required to obtain a specific data point with the importance of that data point. Avoid unnecessary data collection that may overburden participants and research staff.
- Clearly outline the hierarchy of study outcomes so that study staff can assure that the most important outcomes are collected if a participant has limited time or interest.
- Conduct a small pilot study to assess feasibility of the study. Pilot studies can evaluate retention strategies, study burden to participants and research staff, and help determine appropriate frequency and timing of follow-up visits.

that the participant pool remain diverse and representative of the population. The inclusion/exclusion criteria should adequately encompass the intended population of interest. However, exclusion criteria should be set to help reduce the enrollment of patients highly likely to be lost to follow-up, such as individuals with no fixed home address, individuals who do not live in the local area or who plan to move out of the area before the completion of the study, and individuals who are not expected to survive for the length of the study (due to reasons unrelated to the study).[10] However, it is important that the study inclusion/exclusion criteria are not too stringent as to impede recruitment and limit the generalizability of the study conclusions.

Reduction of Study Burden

For successful completion of a clinical study, steps must be taken to reduce the study burden to participants, investigators, and staff. The overall study burden should be considered in the design phase of the study. The study burden to participants can be reduced by aligning study follow-ups and laboratory tests with standard clinical follow-ups or around participant preferred times, limiting data collected from participants to the minimum necessary to meet the specific aims of the study, and predefining outcomes that can be collected via phone or mail versus in-clinic visits.[10] Additionally, Edwards et al found that keeping questionnaires short appeared to increase response rates to postal and electronic questionnaires.[11]

Study staff education on the hierarchy of study outcome importance can also help ensure that the primary outcomes of the study are met. During a study visit, an observant study coordinator can quickly determine if a participant is reaching a point of burnout. In these cases, a knowledgeable coordinator can triage the outcome measures to ensure that the primary outcome measure is obtained. This can be especially important with collecting patient-reported outcome measures. If the primary outcome of the study is the score for a single outcome measure, the coordinator could ensure that the primary measure is completed first, and allow for the less important measures to be skipped on visits in which a participant is too stressed or overwhelmed to complete them all, thus reducing survey burnout.

Defining this outcome hierarchy or other processes for reducing the study burden in the protocol or study manual will help guide multicenter sites and research staff in the priority of data collection. One example to reduce study burden would be to allow for phone or mail collection of patient-reported outcomes if the participant has already met the clinical goals of the study. This would avoid the participant having to return for a follow-up that is not clinically necessary. Additional options could include obtaining permission from the participant to continue to collect information from the medical record even though the patient has withdrawn from active participation in the study.

The overall study burden to the site investigators and study coordinators will also affect study attrition. A high data collection load for an individual participant may reduce the motivation and time available for study staff to adequately build relationships with patients, and track down participants that may appear to be lost to follow-up. When study staff and investigators are overburdened with enrollment, follow-up procedures and data collection, they may also burn out and become more likely to drop out of the study, not enroll, or miss eligible patients in a study.

Sample Size

During the design phase of any clinical study, the sample size calculation is one of the most crucial steps that will determine the overall success of the study. The sample size calculation is completed to determine the minimum number of participants needed to show a difference in the primary outcome. Beyond just the sample size required to reach adequate statistical power, the overall sample size should always be increased to include an estimate of potential loss to follow-up.

Conduct a Pilot Study

A pilot study can be an important step to reduce attrition in a large definitive study. Large clinical studies take significant time, money, and effort to complete successfully. Data from a pilot study can help better define and clarify study outcomes, procedures, and follow-up times for the definitive protocol. Pilot studies can also help determine estimated compliance rate with study procedures and study retention. Specific study-related procedures such as additional follow-ups, additional laboratory or medical images procedures, and patient diaries can be evaluated during a pilot study to determine their effect on study retention. Pilot studies can also help identify subpopulations that may have a higher rate of attrition. This allows for the definitive study to include retention strategies targeted to those specific populations or in some cases include additional exclusion criteria for populations at increased risk of dropout.

Stakeholder Engagement

Early engagement of study stakeholders such as participant representatives (individuals with the medical condition, injury, or demographics of the study population), study site investigators, and study coordinators can help identify and navigate possible barriers to completing study follow-up. This is especially helpful in multicenter studies. As content experts, these stakeholders will have a better understanding of the intricacies of follow-up related to their local cultural, socioeconomic, and medical system barriers. Community engagement has been shown to be affective in the recruitment and retention of clinical study participants, especially in minority[12] and targeted communities.[13]

20.4.2 Methods Center/Sponsor Study Management

During ongoing multicenter clinical studies, there are a number of strategies that can be employed by the Methods/Coordinating Center to assist the study sites with participant retention. ▶ Table 20.2 demonstrates strategies that Methods Center staff should take into consideration while managing multicenter sites to prevent or reduce the impact of loss to follow-up.

Continual Monitoring of Study Data and Outcomes

While data monitoring is obviously important to ensure the accuracy of study data, continual data monitoring by the Methods Center or Coordinating Center is also an invaluable tool in maintaining overall study follow-up rates. Data monitoring should begin as the first clinical data are collected. While sponsors and Principal Investigators must continuously monitor study data to identify

Table 20.2 Coordinating or methods center strategies for reducing loss to follow-up

- Methods/coordinating center staff should continuously and actively monitor electronic data capture systems for missed visits and other signs of participant attrition.
- Staff should routinely contact clinical sites to discuss participants who have missed visits and help locate any patients with overdue visits as applicable.
- Select participating sites with trained research personnel, preferably with a proven track record of participant recruitment and retention
- Send regular updates/newsletters of enrollment and retention to study sites. Include helpful hints for participant retention or innovative ideas to prevent attrition.
- Obtain appropriate funding to offset the costs of the conducting the study and to provide appropriate participant incentives.
- Base study site payments on completion of follow-up visits.

In some cases, newsletters directed at enrolled participants that can be distributed by site study staff, once approved by the appropriate Institutional Review Board. Newsletter topics can include overall study progress, details regarding general patient expectations with the study, and any other appropriate product or study-related information.

potential errors or missing data, they should also be evaluating the data for issues with study follow-up. In the era of advanced electronic data capture systems, data validation can, and should be, conducted by the sponsor/coordinating system in a timely manner. Proactively monitoring study loss to follow-up can allow for protocol adjustments, re-evaluation of inclusion and exclusion criteria, or lead to the identification of innovative ways to maintain study follow-up.

20.4.3 Local Site Study Management to Maintain Follow-Up

While study design strategies and oversite by a methods center can help with participant retention, the bulk of the retention strategies falls on the site research coordinators. ▶ Table 20.3 demonstrates strategies to incorporate into study site management to prevent or reduce loss to follow-up.

Table 20.3 Local site strategies for reducing loss to follow-up

- Ensure that patients are fully informed and understand the expectations and potential burdens of the study prior to enrollment.

- Obtain contact information at the time of enrollment/informed consent from the participant. Also obtain contact information of alternative contacts for the patient, preferably at least one individual who does not live with the patient, but would have contact with the patient.

- Verify patient contact information at each follow-up visit and maintain open communication regarding any planned relocations.

- Continue to re-emphasize how the study will help future patients, the importance of maintaining follow-up, and the follow-up expectations.

- Be as flexible as possible to schedule participant follow-ups at times that are convenient to the participant. This can include scheduling study visits outside of normal work hours or at alternative locations.

- Remind participants of upcoming study visits. Letters can be sent to participants prior to their visit with information on where and when their appointment is scheduled, and contact information if they need to reschedule their appointment. If any special procedures, (e.g., laboratory or imaging studies) are required, this should be included in the communication.

- Make efforts to minimize the amount of time a participant is waiting on study visits. Capitalize on any wait times by allowing participants to complete any study-related forms or questionnaires during any wait times.

- Be familiar with the hierarchy of study outcomes, and prioritize the most important outcome measures to reduce the participant burden.

- Maintain regular contact with participants. Document all attempts to contact participants, including whether the attempt was successful and what contact method (mailing address, phone number, and time of day) was used. If there is a large time period between required study visits, attempt to make contact with participants during this time to ensure correct contact information.
  - Add personalized touches to the participant communication (i.e., birthday cards, holiday card, graduation cards, etc.).

- Make notes of special events for each patient to help maintain a personal connection. These can include upcoming vacations, expected celebrations (weddings, births, etc.).

- Contact participants and alternative contacts by telephone both during normal work hours and afterhours. Use all options for contacting participants and alternative contacts (telephone, SMS messaging, postal mail, e-mail, etc.).

- Depending on the specific study, do not mark patients as loss to follow-up until you have exhausted all options to re-contact the individual and you have reached the end of the study follow-up. Continue to try to call phone numbers that have been disconnected. Continually check participant medical record to determine if any additional visits have occurred, or if patient contact information has been updated. Often in clinical research, a patient who appears to be lost to follow-up may show up in clinics for other reasons.

- Search obituaries and social security death indexes for participants who have missed visits prior to marking them as loss to follow-up. Inmate database searchers may also be helpful. Other internet search engines can also be used to obtain information on missing participants. Some researchers have subscribed to search engines that help track individuals if budgets allow.

- If a participant asks to withdraw from the study because of excess study burden, ask the participant if they are willing to participate in the study in a limited capacity (i.e., allowing for adverse-event monitoring, answering limited study questions). At minimum, ask the participant for consent to access their medical records to monitor for clinical data (as allowed by local regulations/approvals).

- Continue to try to make contact with participants after missed visits even if it does not fall into a study follow-up window. Out-of-window follow-up is generally preferred to a missed follow-up.

- If possible, budget for patient incentives. Monetary incentives such as checks or gift cards can help participants offset the costs of missing work or travel to and from the follow-up visits. Nonmonetary incentives, such as coffee mugs or ink pens with the study logo, can provide a reminder of the study and may help provide a sense of ownership or belonging with the study.

- When possible, assign one investigator and one research coordinator to each patient, and try to keep this consistent throughout the study. This allows the research coordinator and the investigator to build a relationship with the participant.

- Research coordinators and other study staff should have strong interpersonal skills and be culturally sensitive and empathetic toward participants.

- Respectfully inquire with participants who wish to withdraw to determine if there are any obstacles that could be addressed to reduce participant attrition.

Subject Selection and Informed Consent

Individual patient retention strategies begin during the participant screening and informed consent process. During participant recruitment, the potential participant may perceive the benefits of participation in the study, including access to new drugs, innovative devices, or even the prospect of "free" or additional clinical visits or medical evaluations. In situations where the investigator is the patient's current treating physicians, some participants will agree to participate to please their physician or care provider.

The screening process and informed consent process should make it clear to individual that participation is completely voluntary and that if they decide not to participate it will not affect the relationship with their physician or care provider. The potential participant should also completely understand what their participation will entail. The individual obtaining informed consent and enrolling the patient should ask the participant questions to help assess a participant's understanding of the requirements of a study. Will they be able to attend all required follow-up visits? Will they be able to take the drug as prescribed? Do they understand the time and effort that it will take to complete a study diary or required laboratory tests? Will they be able to maintain this schedule for the length of the study? Extra care should be taken with individuals who appear hesitant or uncertain about study participation. Anecdotally, these patients are more likely to not return for study visits. As study staff and investigators, we often feel compelled to enroll as many patients as possible. However, for almost all studies, it is less detrimental to the overall study to not enroll an individual than it is to enroll an individual only for them to become lost to follow-up.

Data Monitoring and Quality Control

While most study staff identify data monitoring and quality control as the sponsor's responsibility, it is also important for site study staff to continuously monitor their own data completion and participant follow-up to ensure the accurate collection of data. As research coordinators, it is very easy to become overwhelmed with too many studies and too many patients to keep close contact with all study patients. Local study staff should have processes in place to stay on top of study follow-up. Multiple current electronic medical record (EMR) systems have the capability to track clinical study participants and notify study staff of research follow-ups or unplanned emergency department visits. Clinical trial management software (CTMS) programs can assist with flagging study windows to help study staff identify which study visits have been completed or missed and when study visits are required. Simple spreadsheet programs can also allow active tracking of study follow-ups. Even without these technological advancements, study staff should be actively tracking study follow-ups to not only ensure that all participants are scheduled and/or contacted during appropriate study windows, but also to ensure that all attempts to contact the participant are documented. Telephone logs or patient contact tracking sheets should accompany local study files to provide documentation of all attempts to reach study participants.

Reducing Study Burden

Reducing the study burden on an individual patient can often be achieved by local study staff. With empathy and understanding, study staff can often identify when a participant is becoming overburdened. By having a strong understanding of the study protocol and study procedures, a study coordinator will understand the hierarchy of study assessments and procedures. This can allow the study coordinator to take steps to reduce the burden to the participant while obtaining primary outcome data. Many times a participant would rather complete any study questionnaire independently if they just do not feel like talking. However, some participants respond better to being verbally asked each question by an interviewer.

Sometimes when a participant is in a hurry, study questionnaires can be sent home with the participant with a preaddressed, stamped envelope for them to return the questionnaires when they have time. While this is not ideal, the delayed return of the questionnaires is better than the questionnaires being completely missed.

An often underestimated point of frustration for study participants is the wait times for study follow-up or inconvenience of available study follow-up times. This is most common in research studies conducted during normal clinical hours. Study staff should also be aware of clinic wait times and schedules, and work to reduce the overall wait time for research participants when possible. Some research clinics have created special office times for research participants, including afterhours visit times to be more convenient for working individuals. When follow-ups are to be conducted over the phone, discussion with the participant regarding the best time to call should occur early on in the study. Laborers, health care workers, and school teachers may be unable to answer a phone call during their normal working hours. This may require afterhours or lunch time phone calls so as not to bother the participant during work or meeting the participant at alternative follow-up locations.

When suitable to the clinic or research setting, patient-reported outcomes can often be completed by the participant during the time that they are in a waiting room or exam room. When study participants are being followed in a standard clinical care setting, study staff should be available to meet with the study participant at (or immediately before) the scheduled clinical visit time. This allows the study staff to take advantage of the down time while the participant is waiting to see the clinician. If appropriate to the study or flow of the clinic environment, certain appointment times can be blocked for research only visits. This may allow for the additional time needed for a research study follow-up.

When possible, allowing for electronic, mail, or phone follow-ups to collect outcome data may reduce the overall study burden for individuals who find it difficult to return for in-clinic visits. Each of these methods may have different follow-up rates that may be affected by the demographics of the study population. In hand surgery research, Nota and colleagues reported a significantly better response rate with phone follow-ups versus electronic or postal mail.[14] In our experience, a mixed method combining multiple available follow-up platforms is almost always necessary to obtain complete follow-up.

Communication Strategies between Participants and Research Staff

A thorough and continued informed consent process is essential to setting up strong communication between study participants and study staff. Continued open communication about study requirements and expectations keeps everyone actively engaged. In addition to reminder letters/phone calls before scheduled study visits, phone calls prior to mailing questionnaires have been shown to increase follow-up and response rates.[11,15]

Research staff should routinely update participant contact information at each visit to ensure that study staff have the correct and most up-to-date phone number, -email address, and mailing address for the participant. It is also important to collect the name and contact information for at least one relative or friend of the participant who does not live with the participant. This allows additional options to help locate an individual if they move or if they are otherwise unable to be reached. One study showed that 51% of orthopaedic patients changed at least one element of their contact information in the last 5 years.[16]

Finding Missing Participants

When study participants begin to miss follow-up visits, and steps have been exhausted in trying to reach the participant through their contact information and their alternative contacts, there are additional steps that a research coordinator can take to attempt to locate missing study participants. A current medical record search should be conducted to determine if new contact information is available or if the participant has returned for an unrelated reason. Online obituary and Social Security Death Index searches should be conducted to see if the participant has died since study enrollment. Many jurisdictions have online databases listing current inmates that are easily searchable if there is reason to believe that the participant may now be incarcerated. Standard search engines can often locate persons through phone and address listings and property searches. Finally, there are a number of more advanced search engines that are available for a fee that can assist in locating these individuals.

Relationships

One of the hardest retention interventions to measure is the relationship between the patient and the investigator and/or study staff. This is where the study coordinators become invaluable. The relationships that we maintain with the participants in our studies must remain professional; however, they should also be genuine. While we are not only asking them to complete diaries and answer personal questions, we are also generally the face of the clinical study to the participant. Depending on the nature of the study, these participants are often scared, confused, frustrated, or hopeful. However, we can provide that listening ear that they need during a potential stressful time in their life. In a qualitative study evaluating retention strategies, study staff that interacted with patients put great value into the interpersonal relationships between study staff and patients.[17]

In today's health care system, patients can feel that they are just a number or a paycheck to clinicians. Study participants also often feel the same way. As clinical researchers, we must acknowledge and promote the autonomy of our participants. Some techniques that have been put in practice to maintain positive relationships with study participants can include follow-up phone calls between study visits to check on the overall status of the participant (not just for data collection or adverse event assessment purposes) or sending birthday cards or holiday cards. It may be helpful to maintain additional notes regarding issues of concern in the participant's life or significant life events. The simple act of asking a participant about their recent vacation or the birth of a grandchild will go a long way in making a participant feel valued as an individual. If a participant is following up with clinical investigators outside of scheduled research visits, the research coordinator should make every attempt to be available for that visit. While attending these visits is helpful to ensure that all adverse events or unanticipated events are documented, it also helps create a continuity of communication.

When approaching a participant during an enrollment or follow-up visit, the research coordinator should always introduce themselves and their purpose in talking with the participant that day. During follow-up visits, after the re-introduction, the research coordinator should use the first few minutes to connect on a personal basis with the participant. Questions such as "How was your vacation?", "How is your new child/grandchild/pet?", "Did you see the game last night?" may help reduce the anxiety that a study participant may have that day. It shows that someone cares about them as an autonomous individual. When research coordinators start the visit by diving in to the required study questions, patients will often feel less engaged and more inconvenienced.

20.4.4 Retention Strategies

Participant Incentives

Both monetary and nonmonetary participant incentives have been used with varying success in clinical research. Participant incentives are usually given at the time of enrollment or after defined events, such as completion of study evaluations, return of study questionnaires, or after completing the entire study. All incentives must be approved by the Institutional Review Board or Ethics Board and the value of the incentive should not be perceived as coercive.

Monetary incentives, such as gift cards, are often used to help study participants cover the costs of travel to study visits or to replace lost wages due to study visits. Monetary incentives are usually in the form of checks or gift cards. Checks can be restrictive in many situations, especially larger institutions, where check processing may take weeks before the participant will receive their incentive payment. Prepaid gift cards can be general and able to be used anywhere credit cards are taken, or they can be specific. Pharmacy or gas gift cards are popular in adult populations, while gift cards to toy stores or book stores may be used in pediatric research studies. When using cash or standard prepaid gift cards, research staff need to be vigilant in both documenting payments and protecting any unassigned gift cards from theft or fraudulent use. Automated participant payment systems allow for automated participant incentive payments on rechargeable gift cards. These automated participant payment systems allow for relatively instant incentive payment with greater regulatory control and reduce the risks of prepaid gift cards including fraudulent use or the participant losing gift cards. However, these systems generally involve an additional charge to the study site for the management and convenience of the system.

Nonmonetary incentives can include other gifts such as ink pens, coffee mugs, t-shirts, and glucose monitors. These nonmonetary incentives often contain the study name logo to also increase a sense of ownership in the study. These incentives can be used as part of the research study to increase study compliance (such as glucose monitors in a diabetes treatment study) or may be unrelated to the research study. Pediatric studies may use nonmonetary incentives that are geared toward their participant populations, including toys, books, notebooks, and journals.

The effectiveness of incentives as a retention strategy has shown mixed results. A systematic review showed that monetary incentives were consistently associated with higher retention and that a higher response rate was generally associated with a higher incentive value.[11,15,18] Conwell et al[8] showed that cash or cash-equivalent incentives were independently associated with a reduction in loss to follow-up. Additionally, non-monetary incentives have not been shown to improve questionnaire response.[18]

Another possible benefit of incentives is that study staff may feel more comfortable maintaining contact and thus more motivated to collect final data from patients who are being incentivized.[17]

20.5 Practical Application

In a research study involving fractures in the hand, research staff worked closely with the Principal Investigator and Subinvestigators to determine the standard follow-ups regarding these injuries to the hand. All investigators agreed to the proposed research study follow-ups and follow-up windows. It was determined that the primary study outcomes would be functional measurements at 3 months postoperative, and patient-reported outcomes at 1 year. These time points were chosen because 3 months reflected the time that most of the surgeons would allow their patients to return to full activity following this injury. One year was chosen because the investigators believed, based on their experience, that a number of participants would request for implant removal between 9 months and 1 year following injury.

Multiple standard retention strategies were put in place. Repeat phone calls, mailings, or e-mail attempts were made to reach the study participants to remind them of their upcoming appointments or to reschedule any missed appointments.

Soon after beginning the study, it was evident that the clinicians did not always follow their standard follow-up sessions. Additionally, it was quickly realized that a large number of individuals with the study injury did not return for the 3-month follow-up. It was hypothesized that these participants were not returning because they were not having any problems. However, without functional outcome measures, this would not be able to be proven. With a high rate of missed 3-month visits, investigators and research staff were worried that the 1-year patient-reported outcomes would also be missed.

Additional recruitment strategies were put in place. The investigators applied for additional research funding to allow for the payment of incentives to the participants for meeting follow-up goals. A modest incentive payment of $30 for follow-up at 3 months and a $10 incentive for completion of the 1-year patient-reported outcomes via mail, e-mail, or phone were decided upon and approved by the Institutional Review Board. Additionally, intermediate study visits were added every 3 months to simply assess for adverse events and verify participant contact information. The protocol was also amended to collect functional outcomes of participants prior to the 3-month follow-up. Participants whose injured hand had reached or exceeded that hand function of the contralateral hand were no longer required to come to an inpatient follow-up visit. Investigators and research staff also added additional follow-up discussion to the initial and follow-up informed consent processes stressing the importance of continued follow-up and that their relationship with the physician would not be affected by refusal to participate in the research project.

20.6 Conclusion

With little evidence to support specific retention strategies, limited budgets, and the vast diversity of populations, medical conditions, and social barriers, researchers must be aware of the problem of participant loss to follow-up and continuously try different methods and look for innovative ways to maintain participant follow-up.

Definitions

- **Attrition:** The loss of participant data (follow-up) over time in a research study. Attrition rates are often used to describe participant dropout.
- **Retention:** Keeping participants enrolled in clinical studies until the primary outcome has been met.
- **Internal validity:** The extent to which the conclusion of a research study is warranted, based on the degree to which bias was minimized.
- **External Validity:** The extent to which the conclusions of a research study can be generalized to populations outside of the study.

References

[1] Schulz KF, Grimes DA. Sample Size Slippages in Randomised Trials: Exclusions and the Lost and Wayward. Lancet 2002;359(9308):781–785

[2] Bush NE, Sheppard SC, Fantelli E, Bell KR, Reger MA. Recruitment and Attrition Issues in Military Clinical Trials and Health Research Studies. Mil Med 2013;178(11): 1157–1163

[3] Janson SL, Alioto ME, Boushey HA; Asthma Clinical Trials Network. Retention of Ethnically Diverse Subjects in a Multicenter Randomized Controlled Research Trial. Control Clin Trials 2001;22(6, Suppl):236S–243S

[4] Parra-Medina D, D'antonio A, Smith SM, Levin S, Kirkner G, Mayer-Davis E; POWER study. Successful Recruitment and Retention Strategies for a Randomized Weight Management Trial for People with Diabetes Living in Rural, Medically Underserved Counties of South Carolina: The POWER Study. J Am Diet Assoc 2004;104(1):70–75

[5] Resnik L, Klinger S. Attrition and Retention in Upper Limb Prosthetics Research: Experience of the VA Home Study of the DEKA Arm. Disabil Rehabil Assist Technol 2017;12(8):816–821

[6] Madden K, Scott T, McKay P, et al. Predicting and preventing loss to follow-up of adult trauma patients in randomized controlled trials: an example from the FLOW trial. J Bone Joint Surg Am 2017;99(13):1086–1092

[7] Kim H, Cutter GR, George B, Chen Y. Understanding and Preventing Loss to Follow-Up: Experiences from the Spinal Cord Injury Model Systems. Top Spinal Cord Inj Rehabil 2018;24(2):97–109

[8] Conwell DS, Mosher A, Khan A, et al. Factors Associated with Loss to Follow-Up in a Large Tuberculosis Treatment Trial (TBTC Study 22). Contemp Clin Trials 2007;28(3):288–294

[9] International Council for Harmonisation of Technical Requirements for Pharmaceuticals for Human Use. Integrated Addendum to ICH E6(R1): Guideline for Good Clinical Practice. November 9, 2016. https://www.ich.org/fileadmin/Public_Web_Site/ICH_Products/Guidelines/Efficacy/E6/E6_R2__Step_4_2016_1109.pdf

[10] Sprague S, Leece P, Bhandari M, Tornetta P III, Schemitsch E, Swiontkowski MF. S.P.R.I.N.T. Investigators. Limiting Loss to Follow-Up in a Multicentre Randomized Trial in Orthopedic Surgery. Control Clin Trials 2003;24(6): 719–725

[11] Edwards SL, Slattery ML, Edwards AM, et al. Factors Associated with Response to a Follow-Up Postal Questionnaire in a Cohort of American Indians. Prev Med 2009;48(6):596–599

[12] Johnson DA, Joosten YA, Wilkins CH, Shibao CA. Case Study: Community Engagement and Clinical Trial Success: Outreach to African American Women. Clin Transl Sci 2015;8(4):388–390

[13] McCullagh MC, Sanon MA, Cohen MA. Strategies to Enhance Participant Recruitment and Retention in Research Involving a Community-Based Population. Appl Nurs Res 2014;27(4):249–253

[14] Nota SP, Strooker JA, Ring D. Differences in Response Rates between Mail, E-mail, and Telephone Follow-Up in Hand Surgery Research. Hand (N Y) 2014;9(4): 504–510

[15] Booker CL, Harding S, Benzeval M. A Systematic Review of the Effect of Retention Methods in Population-Based Cohort Studies. BMC Public Health 2011;11:249

[16] London DA, Stepan JG, Goldfarb CA, Boyer MI, Calfee RP. The (In)Stability of 21st Century Orthopedic Patient Contact Information and its Implications on Clinical Research: A Cross-Sectional Study. Clin Trials 2017;14(2): 187–191

[17] Daykin A, Clement C, Gamble C, et al. "Recruitment, Recruitment, Recruitment": The Need for More Focus on Retention: A Qualitative Study of Five Trials. Trials 2018; 19(1):76

[18] Brueton VC, Tierney J, Stenning S, et al. Strategies to Improve Retention in Randomised Trials. Cochrane Database Syst Rev 2013;(12):MR000032

21 How to Close Out a Study

Kelly Trask

Abstract

Eventually all studies will come to an end and must be officially closed at each site. The process of study closure is shared between the sponsor and investigator; however, the investigator usually delegates closing procedures to the research coordinator. Regardless of whether the study is a large multicenter-regulated clinical study or a small retrospective chart review, the study must be properly closed. The number of steps required to close the study will vary depending on the study. Some of the steps will not be applicable and may be omitted. This chapter describes closing a study with an external sponsor and monitor, but the process is essentially the same for all studies.

Keywords: record retention, termination, final report, closeout visit, participant follow-up care, investigational product accountability

21.1 Introduction

When a study ends at a participating site, it must be officially closed. This process is typically shared between the sponsor and the investigator. The sponsor will conduct a final review or monitoring of the study data, advise the investigator of further follow-up commitments to the study participants, perform a final inventory and accounting of any investigational products (such as drugs, devices, or natural health products), ensure the Trial Master File (TMF) and Investigator Site File (ISF) are in order and all essential documents are filed, and advise the site on the required period to retain the study files.

The site is responsible for ensuring completeness of data for study visits that were conducted and for arranging continued medical care or follow-up of study participants if required. All case report forms (CRFs) must be complete and accurate and submitted to the sponsor. All data queries must be resolved. Study materials, investigational products, and biological samples and specimens must be returned, destroyed, processed, or stored as appropriate.

Study documentation must be complete and organized. Financial obligations must be met and accounts must be closed. All appropriate parties must be notified of the study closure. A final report and notification of closure must be submitted to the ethics committee. And finally, arrangements must be made to store research records in accordance with the contract, protocol, regulations, and/or local policies.

21.2 Reasons for Study Closure

In most cases, closing a study indicates that the study has been completed, that is, enrollment of participants is finished, all participants have completed their involvement, and all data collection is complete. In other cases, however, studies end prematurely for a variety of reasons,[1,2,3] for example:

- Preplanned analyses show that one treatment is better than the other, so it would be unethical to continue.[*]
- The investigational product is unsafe or ineffective.
- An unacceptable risk to participants has been identified.
- Inability to recruit participants.
- Funding is withdrawn.
- The sponsor decides not to pursue marketing and decides to stop the study.
- There are compliance issues at the site (with the protocol, regulations, or local policies).
- The sponsor does not comply with regulations.
- The investigational product becomes unavailable (problems with manufacturing/supply).
- The investigator or other key staff leave the site and there is no replacement.

Studies may be prematurely terminated by the sponsor, the investigator, the ethics committee, or the regulatory authorities. Premature termination may apply to all sites or just your site. If the study is terminated prematurely at your site, the investigator must promptly notify all study participants. The sponsor, the ethics committee, regulatory authorities, other participating sites, and the institution must also be notified of the termination, as applicable.

If the study is terminated while participants are still under treatment (taking study medication,

---

[*] Stopping a study early for this reason is controversial – (Adapted from Bassler D, Montori VM, Briel M, Glasziou P, Guyatt G. Early stopping of randomized clinical trials for overt efficacy is problematic. J Clin Epidemiol. 2008;61(3):241–246.)

using a study device, etc.), arrangements must be made for continued medical care of the participants outside of the study. The investigator may also have obligations for care even if the study treatment has been completed, such as transferring care to another physician or continuing to follow any adverse events that have not yet resolved.

21.3 The Process of Study Closure

Regardless of the reason for study termination, planned or unplanned, the process of study closure is essentially the same. The closure of a study usually involves an on-site closeout visit from a study monitor or sponsor representative. The closure process can therefore be broken down into three stages: preparing for the closeout visit, the closeout visit, and after the closeout visit. It is a good idea to have a standard operating procedure (SOP) and checklist for the study closeout. The SOP should be general enough to suit any study. You can use a generic checklist too, but modifying one to suit your study will streamline the process when the time for closure comes. There is a sample Study Closeout Checklist in the Coordinator's Toolbox at the end of this book (**Toolbox G**).

21.3.1 Preparing for the Closeout Visit

Participants

First and foremost, take care of your study participants. Review all adverse events to confirm they have been resolved or their current status has been documented. For some participants, the last study visit is the end of their follow-up, but others may require further care. Ensure that follow-up care is arranged if necessary. Make sure that all participant payments and compensation are paid in full and receipts are collected (if applicable). Have participants return any study materials to you. This can include unused study medications, medical devices, specimen containers, personal logs, or study diaries. Finally, review contact information for participants in the event that new information becomes available after your site closes.

Data

Make sure that documentation for all visits is complete. Review the CRFs. Ensure that all CRFs are complete and accurately reflect the information in your source documents. Have the investigator sign the CRFs if necessary. Make sure that all CRFs have been submitted to the sponsor. In addition to CRFs, collect and submit any other required data: X-rays, electrocardiograms (ECGs), lab reports, etc. Respond to any open queries and requests for data clarification prior to the closeout visit. Have source documents and medical records available for review during the closeout visit.

Biological Samples

Ensure that all biological samples or specimens have been appropriately processed and analyzed or shipped to the sponsor. Arrange for and document destruction of any unused samples. If samples are to be stored for future use, ensure they are appropriately labeled and stored in accordance with local policies.

Reporting

Ensure that all adverse events have been reported as required to the sponsor and the ethics committee. Also check that any reports from the sponsor (e.g., safety reports, progress reports) have been submitted to the ethics committee and that you have submitted any protocol deviations.

Investigational Product

The investigator is responsible for accountability of investigational products. If the study involved an investigational drug, medical device, or natural health product, ensure that all product has been accounted for, whether it was used, unused, returned, or destroyed. If records have been maintained elsewhere during the study (e.g., pharmacy), notify the responsible person to prepare those documents for closeout.

Trial Master File/Investigator Site File

Ensure that all essential documents are filed. Refer to checklists provided by the sponsor or to applicable Good Clinical Practice standards for a list of essential study documents.[4,5] Presumably the TMF/ISF has been maintained throughout the study, so focus on everything since the last monitoring visit. This would include amendments to study documents and their approvals, the annual approval and other communications from the ethics committee. Correspondence from the sponsor should be filed. Make sure all study logs have been updated (e.g., screening, training, and the delegation of authority log). Also review the previous monitor letter to ensure all action items have been addressed.

Other Parties

Many studies are collaborative efforts within an institution. If other departments have been involved, let them know of the upcoming closeout visit. Ensure that any outstanding study invoices between departments have been paid from the study budget. Facilitate the return of any study equipment that was provided for use during the study (e.g., the lab may have been loaned a centrifuge to process study blood samples). Confirm that equipment and records will be available if necessary during the closeout visit (e.g., calibration and maintenance records for hospital-owned equipment).

Administrative Duties

The research coordinator is typically tasked with arranging the closeout visit, which includes scheduling a time that is acceptable to all required parties—the research coordinator, the investigator, and the monitor at the least. It is possible that others may need to be included, such as pharmacy or laboratory staff and other subinvestigators. Like all monitoring visits, the monitor will need space to review the study files and may need to access participant medical records if there are new participants, visits, or adverse events to monitor.

21.4 The Closeout Visit

The closeout visit is very much like every other monitoring visit, with one exciting difference—it is the last one! If there have been any new participants recruited since the last monitoring visit, the monitor will review informed consents. Any new study visits will be monitored and source documents reviewed. CRFs will be reviewed for completeness and accuracy and to ensure that corrections have been made appropriately. The monitor will confirm that any previous action items or queries have been addressed and will review any new queries that arise.

The monitor will complete a final reconciliation of investigational products (e.g., study drug). The monitor should instruct you on the final disposition of the products. Are they to be destroyed or returned to the sponsor? Product may be packaged and shipped during the visit or instructions may be left for you to do it after the visit. If the product is to be destroyed by the investigator's site, make sure that is documented and filed in the TMF/ISF.

The monitor should also instruct you on what to do with other study materials. Is equipment to be returned or kept? If equipment includes a computer or laptop, be sure to check your local policies—there may be privacy concerns to address before shipping. Also ask about unused materials such as blank CRFs or binders. Are they to be disposed of or returned to the sponsor? If you are disposing of materials, are there any special considerations such as recycling or destruction of confidential information? Other supplies may have been provided, such as blood collection tubes or shipping boxes. Must they be returned or can they be kept for other use?

The monitor will review the ISF to ensure all essential documents are filed. If study documents had not previously been retrieved from other departments (e.g., pharmacy), this is the time to retrieve them and file them in the ISF.

Some documents may have to remain with their respective departments. For example, pharmacy is required to keep a temperature log for drug storage, but they may not keep a separate log for each study. In this case, you may need to obtain a certified copy for your file or ensure that the original will be retained for the required length of time and record the location in the TMF/ISF. Maintenance and calibration records for hospital-owned equipment are another example. You will not likely keep the original records for these in your ISF, but in the event of a regulatory inspection they should be available to you. Know the location and document it in the ISF and discuss the retention period for the original record with the relevant department and your monitor.

Finally, the monitor will meet with the investigator to review the closeout procedures that have been completed and anything else that must be done. The monitor will provide direction from the sponsor to the investigator on follow-up requirements of ongoing adverse events or if participants were still in treatment at termination of the study. The monitor will provide instructions for potential inspections or audits. The monitor should also remind the investigator of the requirements for record retention. Record retention will be discussed later in the chapter.

21.4.1 What if There Isn't a Closeout Visit?

Monitoring of a clinical trial may be conducted in various ways based on the size, scope, and risk level of the trial. If your sponsor has arranged for remote monitoring at your site, there may not be an on-site closeout visit. All the same procedures must still be completed for closeout. The sponsor will advise you of outstanding data, what to do with study materials, and how to submit required information for the sponsor's TMF if there is not an on-site visit.

If your investigator is the sponsor, they are responsible for assisting in the closeout of your site and any others that are participating in the trial.

21.5 After the Closeout Visit

After the closeout visit, you will receive a follow-up letter summarizing the visit. The letter will outline any further steps required from the sponsor's point of view. This would include addressing new queries or perhaps destruction of study materials or disposal of investigational product if it was not already done.

21.5.1 Closing the Study with the Ethics Committee

The final step in study closure is preparing the study closure report for your ethics committee. Your ethics committee will have its own format for the report, but common questions include the following:

- How many participants were enrolled?
- How many participants completed the study?
- How many participants withdrew?
- Why is the study being closed?
- Have all adverse events, protocol deviations, safety reports, etc., been reported to the ethics committee?
- What are the plans for dissemination of the results?

It is important *not* to close the study until your participant data are complete and clean (i.e., no further queries). Once the study has been closed by the ethics committee, you no longer have access

to personal health information in relation to the study. Check with the sponsor that all queries have been closed and all data cleaning is complete before submitting the study closure request to your ethics committee.

Final Report to the Sponsor

The investigator may be required to make a final report to the sponsor (21CFR312.64c).[6] Often, the information required is the same as that in the final report sent to the ethics committee. In some cases, the same report can be used for both.

Administrative Issues

By this point, you have collected all the data, documentation, and equipment from other departments in your institution that have participated in the study with you. You should have received a confirmation letter from your sponsor indicating that your site is closed. You can now notify your collaborators and colleagues that the study is complete. If there are recruiting advertisements, have them taken down. If there were tips or reminders related to the study posted in staff areas, have them removed.

If there are any final invoices or payments due to your site, follow up to see that they are received. Once all accounting is complete, the account may be closed.

21.6 Record Retention

The investigator is responsible for not only maintaining study records during the trial but also archiving them for the required amount of time. The length of record retention may be determined by the sponsor, regulatory authorities, or local policies. For example, ICH-GCP (sections 4.9.5 and 5.5.11)[5] and the United States FDA (21CFR312.57 and 21CFR 312.62)[6] have similar statements on record retention for clinical studies indicating that essential study documents should be retained for at least 2 years after the last approval of a marketing application or at least 2 years after discontinuation if there are no marketing applications pending. Both Health Canada (C.05.12)[7] and the European Union (EU No. 536/2014 article 58)[8] have regulations that require records to be retained for 25 years. Locally, my center requires research records to be retained for a minimum of 7 years.

You must be aware which policies and regulations apply to your research and if there is a discrepancy, you must maintain the records for the longest period of time.

In the earlier examples, the record retention period can be 25 years. That is probably longer than your current study team will be together, so the records must be complete enough to speak for themselves. They need to show that you met all the regulatory requirements during the conduct of the study, that the investigator fulfilled all duties as outlined in contracts and agreements, that you followed Good Clinical Practice in your study conduct, that you were in compliance with the study protocol, and that the rights and safety of the study participants were protected.

When it comes to storing records, space is money. The fewer boxes you have to store, the less it will cost. The ISF may be organized into large three-ring binders with signed informed consents, participant worksheets and CRFs all in separate binders. It may be more economical to remove the paper from the large binders for storage, but you need to ensure that the records remain orderly. Folders, binder clips, binder rings, and zip ties are all options. Remove any duplicate information from your ISF. You only need one copy of each version of a document.

While paper files are easy to store for future viewing, electronic data are a challenge. Hardware and software technology changes with time. The data you save must still be viewable at the end of the retention period. You may need to convert electronic documents to PDF/A, an ISO-standardized electronic document file format for long-term preservation. Other file types may be more difficult than text documents (e.g., CT scan). If you do store files on electronic media, you may also need to include viewing software so they can be opened in the future. Check with your sponsor for guidance.

Not all paper is created equal. Thermal paper is used for some medical device recordings, such as ECGs. Printouts on thermal paper will fade and are not likely to last for the 25 years required in some countries. A certified copy of thermal paper documents should be made and archived with the original source document.

Once the records are packaged for storage, it remains the responsibility of the investigator to ensure their safekeeping. Study records remain confidential records, even after study closure. They must be kept secure, and access to them must be controlled. If the investigator leaves the institution where the study files are stored, the responsibility for their safekeeping must be transferred to an appropriate person and the sponsor must be notified.

Finally, at the end of the retention period, the records must be appropriately destroyed. Always check with the sponsor prior to destruction. Participants' confidentiality must be protected throughout the destruction process. Paper records should be shredded or incinerated. Records stored on a computer hard drive or network should be erased using software designed to remove all data from the storage device. Your institution may have its own procedures for erasing electronic data. It may even include destruction of the hard drive. For data stored on USB drives, tapes, CDs, or DVDs, the storage devices should be physically destroyed. You should keep records describing what records were destroyed, when, and how they were destroyed.

An SOP for record retention is recommended to ensure consistency across all studies. SOPs are updated as procedures change, and previous versions are kept. Even if the process for record retention changes 20 years from now, any future research coordinator should be able to look back at the SOP that was in place at the time of the study closure to understand how it was done.

21.7 After the Study Closure

Although not a requirement, it is a good idea to have a study debrief with your investigator and the rest of your research team. There are lessons to be learned from every study. Were there any challenges that were overcome and how can that be used in the next study? Was the workload as expected and was the budget sufficient to cover all study costs? Maybe there were checklists or templates provided by the sponsor that were particularly helpful that you can adapt to other studies. This is also a time to discuss how the study results will be disseminated to those who participated at your site once the results become available (e.g., presentations or a newsletter). Seeing the results of everyone's hard work keeps the enthusiasm going for current and future studies.

Study closure is the end of the study, but if your investigator is also the sponsor it is not the end of responsibility. The study results must be analyzed and a final report must be submitted to regulatory authorities, if applicable. If the study was a clinical trial, the clinical trial registry listing must be updated with the results. The final stage is publication and dissemination of results.

21.8 Practical Application

A number of years ago, I was asked to retrieve some data from an old study that had been archived. My investigator was the only remaining staff person that had been involved in the study but he could not remember the ethics reference number or even the exact study name. He knew approximately when the study had ended and that it had been archived but not how many boxes or what was in each box. Someone had completed all the forms to store the boxes in accordance with our institution's policy, but no one in my office could find copies of the forms. Thankfully the institution had a defined process and the research office was able to help me find the boxes I needed. Of course that was only half the battle!

All of the files in the boxes had been removed from their binders and fastened together with elastic bands, which had essentially disintegrated over time, so that I had five boxes of paper with no separation between ISF documents and participant records and no idea what was in each box. I eventually found what I needed, and learned how NOT to store research records!

My office now has a better process for record retention. Much of it is dictated by my institution's guideline for record retention, which defines the process of preparing records for storage, transferring the records to the storage area, access to records after storage, and destruction of records at the end of the retention time. But the most important thing I learned during my search was to carefully complete a "Storage Box Content List" (▶ Fig. 21.1) and have a designated location to store the document. I also put a copy into each storage box. It simply lists in which box to find each document. It is especially helpful when participant CRFs are spread over a number of boxes to know the range of participant numbers in each box, or to know that correspondence prior to a certain date is in one box and after a certain date is in the next. I hope that means that someone coming behind me will have an easier time finding what they need.

21.9 Conclusion

Studies close for a variety of reasons, but the process of study closure remains largely the same regardless of the reason for the closure. First and foremost in any study closure is to communicate with your study participants and ensure that they are provided with the follow-up care they need. Collect and submit all of your data. Work with your sponsor to return or dispose of study materials and investigational products. Finally, organize all study documents and arrange for long-term storage.

Definitions

- **Adverse event:** Any untoward medical occurrence in a study participant, whether or not there is a causal relationship with the study treatment.
- **Case report form:** A document (written or electronic) designed to capture all protocol-required information on each study participant.
- **Certified copy:** A copy (irrespective of the type of media used) of the original record that has been verified (i.e., by a dated signature or by generation through a validated process) to have the same information, including data that describe the context, content, and structure, as the original.
- **Essential documents:** Study documents that permit evaluation of the conduct of a study and the quality of the data produced.
- **Ethics committee:** An independent committee, board, or group that reviews research involving human participants. The ethics committee approves the initiation of studies and provides periodic review for the purpose of protecting the rights, safety, and well-being of human participants in research. The ethics committee may be known locally as an Independent Ethics Committee (IEC), Institutional Review Board (IRB), Medical Research Ethics Committee (MREC), or Research Ethics Board (REB).
- **Good Clinical Practice:** Regulations and guidelines that describe the responsibilities of sponsors, investigators, and ethics committees involved in clinical studies. Their purpose is to protect the safety, rights, and welfare of participants and ensure accuracy of data collected during the study.

Storage box content list

Study:_____ Closure date:_____ # Of boxes: _____

Document	Box #
Protocol, all approved versions and amendments	
Product information (investigator's brochure, product monograph, instructions for use, etc.)	
Product storage and accountability (shipping, receiving, temperature logs, dispensing, final disposition)	
Ethics documentation (approvals, correspondence, membership)	
Blank copies of approved forms (informed consent, CRFs, questionnaires, surveys)	
Laboratory documents (accreditation, lab normal, staff training)	
Specimen records (processing, storage, shipping)	
Staff qualifications (CVs, licenses, training documents)	
Site logs (monitoring logs, delegation of authority, screening and enrollment)	
Regulatory documents (FDA form 1572, health canada authorization, etc.)	
Contracts and agreements	
Financial disclosures	
Sponsor correspondence	
Monitoring reports	
Safety reports	
Signed informed consents	
Participant files (source documents and completed CRFs) _____ to _____	
Participant files (source documents and completed CRFs) _____ to _____	

Fig. 21.1 Sample storage box content list.

- **Informed consent:** The process by which a participant confirms their willingness to participate in a study. It also refers to the written documents that accompany this process, namely, the participant information and informed consent signature form.
- **Investigator:** A person responsible for conducting the study at a study site. The lead investigator who holds the overall responsibility is referred to as the Principal Investigator (PI) or Qualified Investigator (QI) and the others may be referred to as subinvestigators.
- **Investigator Site File:** The collection of essential documents for a study, which are held by the investigator. It is sometimes referred to as the site "regulatory binder" or the site master file.
- **Monitor:** A person who is appointed by the sponsor to monitor the study by overseeing its progress and ensuring it is being conducted in accordance with the protocol, good clinical practice, written procedures, and regulatory requirements. The monitor is sometimes called the Clinical Research Associate (CRA).

- **Participant:** A human subject participating in a study.
- **Protocol:** A document that describes the rationale, objective(s), design, methodology, statistical plan, and conduct of a study. It is sometimes called a Clinical Investigation Plan (CIP).
- **Protocol deviation:** A planned or unplanned change from, or noncompliance with, the approved research protocol.
- **Query:** A request for clarification on a data item collected for a study to resolve an error or inconsistency discovered during data review.
- **Source documents:** Original documents, data, and records, that is, a document where the data are first recorded.
- **Sponsor:** The person, company, or institution that is responsible for the initiation of a study.
- **Standard operating procedure:** A set of step-by-step instructions that describe the activities required to complete a task.
- **Trial Master File (TMF):** The collection of essential documents for a study. The TMF is normally composed of a sponsor master file, held by the sponsor organization, and an investigator site master file, held by the investigator (often called the Investigator Site File or ISF). These files together comprise the TMF for the study.

References

[1] Pak T, Rodriguez M, Roth F. Why Clinical Trials are Terminated. 2015; https://www.biorxiv.org/content/early/2015/07/02/021543. Accessed May 30, 2018

[2] Klimt CR, Canner PL. Terminating a Long-Term Clinical Trial. Clin Pharmacol Ther 1979;25(5, Pt 2):641–646

[3] Williams RJ, Tse T, DiPiazza K, Zarin DA. Terminated Trials in the ClinicalTrials.gov Results Database: Evaluation of Availability of Primary Outcome Data and Reasons for Termination. PLoS One 2015;10(5):e0127242

[4] International Organization for Standardization. Clinical Investigation of Medical Devices for Human Participants–Good Clinical Practice (ISO Standard No. 14155). Geneva: International Organization for Standardization; 2011

[5] International Council for Harmonisation of Technical Requirements for Pharmaceuticals for Human Use (ICH). ICH E6(R2) Good Clinical Practice (GCP) Guideline. http://www.ich.org/products/guidelines/efficacy/article/efficacy-guidelines.html Accessed May 30, 2018

[6] US Food and Drug Administration. Code of Federal Regulations, Title 21, Vol. 1: Part 312. Investigational New Drug Application. Silver Spring, MD: FDA; 2018

[7] Health Canada. Part C, Division 5 of the Food and Drug Regulations (Drugs for Clinical Trials Involving Human Subjects). https://www.canada.ca/en/health-canada/services/drugs-health-products/drug-products/applications-submissions/guidance-documents/clinical-trials/links.html. Accessed November 16, 2018

[8] Clinical Trial Regulation EU No. 536/2014 of the European Parliament and of the Council of 16 April 2014 on clinical trials on medicinal products for human use, and repealing Directive 2001/20/EC. https://ec.europa.eu/health//sites/health/files/files/eudralex/vol-1/reg_2014_536/reg_2014_536_en.pdf. Accessed November 16, 2018

Further Reading

Woodin KE. Study closure. In: Gambrill S, Gualdoni Paul Jr, eds. The CRC's Guide to Coordinating Clinical Research. Boston, MA: CenterWatch; 2004:139–145

22 Knowledge Dissemination: Getting the Word Out!

Cheryl Kreviazuk, Darren M. Roffey

Abstract

The objective of this chapter is to provide research coordinators with the necessary information and tools to disseminate knowledge to the appropriate audience. Along with providing advice as to how to construct a dissemination plan, we present two methods of knowledge dissemination: "traditional" and "nontraditional." Various mediums of knowledge dissemination are discussed in detail under the construct of each of the two methods, along with the pitfalls and barriers to implementation that are most commonly encountered. Our aim is to provide practical information to researchers as to the importance of effective knowledge dissemination in an effort to bridge the knowledge-to-action gap.

Keywords: knowledge dissemination, knowledge translation, knowledge-to-action, publication, journal, conference, social media, knowledge user

22.1 Introduction

Increased interest surrounds the knowledge-to-action (KTA) gap that currently exists in science and medicine. The KTA gap refers to the notion that despite the plethora of evidence being supplied on a daily basis from research study findings, knowledge is not being accepted and/or introduced into real-life scenarios and applications.[1] Graham et al emphasized that despite all the resources available to the modern researcher, there remains significant apprehension as to how much published research data are being translated into practice, and when it does, the length of time it takes to reach this final stage.[2] Unfortunately, the worst-case scenario is that, because of this KTA gap, patients may be deprived of optimal care and treatment options. While KTA and knowledge translation have previously been described as a process of "creation" and "action,"[1,2,3] the focus of this chapter will be on the "action" cycle, which is analogous to knowledge dissemination (► Fig. 22.1).

Knowledge dissemination refers to the process of disclosing knowledge in a manner that is tailored to the respective audience.[3] The audience may be a group of patients, the general public, or even what is termed a knowledge user (i.e., an individual who could use this knowledge to create policy change or make informed decisions regarding care and treatment).[3] Knowledge dissemination generally occurs at the end of a research study once the authors have decided upon what information should be shared and where, or, ideally, may be integrated into the project itself if deemed appropriate by the researchers.[4] Granting agencies often require applicants to disclose their knowledge dissemination plans in their application submission. Example guidelines often stipulate that while research findings may be diffused via unplanned and uncontrolled platforms (i.e., disclosed by peers), applicants must identify the strategies that will be used to actively disseminate the knowledge to a purposeful audience.[4]

The purpose of this chapter is to outline and review the "traditional" and "nontraditional" methods of knowledge dissemination. The goal is to provide research coordinators with the pros and cons of each method so that it is possible to make the best-informed decision regarding knowledge dissemination for any particular type of research study. A practical application will seek to enlighten research coordinators on how to practically disseminate knowledge in a modern research environment. The aim is to provide research coordinators with the necessary tools to close the KTA gap and make informed decisions about knowledge dissemination.

22.1.1 Knowledge Dissemination

Knowledge translation is engrained in the official mandate of granting agencies the world over.[5] While knowledge dissemination is but one key element of knowledge translation, its importance should not be diminished. As opposed to diffusion ("just let it happen"), which is typified as passive, unplanned, uncontrolled dissemination where potential users need to seek out the information, dissemination ("make it happen") is an active process to communicate results to potential users by targeting, tailoring, and packaging the message for a specific target audience. In order to assist the principal investigator, the research coordinator should be aware of the following key

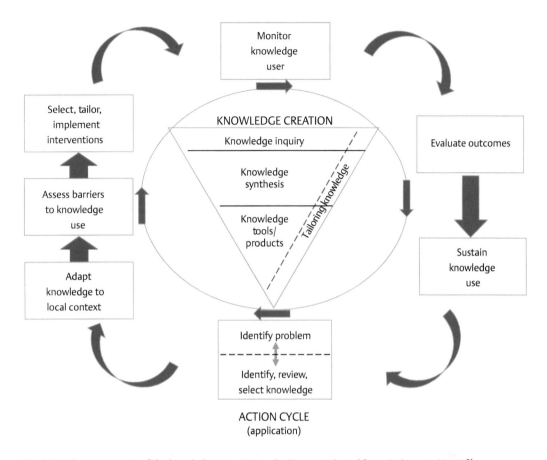

Fig. 22.1 The components of the knowledge-to-action cycle. (Source: Adapted from Graham et al 2006.[2])

points with regard to the basic tenets of knowledge dissemination[6]:

- Strategies informed by high-quality evidence that consider applicable factors critical to successful knowledge translation should be outlined in a dissemination plan created during the development phase of the research study.
- Researchers should engage multiple knowledge users and stakeholders to aid with planning and executing their dissemination plan.
- Disseminated messages should be clear, concise, action oriented, and tailored to the targeted audience.
- Individuals or organizations who disseminate knowledge should be credible messengers.
- Researchers should engage in discussion to evaluate the strengths and weaknesses of their dissemination plan for future reference and improvements.

22.1.2 Maximizing Uptake of Knowledge Dissemination

To maximize the uptake of knowledge dissemination, it is important that the research coordinator answer the following five questions originally posed by Reardon and Gibson.[7] In doing so, it will provide the necessary information to adequately and efficiently work with the principal investigator to develop a dissemination plan. Ideally, this task should be completed in the planning phase of the project so that it can be included in any granting application submissions.

1. What is the message?
   a. While a research project may generate many findings, for the purposes of disseminating the results, what key message should readers take home with them?

2. Who is the audience?
   a. Be specific. If it is a patient cohort, what is the basic demographic information? If it is a group of physicians, is the aim to target family doctors or surgeons?
3. Who is the messenger?
   a. Knowledge uptake is greater when it is disseminated by individuals who are seen as credible and trustworthy with the target audience.
4. How will the knowledge be disseminated?
   a. The manner in which knowledge is disseminated will greatly impact uptake, so it is important to adjudicate all possible methods and ensure the message is clear, concise, and tailored to the target audience.
5. What is the expected outcome?
   a. What information do you want your audience to retain? Three potential outcomes are of most importance: (1) awareness of a topic (indirect use), (2) changes in behavior (direct use), and (3) supporting a current decision (tactical use).

Suffice to say, how each preceding question is answered will greatly impact the subsequent question thereafter. Research coordinators are encouraged to involve all relevant stakeholders to ensure their learned views are considered to ascertain the most complete answers.

22.1.3 Developing an Effective Dissemination Plan

Lomas first defined dissemination as an active concept where knowledge is launched in a manner that is personalized to the anticipated audience.[8] In the years since, interest has piqued with regard to knowledge dissemination and an increased value has been placed on an effective dissemination plan.[9] As research coordinators and principal investigators are preparing ideas related to upcoming research studies, it is of value to identify the goals of knowledge dissemination and what methods will be taken to ensure maximum knowledge uptake. Completing this process will not only help orient the research team toward their ultimate goal, but also serve as a valuable addition to any submission for granting agencies to determine where support is needed.

The National Center for the Dissemination of Disability Research has identified 10 steps that can act as a guideline for developing an effective knowledge dissemination plan (▶Table 22.1).[9] The amount of time required to plan for effective dissemination should not be underestimated. It is worth repeating that principal investigators and research coordinators are encouraged to consider the proposal development phase as the best time to begin this planning. Although several characteristics of effective dissemination plans are worthy of discussion, for the purposes of this chapter, the focus will be upon step 6 in ▶Table 22.1: determine the medium that will best deliver the content/message to potential users.[9] In discussing this concept, the choice of medium will be further broken down into what has been termed "traditional" and "nontraditional" methods of knowledge dissemination.

Table 22.1 Key elements to consider when designing a knowledge dissemination plan

1.	Establish feasible goals for the dissemination plan
2.	Articulate specific objectives required to achieve each goal
3.	Define the scope and characteristics of potential knowledge users/target audiences
4.	Determine what content/information will be disseminated (comprehension level, language, framing to meet the needs of defined user groups, etc.)
5.	Identify sources that potential user groups view as being credible, and consider ways to partner with these sources, such as accessing a group's network
6.	Determine the medium that will best deliver the content/message to potential users
7.	Decide how to determine the success of the dissemination activities; what measures or indicators will be used and how will these be collected and analyzed as part of this evaluation?
8.	Describe what steps will be taken to promote ongoing access to project-related content, and consider how users will access this information in the future
9.	Identify strategies to inform potential users about the availability of project-related information, including accessible format(s)
10.	Identify potential barriers that may interfere with users' access to or application of the knowledge, and develop targeted strategies to reduce these barriers

Source: Adapted from the National Center for the Dissemination of Disability Research.[9]

22.1.4 Traditional Knowledge Dissemination

Traditional methods of knowledge dissemination refer to the most commonly recognized and employed forms of circulating research ideas and findings. Pros and cons of various methods falling under this category are discussed in the following.

Journal Publication

Commonly regarded as the "gold standard" for knowledge dissemination, researchers often consider publication of their results in a high-impact factor journal to be the definition of a successful project.[10] Once a study has been completed and researchers have decided to pursue publication, careful consideration should be taken to decide which journal could serve as the best platform. Examining the scope of the journal and previously published content from past issues should provide researchers with an idea as to whether the journal is the most appropriate platform for reaching the target audience. It is worth noting that focusing solely on journal impact factor alone is becoming increasingly eschewed as the gaming of this metric has biased journals against publishing important papers in fields that are much less cited than others.[11] The advent of open-access publication has also mired the decision as to which journal will be most suitable. Open access allows knowledge users unrestricted free access to the content, and sometimes permits re-use and distribution on different platforms (e.g., ResearchGate).[12] Whereas typical subscription-based journals are accessible only to readers who pay for a subscription or have institutional access, the greatest advantage of open-access journals is that they allow for a larger audience to view the content for free, thereby potentially increasing the reach of the work to new readers and users.[13] The biggest con regarding open access is the financial cost associated with article-processing fees, which can get into the thousands of dollars (USD). Alas, in order to provide knowledge free to the general public, open-access journals have to charge processing fees to recoup the costs for each issue. While publication in a high-impact factor journal can afford researchers credibility and increased standing among their peers, Young et al declared it but a single step on a long journey, and more importantly, it should not be assumed that publication will automatically lead to implementation into practice.[10] Research coordinators can play an integral role in formatting, finalizing, and submitting the manuscript and affiliated files to the chosen journal, and then corresponding with the editorial staff throughout the review process up until the point of acceptance or rejection.

Conference Presentation

Medical and scientific conferences present an opportunity for academics and researches to quickly share knowledge, create discussions, and foster new collaborations.[14] In the months preceding a conference, a call for abstracts is sent out, requesting submissions from authors to discuss their research study in the field of interest. Studies do not have to be completed to be eligible (i.e., interim analysis is acceptable); however, all work must be original and the information cannot have been published previously. To clarify, these studies can subsequently be written up and published in journals of the author's choosing. Abstracts will be peer reviewed by the conference committee and, if successful, designated as a poster or podium presentation.

- Poster presentations are a visual display of the objectives, methods, results, and conclusions of a research study. Poster presentations allow attendees to view at their own pace and also engage in conversation with the author during designated time periods. A great deal of time and effort goes into creating a visually arresting poster, and research coordinators are normally primarily responsible for their design, modifications, and printing. To ensure maximum dissemination of knowledge, posters must be clear, concise, and visually appealing. Researchers are encouraged to stand beside their poster during breaks in conference proceedings to answer questions and facilitate discussions with readers.

- Podium presentations are oral presentations consisting of a slideshow outlining the objectives, methods, results, and conclusions of a research study. Podium presentations allow researchers to verbally showcase their findings in real time in front of an audience with visual aids. An effective podium presentation is the most efficient manner afforded to a researcher to disseminate their results to knowledge users; more than that, it can foster follow-up discussions and feedback among viewers with a wide array of expertise. Research coordinators can assist the principal investigator with preparing the slideshow, ensuring that the slides are easy to follow, are not too busy with too much information per slide, and the presentation fits within the requested time allotment. Handouts available for the audience postpresentation are not mandatory, but they can serve as valuable take-home material for future correspondence. Recently, conferences have begun to shift toward embracing alternative mediums, in that they are now commonly promoted through social media sites and have been using hashtags and e-posters in the hopes of attracting a greater online audience.[15]

It is worth noting that conference attendance can be prohibited by financial costs, travel requirements, and time demands. Trainees, juniors, single parents, and people with immigration challenges sometimes are not in a position to attend.

Press Release

Press releases can occur via television, radio, newspaper, and podcasts, among a myriad of available mediums. Press releases facilitate quick dissemination of information to a wide audience, allowing researchers to communicate with more knowledge users and the general public faster and easier than journal publications or conference presentations. Research coordinators can work with the principal investigator, in coordination with the press office or communications team of the hospital or research institution, to craft the message to be conveyed via press release. Press release issuance and the subsequent actual coverage it receives can be fickle and hard to predict, although studies concerning common behaviors (e.g., alcohol consumption) tend to receive media attention.[16] Furthermore, there is growing concern that the media may have too powerful a voice[12] and that this voice can sometimes misinterpret information, create inaccurate or bold statements, and may even neglect to disclose imperative information.[17]

Institute Website and Newsletter

Hospitals and research centers often use online platforms to highlight research progress at their institution. For example, the Ottawa Hospital Research Institute website (http://www.ohri.ca/home.asp) enables researchers and patients alike to read about studies conducted in various research programs, recent research news, and upcoming seminars and events.[18] Independent researchers can benefit from visiting such websites when seeking collaboration with institutional members. Researchers within the same institute, but conducting studies in different fields, may see opportunities for collaboration from study write-ups in weekly newsletters. This is an ideal scenario wherein dissemination pertaining to a research study attracts the attention of a knowledge user, who then contacts the research coordinator or principal investigator about the study for future discussion. Patients may also benefit by learning about research studies that are currently underway, and medical and scientific advancements derived from studies conducted by the institution.

Departmental Research Day

Departments hold annual research days to promote the advancement of research made by their students, residents, researchers, etc. Similar to a 1-day conference, members within the department present their research to their peers and engage in conversation surrounding their findings. Department members are encouraged to advance their public speaking abilities, critical-thinking skills, and to use the occasion to foster relationships and collaborations among colleagues. Mills et al found that participation in an annual departmental research day for pediatric trainees was significantly correlated with future publications.[19] Internal sharing of research study results encourages researchers to disseminate knowledge throughout the broader research community, and not to simply safeguard their results (or shortcomings) within the walls of their department.

Policy Brief

Researchers who wish to present their research to a nonspecified audience may choose to do so using policy briefs. The purpose of these short briefs is to bring attention to the impact of their research study by challenging or defending current policies. Policy briefs are intended to be concise and have a clear message, allowing the audience to quickly obtain enough information to elicit conversation between policy makers.[12] While policy briefs can elicit change at a high level, they must be extremely well thought out so as to not exclude any necessary information. As researchers can only control what is written, and not what is interpreted by policy makers, messages must be clear and researchers cannot assume the audience is familiar with everything that is discussed.

Research Report

Researchers with projects that are funded by granting agencies or sponsors are required to complete end-of-grant research reports.[20] These reports serve as a summary of the findings, and act as a critical evaluation of the project. Format and structure of the reports are often clearly laid out in the original research study agreement. The greatest advantage to completing a research report is that the information that is entered can serve multiple purposes (along with potentially being posted on the agency or sponsor website). The World Health Organization suggested that authors who generate research reports can re-use the tables and figures in future conference presentations. The abstract for the report can also serve as a press-release precursor. Finally, the entire report can be used as a template for a future journal publication.[12]

22.1.5 Nontraditional Knowledge Dissemination

Nontraditional methods refer to new and novel techniques and applications to disseminate knowledge that embrace modern technologies. With the constant evolution of social media, these methods are growing and expanding every day. When transitioning from traditional to nontraditional methods of knowledge dissemination, researchers must be careful that messages and mediums are customized to the targeted audience.[20]

Academic Social Networks

Academic social networks are becoming more and more popular.[21] Sites such as LinkedIn, ResearchGate, and Academia.edu allow researchers an online platform to share their findings, connect with other researchers, and find related work.[22] Researchers are encouraged to explore which platform is most used at their respective institution and among their colleagues. One recent study indicated that approximately 37% of researchers at the University of Bergen in Norway had at least one profile from the following sites: ResearchGate, Academia.edu, Google Scholar Citations, ResearcherID, and ORCID.[23] Many sites are free to use and provide users with the freedom to choose how much or how little they disclose on their profiles. ResearchGate allows users to post their contributions under the following categories: Article, Chapter, Conference Paper, Data, Research, Presentation, Poster, Preprint, and Full texts. ResearchGate also allows users to pose public questions, request and share their work, and openly discuss ongoing research—all under the guise of disseminating knowledge and fostering a collaborative and sharing environment. One caveat is that researchers must be cognizant of copyright infringement and the legalities behind re-publishing work. Elsevier, one of the largest academic publishers, sent out warning notices to members on Academia.edu who were republishing their own work and were seemingly unaware of the copyright policies.[21] As such, researchers are encouraged to review publishing contracts for their rights as authors.

Twitter

Twitter launched in 2006 and although the platform has evolved since its initiation, what remains is its ability to quickly disseminate information to a wide range of individuals and users across many socioeconomic and racial backgrounds.[24] Granted, while it is mainly used to convey ideas and thoughts in short condensed messages, the inclusion of hashtags has allowed for the search and retrieval of related information at the click of a button.[25] Alternative metrics measure the number of online mentions that an academic paper receives and is an increasingly important outcome in terms of ascertaining the scope of online dissemination.[26] In the event of fast-spreading illnesses, social media such as Twitter and Facebook can play a vital role in disseminating knowledge to a large body of people.[27] During the H1N1 outbreak in 2009–2010, the Centers for Disease Control and Prevention used Twitter to share up-to-date knowledge and findings with physicians across the world. The greatest advantage to Twitter is the speed at which information can be spread. However, countering this positive element is the fact there is also a high risk that false information could be sent out and then perpetuated among a wide array of readers without any easy recourse for correction (#FakeNews). Another concern with using Twitter to disclose research findings is the risk of violating health information privacy rules and patient confidentiality. Principal investigators and research coordinators posting on social media must take extra precautions to protect themselves and their institution from the risk of being misquoted or violating patient rights.

Preprints

Preprint servers host drafts of manuscript that have not yet undergone peer review or are in the final stages of the publication process. Preprint servers cater for a wide variety of research interest, with some of the more popular options being arXiv,[28] PeerJ Preprints,[29] Open Science Framework,[30] and Social Science Research Network.[31] The benefits of preprints are clear, in that they allow for work to be made publicly available freely and very quickly, and without significant barriers. In fields that move rapidly, they can be a means to establish precedence of findings. Many preprint servers also enable commenting, which allows for public discussion of the work. In comparison, Powel found that manuscript submission to publication takes on average 100 days,[32] and the journal publication process is often plagued with delays from rejection letters to major revisions, minor revisions and formatting requests, to numerous correspondence requirements. Alas, authors may question the authenticity of preprints for fear of rejection in future journals submission. However, very rarely do journals acknowledge preprints as a form of prior publication, which would normally result in rejection.[33] Researchers also need not fear about being "scooped" (i.e., inadvertently or purposely neglecting to disclose the original author); rather principal investigators and research coordinators are encouraged to use licenses and format permits that retain copyright to their own work. As preprints are not peer reviewed, tenure and granting agencies will review any inclusion of preprints with greater scrutiny, so there is a distinct need to ensure the work is critically appraised before posting. Fortunately, many preprint servers enforce policies that will not allow work to be published that could be potentially damaging to human health (e.g., a study that reports on the negative effects of vaccines).[33]

Free Open Access Medical Information

Free open access medical information (FOAM) has recently been embraced by numerous practitioners.[34] The purpose of FOAM is to provide free resources to individuals involved in health care around the world. FOAM is a transformative disruption in knowledge dissemination, delivering massive collections of free resources on medical practices via blogs, podcasts, photographs, Facebook pages affiliated with institutions, YouTube channels, etc. FOAM can provide individuals with greater access to medical information, as well as facilitate collaborative online discussions and the sharing of knowledge and resources between users. The concern is the risk of breaching health information privacy rules and violating patient confidentiality. While some have argued that FOAM should replace the process of peer reviewing studies prior to publication, others have contended that because FOAM occurs postpublication, this may lead to the dissemination of deceptive research.[34] Further, the ease with which FOAM can be posted online, combined with the savvy use of graphics, means that any researcher is now able to create content that looks authoritative.[35] Although FOAM can serve as a tool to facilitate online discussions that are easily accessible and freely available, FOAM may be best served to complement traditional methodologies.

Blogs and Podcasts

Blogs and podcasts have recently begun to emerge as alluring platforms for individuals to learn about various topics in an innovative and arguably easily digested manner.[36] A blog refers to a website where the host creates posts that appear in reverse chronological order. Each blog post may have a new topic or be a continuation of the previous entry. Podcasts are similar in many ways, but instead of being posted online to be read, they are recorded with intent of being listened to. Both platforms allow for quick dissemination of research findings in a nontraditional manner that differs from the standard introduction, methods, results, and discussion format. Blogs and podcasts provide the authors with a medium to express themselves openly. Most blogs and podcasts are available for free; however, some require a subscription fee to access their content. While blogs encourage public contribution with the inclusion of a comments section, many criticize the credibility as the expertise behind the input may be limited.[37] Readers must also be cautious before accepting the research in blogs and podcasts as fact as, with many of the nontraditional methods, no peer-review process has been undertaken to vet the study data. Nonetheless, health care blogs created by patients have been gaining popularity in recent years, with data showing they can have tremendous positive impacts on the psychological health and well-being of other patients by creating a network of supportive members.[37]

Digital Storytelling

Digital storytelling can be a powerful and unique tool to disseminate knowledge. Also referred to as web comics, researchers can create engaging stories that are easy to read and can actively engage viewers in a way that is visually appealing.[38] Infographics are another tool with which to engage viewers using powerful images (e.g., warning labels on cigarette packaging). Infographics can provide powerful messages that, importantly, can be easily understood regardless of social status or educational background. Visual art and theater can also serve as very engaging methods to disseminate knowledge that can be appropriate for individuals of all ages.[39] One of the most appealing aspects of live performances is it often encourages the audience to create their own interpretations of the work that may then facilitate further conversation between the audience and the presenter.[38]

22.1.6 Traditional versus Nontraditional Knowledge Dissemination: Which Is Better?

With all of the available traditional and nontraditional methods of knowledge dissemination, a growing consensus purports that a combination of the two is the best way forward.[3,12,20] The Canadian Institutes of Health Research and the World Health Organization agree that when it comes to knowledge dissemination, stakeholders should learn to work together with a mutual goal to eliminate the KTA gap.[3,12] This is where the importance of a knowledge dissemination plan comes into action. While most granting agencies require researchers to provide them with a dissemination plan before beginning the work, many investigator-initiated projects overlook its importance.[20] Evaluating previous plans and their effectiveness can allow researchers to choose the best combination of methods to disclose and announce their work.[12] Regardless of the mediums chosen, evaluating and critiquing knowledge dissemination is becoming more important in academia too. Recently, the Mayo Clinic Academic Appointments and Promotions Committee incorporated "social media" into their consideration for academic advancement or tenure.[40] As such, researchers seeking to obtain tenure are encouraged to incorporate many of the available nontraditional social media platforms to disseminate their research findings.

22.1.7 Barriers to Implementation

While this chapter has focused on ways to disseminate knowledge and the various platforms that enable it, a concern for many researchers are the various known barriers to implementation. Such barriers can exist between knowledge users, among the audience, between the researcher and the institution, and within the research team itself.

Knowledge Users

The sheer volume of articles being published each and every day means it is impossible for clinicians to keep on top of all the new material.[1] Not only that, but physicians are not always well versed on how to sift through "good" versus "bad" research. Ambiguous findings may add to the confusion and make deciphering trustworthy evidence significantly harder.[12]

Audience

Depending on the audience, a healthy dose of skepticism and doubt may be present. Doubt may derive from several of the new nontraditional methods allowing researchers to publish material without peer review. Allowing the general public to edit resource material is also seen as troubling (i.e., Wikipedia).[40] As the audience is directly affected by policy changes stemming from the disseminated research, the risks and benefits to any changes in policy or practice must be clearly laid out.

Institutions

Researchers in institutions may fall victim to "group-think," which is a thought pattern process that can cause individuals to think "what would the group do?" rather than what they, as an individual, would do in any particular situation when presented with the evidence at hand.[12] Having an awareness of group-think and providing avenues for open and nonjudgmental discussion may help overcome this barrier to progress at institutions.

Researchers

Despite their knowledge user status, significant barriers to knowledge dissemination can exist within the research community. A minority of researchers believe that sponsored studies come with restrictive intellectual property rights and as such, they do not attempt to replicate studies.[41] This can have a detrimental effect whereby researchers do not attempt to challenge recently published findings, which in and of itself is a vital step in verifying the authenticity of results within science and medicine. In addition, authors fear that disseminating their knowledge may lead to "being scooped" and, consequently, will purposefully neglect to disclose all relevant methodological steps that are crucial to reproduction.[41] Researchers should not be viewed as competition, but rather as a member of the larger team. On a separate note, researchers wishing to disseminate knowledge creatively may be faced with the financial strains of creating brochures, online videos, and conference presentations.[10] The preparation of such materials should be carefully considered as they can be time-consuming and costly.

Predatory Journals

While many cite the advantages to open-access publishing, there is a growing concern relating to the proliferation of what have been deemed "predatory journals."[42] The term "predatory" derives from the idea that researchers are being tricked into believing the journal is legitimate and credible. Instead, researchers often pay a hefty fee to publish in a journal that lacks an arduous peer-review process and is rarely indexed in respected databases (e.g., PubMed). The uptick of predatory journals has also had a cascading impact on the legitimacy of knowledge dissemination sites like ResearchGate too.[43] It is important for principal investigators and research coordinators to be able to identify and avoid predatory journals (see ▶ Table 22.2).[44]

22.2 Practical Application

In this section, by using the aforementioned outline proposed by Reardon and Gibson,[7] we will attempt to guide research coordinators on how they can help put together a plan for maximizing knowledge dissemination using a hypothetical research scenario.

Dr. Millar from the Division of Orthopaedic Surgery has recently completed a research study where she and her team recruited 180 participants who

Table 22.2 Red flags to consider in order to avoid predatory journals

1. The scope of interest includes nonbiomedical subjects alongside biomedical topics
2. The website contains spelling and grammar errors
3. Images are distorted/fuzzy, intended to look like something they are not, or which are unauthorized
4. The homepage language targets authors
5. The Index Copernicus Value (a bogus metric) is promoted on the website
6. Description of the manuscript handling process is lacking
7. Manuscripts are requested to be submitted via email
8. Rapid publication is promised
9. There is no retraction policy
10. Information on whether and how journal content will be digitally preserved is absent
11. The article processing/publication charge is very low (e.g., <US$150)
12. Journals claiming to be open access either retain copyright of published research or fail to mention copyright
13. The contact email address is nonprofessional and not journal affiliated (e.g., @gmail.com or @yahoo.com)

Source: Adapted from Shamseer et al.[44]

had fallen and suffered a femoral neck fracture (broken hip). Through semistructured interviews conducted postoperatively, Dr. Millar found that 80% of patients were afraid of falling again.

1. What (is the message):
   a. After evaluating her research, Dr. Millar identifies several key points. After a discussion with her coauthors, the research group agrees that the key message they wish to disclose is that patients who experience a fall are afraid of suffering further falls.
2. To whom (audience):
   a. While Dr. Millar acknowledges the importance of disclosing this information to her peers in the field, the research group feels that the users most affected by this knowledge are (1) the patients who have experienced a fall and (2) the physiotherapists who end up treating this patient cohort.

3. By whom (messenger):
   a. Dr. Millar has only been working at her institution for 2 years, so she decided, upon consultation, to collaborate on this study with the Chief of the Division of Orthopaedic Surgery, Dr. Miles. Dr. Miles is the most senior author on the project and as such, Dr. Millar has enlisted her to help disseminate the research to the target audiences. In addition, Dr. Millar has enlisted the help of the Head of the Clinical Physiotherapy Program at their institution, Dr. Walsh. Altogether, Dr. Millar strongly believes that the knowledge stemming from her research study will be best disseminated as a collaborative effort between the Division of Orthopaedic Surgery and the Clinical Physiotherapy Program.

4. How (transfer method):
   a. Dr. Millar arranges for a meeting between herself and the two "messengers." During this meeting, Dr. Miles suggests that the group seek publication in a well-known and high-impact journal focusing on orthopaedic surgery and rehabilitation. These three coauthors agree that the research coordinator should examine several potential journals and then pitch the findings to them to ensure they choose the journal appropriate to disseminate their findings. Dr. Millar will contact the communications manager for the institution to request that details about her study findings be included on the website and included in the next newsletter. Dr. Walsh requests that the research group arrange for an in-service with the physiotherapists who work with orthopaedic surgery patients to educate them on the findings and to elicit conversation around the topic of fear of falling and what can be done to reassure the patients. Finally, Dr. Millar recommends that patient education materials in the form of pamphlets be designed and disseminated to patients to take home with them at discharge for further reading.

5. With what expected impact (evaluation):
   a. By deciding to pursue multiple distinct methods of knowledge dissemination, the doctors agree that they will hopefully serve a different yet combinatorial purpose,

with each method just as important as the next. Seeking publication in a high-impact journal will provide the research findings with credibility and elicit conversation among their peers. Posting the findings on the website and in the institutional newsletter should help foster discussion among clinicians from different programs, and facilitate future collaborative projects. An in-service with physiotherapists will stimulate conversation between clinical professionals and allow for a mutual approach on how to treat and manage this cohort of patients. Finally, patient education materials will serve as visual reminders that their fear of falling again is normal and actually quite common and that there are ways to minimize this reoccurrence. Ensuring the pamphlet handout is clear, concise, and easy to read independent of education level is extremely important.

22.3 Conclusion

The end goal of a research study for many principal investigators is publishing their results in a high-impact factor journal. While this is important to gaining credibility and fostering conversation between peers, it does not necessarily guarantee that knowledge will be disseminated to the applicable target audience. With the creation of new technologies and the advent of many nontraditional methods, it is necessary to consider both the message and the medium when planning how to disseminate knowledge. With that in mind, it may prove beneficial to create a dissemination plan during the early phases of the research study. By employing the steps and information outlined in this chapter, researchers can ensure that all elements have been adequately thought out when preparing to disclose and disseminate knowledge. The collaboration of various stakeholders and the incorporation of both traditional and nontraditional methods of knowledge dissemination should permit for the greatest uptake of information. Finally, it is important that researchers critically evaluate their efforts at disseminating knowledge to ensure the appropriate mediums were used and to help improve upon their planning for future research endeavors.

Definitions

- **Knowledge dissemination:** Process of disclosing and disseminating knowledge in a manner that is tailored to best reach the respective target audience.
- **Traditional knowledge dissemination:** Classic, tested, acceptable forms of circulating research ideas and findings (e.g., journal publication, conference presentations, press releases).
- **Nontraditional knowledge dissemination:** New and novel methods to circulate research ideas and findings that embrace developing technologies (e.g., Twitter, FOAM, blogs, preprints).
- **Knowledge-to-action gap:** An acknowledge phenomenon whereby knowledge is not being accepted and introduced into clinical practice despite a plethora of evidence provided by continually evolving research findings.

References

[1]   Straus SE, Tetroe J, Graham I. Defining Knowledge Translation. CMAJ 2009;181(3–4):165–168

[2]   Graham ID, Logan J, Harrison MB, et al. Lost in Knowledge Translation: Time for a Map? J Contin Educ Health Prof 2006;26(1):13–24

[3]   Canadian Institutes of Health Research. Knowledge Translation. 2016. Accessed July 25, 2018. Available from: http://www.cihr-irsc.gc.ca/e/29418.html

[4]   Canadian Institutes of Health Research. Section 5.1 Knowledge Dissemination and Exchange of Knowledge. 2010. Accessed August 15, 2018. Available from: http://www.cihr-irsc.gc.ca/e/41953.html

[5]   McLean RK, Graham ID, Bosompra K, et al. Understanding the Performance and Impact of Public Knowledge Translation Funding Interventions: Protocol for an Evaluation of Canadian Institutes of Health Research Knowledge Translation Funding Programs. Implement Sci 2012;7:57

[6]   Canadian Institutes of Health Research. CE Handbook - Chapter 7: Knowledge Dissemination and Public Outreach (Focus Area 4). 2010. Accessed August 15, 2018. Available from: http://www.cihr-irsc.gc.ca/e/42212.html

[7]   Reardon RLJ, Gibson J. From Research to Practice: A Knowledge Transfer Planning Guide. Toronto, ON: Institute of Work and Health; 2006

[8]   Lomas J. Diffusion, Dissemination, and Implementation: Who Should Do What? Ann N Y Acad Sci 1993;703:226–235, discussion 235–237

[9]   National Collaborating Centre for Methods and Tools. Developing an Effective Knowledge Dissemination Plan. 2001. Accessed August 15, 2018]. Available from: http://www.nccmt.ca/knowledge-repositories/search/49

[10] Young PJ, Nickson CP, Gantner DC. Can Social Media Bridge the Gap Between Research and Practice? Crit Care Resusc 2013;15(4):257–259

[11] Alberts B. Impact Factor Distortions. Science 2013; 340(6134):787

[12] World Health Organization. Implementation Research Toolkit Participants Manual. 2014. Accessed July 25, 2018. Available from: http://www.who.int/tdr/publications/year/2014/participant-workbook5_030414.pdf

[13] Ottawa Hospital Research Institute. Deciding Where to Submit August 10, 2018. Available from: http://www.ohri.ca/journalology/submission.aspx

[14] Pellecchia GL. Dissemination of Research Findings: Conference Presentations and Journal Publications. Top Geriatr Rehabil 1999;14(3):67–79

[15] Wilkinson SE, Basto MY, Perovic G, Lawrentschuk N, Murphy DG. The Social Media Revolution is Changing the Conference Experience: Analytics and Trends from Eight International Meetings. BJU Int 2015;115(5):839–846

[16] Zhang Y, Willis E, Paul MJ, Elhadad N, Wallace BC. Characterizing the (perceived) newsworthiness of health science articles: a data-driven approach. JMIR Med Inform 2016;4(3):e27

[17] Lee E, Sutton RM, Hartley BL. From Scientific Article to Press Release to Media Coverage: Advocating Alcohol Abstinence and Democratising Risk in a Story about Alcohol and Pregnancy. Health Risk Soc 2016;18(5–6): 247–269

[18] The Ottawa Hospital Research Institute. The Ottawa Hospital Research Institute August 11, 2018. Available from: http://www.ohri.ca/home.asp

[19] Mills LS, Steiner AZ, Rodman AM, Donnell CL, Steiner MJ. Trainee Participation in an Annual Research Day is Associated with Future Publications. Teach Learn Med 2011;23(1):62–67

[20] Gagnon ML. Moving Knowledge to Action Through Dissemination and Exchange. J Clin Epidemiol 2011;64(1): 25–31

[21] Ovadia S. ResearchGate and Academia.edu: Academic Social Networks. Behav Soc Sci Librar 2014;33(3): 165–169

[22] Batooli Z, Ravandi SN, Bidgoli MS. Evaluation of Scientific Outputs of Kashan University of Medical Sciences in Scopus Citation Database based on Scopus, ResearchGate, and Mendeley Scientometric Measures. Electron Physician 2016;8(2):2048–2056

[23] Mikki S, Zygmuntowska M, Gjesdal OL, Al Ruwehy HA. Digital Presence of Norwegian Scholars on Academic Network Sites: Where and Who are They? PLoS One 2015;10(11):e0142709

[24] Scanfeld D, Scanfeld V, Larson EL. Dissemination of Health Information Through Social Networks: Twitter and Antibiotics. Am J Infect Control 2010;38(3):182–188

[25] Gai N, Matava C. Twitter Hashtags for Anesthesiologists: Building Global Communities. A A Pract 2019;12(2): 59–62

[26] Madden K, Evaniew N, Scott T, et al. Knowledge dissemination of intimate partner violence intervention studies measured using alternative metrics: results from a scoping review. J Interpers Violence 2019;34(9):1890-1906

[27] Eytan T, Benabio J, Golla V, Parikh R, Stein S. Social Media and the Health System. Perm J 2011;15(1):71–74

[28] arXiv.org e-Print archive. August 15, 2018. Available from: https://arxiv.org/

[29] Peer J. Preprints. August 15, 2018. Available from: https://peerj.com/preprints/

[30] Framework OS. Open Science Framework. August 20, 2018. Available from: https://osf.io/

[31] Social Science Research Network. SSRN. August 20, 2018. Available from: https://www.ssrn.com/en/

[32] Powell K. Does it Take too Long to Publish Research? Nature 2016;530(7589):148–151

[33] Bourne PE, Polka JK, Vale RD, Kiley R. Ten Simple Rules to Consider Regarding Preprint Submission. PLOS Comput Biol 2017;13(5):e1005473

[34] Nickson CP, Cadogan MD. Free Open Access Medical Education (FOAM) for the Emergency Physician. Emerg Med Australas 2014;26(1):76–83

[35] Murray H. Finding FOAM and not Froth. CJEM 2018; 20(2):162–163

[36] Cadogan M, Thoma B, Chan TM, Lin M. Free Open Access Meducation (FOAM): the rise of emergency medicine and critical care blogs and podcasts (2002–2013). Emerg Med J 2014;31(e1):e76–e77

[37] Joshi A, Wangmo R, Amadi C. Blogs as Channels for Disseminating Health Technology Innovations. Healthc Inform Res 2017;23(3):208–217

[38] Luesby D, Lusk E, Harris, M. Knowledge Transfer and Exchange in Action. Toronto, ON: BrainXchange; 2011

[39] Alberta Addiction & Mental Health Research Partnership Program. Creative Knowledge Translation: Ideas and Resources Edmonton, AB2015. August 20, 2018. Available from: https://www.albertahealthservices.ca/assets/info/res/mhr/if-res-mhr-creative-kt.pdf

[40] Cabrera D, Vartabedian BS, Spinner RJ, Jordan BL, Aase LA, Timimi FK. More than Likes and Tweets: Creating Social Media Portfolios for Academic Promotion and Tenure. J Grad Med Educ 2017;9(4):421–425

[41] Evans JA; Industry Collaboration. Scientific Sharing, and the Dissemination of Knowledge. Soc Stud Sci 2010;40(5):757–791

[42] Moher D, Moher E. Stop Predatory Publishers Now: Act Collaboratively. Ann Intern Med 2016;164(9):616–617

[43] Memon AR. ResearchGate is no Longer Reliable: Leniency Towards Ghost Journals may Decrease its Impact on the Scientific Community. J Pak Med Assoc 2016; 66(12):1643–1647

[44] Shamseer L, Moher D, Maduekwe O, et al. Potential Predatory and Legitimate Biomedical Journals: Can you Tell the Difference? A Cross-Sectional Comparison. BMC Med 2017;15(1):28

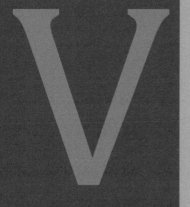

Part V

Advanced Principles of
Research Coordination

23 Regulatory Trials: Key
Differences from
Standard Trials   236

24 How to Survive a
Site Audit   251

25 Monitoring in a Clinical
Study: Why and How?   258

26 Managing Large Studies:
Organization and
Committees   267

27 International Research:
Challenges and Successes   276

V

23 Regulatory Trials: Key Differences from Standard Trials

Deborah J. Carr

Abstract

Regulatory trials are clinical trials that are overseen by a national regulatory agency through all phases of study. Results from such trials play a vital role in providing evidence used to approve the use of new medicines and devices in patient care. Key aspects of regulatory trials include Good Clinical Practice, the development and adherence to a protocol, trial registration, prompt disclosure of trial results, safety reporting, documentation, audits, investigator qualifications, and the clinical study report. Worldwide harmonization of standards related to these aspects of clinical trials has shaped regulatory frameworks with a view to promote public health and ensure that the information used to guide approvals is based on the foundations of safety, efficacy, and quality.

Keywords: regulatory agency, International Conference on Harmonisation, protocol, adverse event, Good Clinical Practice

23.1 Introduction

23.1.1 What Are Clinical and Regulatory Trials?

Clinical trials are preplanned research studies conducted in humans to determine safety, quality, and efficacy of health-related interventions that may include drugs, cells, and other biological products, surgical procedures, radiologic procedures, devices, behavioral treatments, process-of-care changes, and preventive care. This definition includes phase I to IV trials.[1]

Regulatory trials provide evidence used to evaluate the safety and efficacy of interventions and play key role in the approval to use new devices in patient care. Regulatory authorities worldwide ensure that regulatory trials of both registered and nonregistered medicines and devices comply with established standards for safety, quality, and efficacy prior to use. Regulatory trials are time intensive and involve extensive and prescriptive documentation, and detailed protocols that are also under strict regulation. The regulatory submission process is the rate-limiting step of any clinical trial and significantly impacts trial timelines.[2]

In this chapter, the unique data management, trial design, execution, monitoring, and reporting considerations that are key to the conduct of regulatory trials are outlined and examples are provided from the author's experience. The following are discussed in the chapter: some of the processes involved before, during, and after regulated trials; key regulatory authorities and frameworks worldwide; the overarching principles critical to the framework used in trial design; and what regulatory authorities require from research coordinators and study teams during the conduct of trials under regulation.

23.2 History of Regulation and International Harmonization

The International Council for Harmonisation (ICH), formerly the International Conference on Harmonisation, held its first meeting in October 2015 to establish ICH as an international association and legal entity under Swiss law. By this time, it became clear through marked events in history and in multiple geographic regions that autonomous evaluation of medical interventions is necessary before distribution to ensure a globally safe market. Such events include the Elixir Sulfanilamide disaster in the United States in 1937,[3] the thalidomide tragedy in Europe in the early 1960s that expanded to North America and South America over the next few decades,[4] the controversial safety testing of Opren in the United Kingdom in the 1970s,[5] and untested efficacy of diethylstilbestrol (DES) approved for use in pregnant women in the United States.[3] Although many guidelines have been standardized globally, they are implemented using country-specific legislation that can result in differing, and often confusing, regulatory environments.[4]

Worldwide, the 1960s and 1970s marked a period of increased legislation and guidelines for rigorous testing on the safety, quality, and efficacy of medicinal products. This is, in large part, due to the awareness generated by the thalidomide tragedy concerning the lack of regulation in the pharmaceutical industry. While markets expanded globally beyond traditional boundaries and the industry recognized the need for proper evaluation of medicinal products, divergent technical requirements from country to country created confusion, the necessity to duplicate resource-intensive clinical trials and, resultantly, increasingly prohibitive costs for research and development.[6]

In the 1980s, the European Commission (EC) demonstrated that harmonization of regulatory requirements for pharmaceuticals was possible by unifying regulatory authorities across Europe. Similar transnational efforts took place at this time involving select European countries, Japan, and the United States. In 1989, at the World Health Organization (WHO) International Conference of Drug Regulatory Authorities (ICDRA), in Paris, implementation plans were set in motion. Subsequently, this group approached the International Federation of Pharmaceutical Manufacturers and Associations (IFPMA) to establish a regulatory industry initiative that would lead to the international harmonization of the pharmaceutical industry, resulting in the formation of ICH.[7] Its mission is to promote public health, which remains true today.

One of the ways in which ICH has demonstrated commitment to promoting public health was to steer international harmonization. This has been accomplished through the development and promotion of technical guidelines that are implemented by regulatory authorities worldwide and produced in collaboration with regulatory authorities, regional harmonization initiatives, international industry pharmaceutical organizations, and international organizations with an interest in patient care. The standards laid out through ICH have been adopted for research in medical products and device, making it relevant to all researchers involved in regulatory trials. More details about the ICH, including work products and guidelines, meetings, and training can be accessed at http://www.ich.org. More details about the ICH and its relation to good clinical practice (GCP) can be found in Chapter 10.

23.2.1 Role of the Regulatory Agency

A regulatory agency (also referred to as regulatory authority, regulatory body, or regulator) is a federal organization responsible for approving the import, sale, and distribution of drugs and medical products for clinical trials with the ultimate mission to ensure public health. This is achieved by reviewing clinical trial applications (CTAs) for phase I, II, and III clinical trials filed by clinical trial sponsors. Decisions to approve drugs and medical products are evidence based to ensure safety, quality, and efficacy.[2]

The ICH is the main regulatory agency in the world, with both member and observer states. Health Canada, for example, is the federal regulator in Canada and a member of the ICH responsible for authorizing distribution of medicinal products for clinical trials and into market. Regulatory bodies review CTAs for phase I, II, and III clinical trials, filed by clinical trial sponsors, and determine when medicinal products are deemed safe, efficacious, and of adequate quality to be used in patient care. Health Canada uses evidence in CTAs to determine, for example, that subjects participating in trials will not be exposed to undue risks. Every year, Health Canada authorizes over 900 clinical trials in patients.[8] Other key similar governmental authorities exist in most nations around the world and oversee clinical trial activities within their jurisdiction. Members of the ICH include the Food and Drug Administration (United States), EC (Europe), and China Food and Drug Administration (China).

Technischer Überwachungsverein (TUV) is one of the world's leading and longstanding technical service providers of testing and product certification, inspection, auditing, and system certification. Similar to regulatory bodies, TUV's purpose is to protect people, but goes further to protect the environment and assets from technology-related risk. By defining standards and going beyond regulatory compliance, medical devices often go through an additional application for certification from TUV.

As a research coordinator, you may find it confusing to navigate through regulatory affairs, particularly when working on multicenter and transnational clinical trials. You are not alone. There is limited information available that clearly describes how regulatory agencies, sponsors, and researchers work together to satisfy competing national and international demands. Resources that provide some support in this area are available at universities, through government agencies, and industry-sponsored associations.

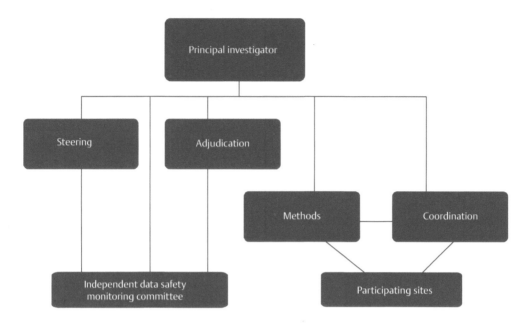

Fig. 23.1 Conventional clinical trial structure. (Adapted from Sprague and Bhandari 2009.[9])

23.2.2 Structure of Regulatory Trials

One of the most significant features of regulatory trials is the complexity of its organizational structure. Conventional clinical trials have a "flat" structure, where the principal investigator is directly involved in all aspects of trial management. ▶ Fig. 23.1 displays an organizational chart for a standard clinical trial. The principal investigator is responsible for communicating with each stakeholder, at times independently, in addition to communicating with the ethics committee.[9] Some of the communication activities can be delegated to research coordinators.

Regulatory trials have a specific structure that is complicated and has a distinct division of labor. In such trials, the principal investigator, who often holds a current medical license, is often responsible for the investigational new drug/product application and for ensuring that the trial is conducted properly.[10] Sometimes, the sponsor holds this responsibility. ▶ Fig. 23.2 shows the clinical structure of the late infantile neuronal ceroid lipofuscinosis (LINCL) regulatory trial, which is a phase I regulatory clinical trial

of gene medicine–based therapy for a fatal neurodegeneration disease in children. In this study structure, the principal investigator has no direct contact with site investigators and clinicians, completely removing possible conflicts of interest between patient care, the study sponsor, and clinical trial objectives. At the same time, regulatory authorities (e.g., FDA, National Institutes of Health [NIH]) have direct access to clinical operations for auditing and regulatory reporting purposes.[11] The principal investigator is still responsible for overseeing study operations, but direct access to clinical operations by regulatory authorities and ethics committees ensures that safety reporting, participant rights, and efficacy results used by the regulatory authorities for approvals are independently considered.

23.2.3 Key Differences between Standard Clinical Trials and Regulatory Trials

There are a lot of differences between standard clinical trials and regulatory trials. Perhaps the most significant and obvious difference is oversight by a national regulatory agency on the

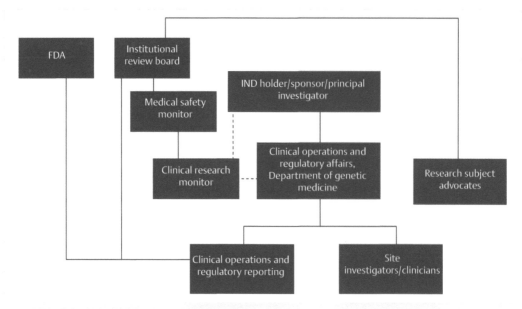

Fig. 23.2 Clinical organizational chart for the LINCL study. (*Abbreviations:* FDA, Food and Drug Administration; IND, Independent New Drug/Device application holder.) (Adapted from Arkin et al 2005.[11])

conduct of the trial before the trial starts, during the trial, and after the trial is completed or terminated. This constant involvement is the largest component in the lengthy timelines of regulatory trials and a key component in associated study costs. Other key features of regulatory trials are listed and described in the following section.

23.2.4 Good Clinical Practice Relevant in Regulatory Trials

GCP is a set of ethical standards laid out by the ICH to ensure that medicinal products, including pharmaceuticals, medical devices, blood products, alternative medicines, and other products along the patient care pathway, are evaluated and introduced into the global marketplace based on the highest level of evidence available. Not all clinical trials have to follow GCP ethical standards, but regulated clinical trials must be GCP compliant, to guarantee safety, efficacy, and high quality. While these standards support the use of medical products in the marketplace, they also serve to protect the rights, safety, and well-being of trials subjects.[12] Further details about GCP can be found in Chapter 10.

Below is a summary of GCP principles that may be applied to nonregulatory clinical investigations, but must be applied when generating clinical trial data that are intended to be submitted to regulatory authorities in the United States, European Union, and other ICH member states.[13,14] Many of these principles are also required by ICH observer states. There are 13 core principles in total, but 8 that are key to concepts discussed in this chapter (truncated from *Guideline for Good Clinical Practice, Integrated Addendum to ICH E6 (R1)*) have been paraphrased here:[1]

1. Clinical trials should be carried out in the spirit of the Declaration of Helsinki, that is, with the highest standard of ethical principles for medical research involving human subjects.
2. When planning a trial, risks to individual subjects and society, including animal and human public health, need to be considered against the potential benefits to patient care and future research. Literature reviews, feasibility studies, and pilot studies are helpful in this area.
3. Clinical trials should be developed using evidence-based approaches, and laid out in a clear, easy-to-follow format, referred to as a protocol.

4. A protocol must be submitted to and approved by an institutional review board (IRB) or independent ethics committee (IEC) before it begins. Once approved, a trial must be conducted exactly as stated in the protocol.
5. All members of a clinical trial team must demonstrate adequate education, training, and experience to fulfill their role in the study.
6. Information collected, exchanged, reported, analyzed, and interpreted during the course of a clinical trial must be handled with high-level data standards.
7. Subject confidentiality and, when necessary, anonymity must be protected and respected in the course of a clinical trial, and implemented according to relevant regulatory requirements.
8. Clinical trials involving investigational new products should use current good manufacturing practice (CGMP) to protect subject safety.

23.2.5 Follow a Detailed Protocol

Clinical trials should be developed using evidence-based approaches, and laid out in a clear, easy-to-follow format, referred to as a protocol. Regulatory trials must adhere to the protocol agreed to by the sponsor and investigator, which will be registered through one of the below-mentioned trial registries.

Deviations from regulatory trial protocols are not permitted without agreement by the sponsor, review by the IRB, and without a good reason, except when the safety of trial subjects is in question or if the deviation is considered a minor administrative change. Deviation forms are completed and retained to document important deviations from protocols.[15]

The requirement to follow a protocol also extends to planned analyses. Part of the protocol development process is identifying what information will be collected during the trial and how it will be analyzed. This involves describing outcome measures and listing primary and secondary endpoints that will be evaluated to draw conclusions about safety, efficacy, or quality of the intervention. Poorly planned analyses may bias the results of a trial and weaken confidence in the conclusions drawn. For example, conducting analyses on endpoints not originally outlined could lead to questions surrounding fishing for significance. Omitting analyses of identified endpoints can cause questions around safety to arise. If an unplanned analysis is conducted, the clinical study report should explain why it was necessary and how this change could impact the interpretation of the results.

Required elements of a clinical trial protocol and protocol amendments are detailed in the Guideline for Good Clinical Practice E6(R2).[1]

23.2.6 Trial Registration

Trial registration is the reporting of clinical trial design and methods by investigators to an accepted registry that makes this information publicly available. The WHO and International Committee of Medical Journal Editors (ICMJE) have been strong in this area, sending the consistent message that trial registration is a responsibility that ensures honest reporting.[16,17,18] The WHO has worked extensively on developing internationally accepted standards for trial registry and sharing this information with the research and patient community.[33] The ICMJE has supported this work through publication processes by requiring authors of manuscripts reporting regulated clinical trial results to provide their clinical trial registration number with any submissions.

There are many trial registries worldwide and the ICMJE does not give preference to any registry over the other. However, trial registries must be publicly accessible, available at no charge, and managed by a nonprofit organization.[16] The purpose of making this information available is to support a transparent research process that aids subjects, researchers, sponsors, and patient care. Public registration allows potential subjects to review similar studies and gauge potential risks to their own health before agreeing to participate. Registration or study design and investigational products allow researchers and sponsors to prevent unnecessary duplication of efforts, creating an environment where research can build on previous successes and mitigate previously reported safety risks. Finally, it provides regulatory agencies the opportunity to evaluate the risk of proposed clinical trials against an important body of evidence that is available prior to publication.

The WHO Registry Network is a network of prospective trial registries established in 2006 that help make all information about clinical trials involving humans freely available. For a clinical trial registry to be considered part of the WHO Registry Network, it must meet the WHO Registry Criteria. In November 2018, WHO published a set of international standards for clinical trial registries, and listed the minimum amount of trial information that must appear in a registry to meet these standards.[18] ▶Box 23.1 outlines the Trial Registration Data Set (TRDS), which is the minimum set of data required to meet the standards for content, quality and validity, accessibility, unambiguous identification, technical capacity, and administration and governance.

Box 23.1 Trial Registration Data Set (TRDS) (World Health Organization 2018)

Primary Registry and Trial Identifying Number
Date of Registration in Primary Registry
Secondary Identifying Numbers
Source(s) of Monetary or Material Support
Primary Sponsor
Secondary Sponsor(s)
Contact for Public Queries
Contact for Scientific Queries
Public Title
Scientific Title
Countries of Recruitment
Health Condition(s) or Problem(s) Studied
Intervention(s)
Key Inclusion and Exclusion Criteria
Study Type
Date of First Enrollment
Sample Size
Recruitment Status
Primary Outcome(s)
Key Secondary Outcomes
Ethics Review
Study Completion Date
Summary Results
Data Sharing Plan

More details on each of these data elements and primary and partner registries in the WHO Registry Network worldwide that meet these criteria can be found at http://www.who.int/ictrp/network/criteria_summary/en/ and http://www.who.int/iris/handle/10665/274994

23.2.7 Prompt Reporting and Public Disclosure of Interventional Clinical Trial Results

There are many examples of safety data being withheld from the public and regulatory bodies, where perhaps the most tragic and transformative example is the thalidomide disaster that affected public health across the globe for decades and continues to affect public health today.[20] More information about this tragedy and dark area in pharmaceutical history will be discussed in the practical example at the end of this chapter. A key principle in GCP is that the trial protocol be made available and that results are reported publicly as soon as possible.

The WHO has also been strong in the area of timely reporting of clinical trial results. With time, guidance in this area has become more prescriptive and less ambiguous in the interest of public health and safety. In addition to reaffirming the ethical imperative of reporting clinical trial results, the WHO's latest statement defines reporting timeframes, calls for reporting past study results that remain unpublished, and outlines how to link trial registry entries with published results.[21] Main features of this statement include that clinical trials must be reported within 24 months of completion but ideally within 12 months and that publications should be open access where possible.

Measures to enhance clinical trial transparency and reduce selective reporting continue to evolve and expand globally. The new EU Clinical Trials Regulation No. 536/2014 will harmonize how clinical trials are reported and disclosed across the EU, providing even greater transparency. In the United States, the Department of Health & Human Services (HHS) and NIH have issued new policies to expand the scope of clinical trial registration and sharing findings. The government of Canada has recently announced that the health science industry is one of the sectors targeted for regulatory reform. One area under review is working to make clinical information about the safety and efficacy of drugs and medical devices available to the public, assuring consistency across regulatory bodies in other regions and across investigational products used in clinical trials.[13]

Despite recent national and international initiatives, existing regulatory requirements, and coordinated efforts by the ICMJE, studies on clinical trial transparency rates show that there is still work to be done in this area. Not all trial results are reported through manuscript submissions or registries and some who do fail to do so within established timelines.[22,23] The public availability of clinical trial results through trial portal registries and moves toward universal mandatory registration will hopefully improve public access to this information.

23.2.8 Safety Reporting

Clinical trials provide the quality, safety, and efficacy evidence used by regulatory agencies to approve the use of medical products in humans. Since these trials often involve experiments using human participants, they must adhere to established standards to protect the rights, safety, and well-being of participants.[24] Some of the established international standards for safety include the ICH-GCP,[15] International Ethical Guidelines for Biomedical Research Involving Human Subjects issued by the Council for International Organizations of Medical Sciences (CIOMS),[25] and the ethical principles set forth in the Declaration of Helsinki.[12]

As sponsors in pharmaceutical, medical device, biological products, and other health science innovation sectors move into an ever-expanding global marketplace, so, too, does their responsibility to ensure safety and to be accountable to a multitude of regulatory requirements, in a process known as pharmacovigilance. Pharmacovigilance is the science and activities related to the detection, assessment, understanding, and prevention of adverse effects or any other drug-related problems.[26] Recently, this definition has been expanded to include herbal medicine, traditional medicines, biological products, medical devices, and vaccines. Safety evaluation is critical to all stages of the medical product life cycle and provides a foundation for pharmacovigilance efforts. Prior to market authorization, safety needs to be assured, and this occurs through the process of rigorous testing, safety monitoring, developing a safety profile, and reporting these results to the medical community at large, including patients.

23.3 The Research Coordinator's Responsibilities

Research coordinators may be tasked with recording and/or reporting clinical safety data information. Two main areas within clinical safety data include standard terminology[5] and reporting mechanisms.[27] This information is laid out in detail in the Clinical Safety Data Management: Definitions and Standards for Expedited Reporting E2A,[28] but it is summarized in the following section.

23.4 Standard Definitions

There are very important basic terms that need to be understood and used internationally when discussing safety during regulated clinical trials. These terms are used by sponsors, regulatory agencies, IRBs, universities, in the literature, and other relevant stakeholders worldwide, and have been agreed upon through international collaboration. Key terms that are important when recording and reporting safety information to sponsors and ethics committees, particularly when regulatory authorities are involved, and how they should be used, are the following:[28]

- *Adverse event (or adverse experience)*: Any untoward medical occurrence in a patient or clinical investigation subject administered a pharmaceutical product and which does not necessarily have to have a causal relationship with this treatment.
- *Adverse drug reaction (ADR)*: During the pre-approval clinical experience, all noxious and unintended responses to a medicinal product related to any dose should be considered ADRs. Regarding marketed medicinal products, a response to a drug that is noxious and unintended and that occurs at doses normally used in man for prophylaxis, diagnosis, or therapy of disease or for modification of physiological function.
- *Unexpected ADR*: An adverse reaction, the nature or severity of which is not consistent with the applicable product information (e.g., Investigator's Brochure for an unapproved investigational product).
- *Severe:* Note that "severe" and "serious" have two very different meanings. "Severe" describes the intensity of a specific event.
- *Serious adverse event or ADR:* A serious adverse event (experience) or reaction is any untoward medical occurrence that at any dose:
  - Results in death.
  - Is life-threatening.
  - Requires inpatient hospitalization or prolongation of existing hospitalization.
  - Results in persistent or significant disability/incapacity.
  - Is a congenital anomaly/birth defect.

Such reactions must be reported promptly to regulators.

23.5 Expedited Reporting: When, What, Why, and How?

23.5.1 What and Why?

All adverse events that are serious and unexpected must be reported immediately. Expected serious reactions and serious reactions that are not considered related to the investigational product are not subject to expedited reporting. In some situations, rapid communication to regulatory authorities is necessary, simply based on medical and scientific judgment. This includes the following: an increase in an "expected" severe adverse event; a significant hazard to a patient population, such as reduced efficacy of a life-saving intervention; and a major safety finding from a recently completed preclinical trial. Regulatory agencies must be notified by the sponsor by telephone, facsimile transmission, or in writing. They should never be informed by email, as email is not considered a safe way to transfer identifiable health information.

23.5.2 When?

A research coordinator should inform the principal investigator of a serious adverse event right away, who will then report this information to the IRB and any other relevant stakeholders. There are internationally accepted timeframes for reporting adverse events, particularly for serious and unexpected adverse events, to regulatory agencies. These are listed in the following section.

23.5.3 Event Time Frame

Fatal or life-threatening unexpected ADRs: 7 calendar days after first notification.

Other serious, unexpected ADRs: 15 calendar days after first notification.

23.5.4 How?

For regulatory purposes, initial reports of serious or unexpected adverse events should be reported within the above timeframe and contain the following minimum set of criteria:
- An identifiable patient.
- A suspect medicinal product.
- The reporting source.
- An adverse event or outcome that is considered serious and unexpected, and for which a causal relationship is expected.

There are a variety of ways that expedited reporting of adverse events can take place. Attachment 1 of the Clinical Safety Data Management: Definitions and Standards for Expedited Reporting E2A[28] has the criteria above broken down by each element. The CIOMS-I form is a widely accepted standard for collecting and reporting this information. The form is not required, but the information is. This form can be accessed through the link "https://cioms.ch/cioms-i-form/," in case you or your research team ever need to collect and report this information.

23.5.5 Documentation

One of the main features of regulatory trials is the volume and breadth of the essential documents required to ensure that quality data are produced through the trial. Documents are required to indicate compliance with regulatory processes; detail the product under investigation; guarantee adequate training of the study team; confirm adequate data safety standards are in place; and confirm that an evidence-based protocol will be, is, and was followed to completion or study termination. These documents are audited by the sponsor's independent audit team and inspected by regulatory authorities to confirm the validity and integrity of the study being conducted.

Essential documents for a regulated clinical trial can be understood by being grouped according to the stage of the trial for which they are typically generated: (1) before the clinical phase of the trial begins, (2) during the clinical conduct of the trial, and (3) after completion or termination. These documents are summarized in ▶ Table 23.1 and are typically housed in trial master files (see Chapter 13 for more details about the trial master file):

23.5.6 Audits

All regulatory clinical trial sites need to be prepared for an audit by a sponsor, ethics committee, or regulatory agency. The purpose of audits is to evaluate trial conduct and compliance with the protocol, standard operating procedures (SOPs),

GCP, and applicable regulatory requirements using a systematic approach.

Details about the components of an audit, and how to prepare for and survive an audit, are presented in Chapter 24.

23.5.7 Investigator Qualifications and Agreements

All study trials that are GCP compliant require that investigators and all members of the research team have adequate education and skills to complete their role in the study. There are regulatory requirements that outline the necessary education, training, and experience of members of the clinical trial team, including what documents are required for their confirmation. During a regulatory audit, evidence of adequate qualifications, training, and experience of all site staff is one of the most important sets of essential documents reviewed. It is important that all of this information is up-to-date, including signed and dated updated curriculum vitae for each research team member, document training logs, evidence of current CGP training, evidence of current and relevant professional certifications, a copy of current license to practice, and evidence of any other training or credentials required to confirm that those involved in the clinical study are qualified to do so. An example of this is a listing of when and how each team member was trained on the study protocol. If relevant, training performance should also be documented (e.g., if a quiz was administered). This information must be easily accessible through the Trial Master File.

23.5.8 Clinical Study Report

There has been international agreement to assemble all the quality, safety, and efficacy information for clinical trials in a common format called the Common Technical Document (CTD). The harmonization of the CTD, led by the ICH, has drastically simplified regulatory review processes, particularly where multicenter trials are conducted internationally and there was the previous need to reproduce, submit, and review multiple regulatory submissions.[29] All of the results obtained through regulated clinical trials must be presented in the clinical study report, which is the fifth module of the CTD. Details on how to complete a clinical study report for regulatory trials can be found at

https://www.ich.org/fileadmin/Public_Web_Site/ICH_Products/Guidelines/Efficacy/E3/E3_Guideline.pdf.

23.5.9 Practical Application

Regulating trials is about much more than the conduct of clinical trials. It is also about transparency and credibility and extends to how results are applied to the development of interventions, reported in scientific literature, and shared with the public, be it through formal knowledge translation channels, marketing materials, or product labeling.

The thalidomide tragedy in the late 1950s was a seminal moment in pharmaceutical history sparking international recognition of the need for regulation reform in the industry. Because of the serious and long-lasting impacts of the thalidomide that spread worldwide and into subsequent generations, thalidomide is considered one of the most important drugs of the 20th century in terms of mobilizing health legislation and starting a movement for pharmacovigilance for medications. It represents a dark period in pharmaceutical history and was the impetus for transforming state authority over the pharmaceutical industry across the world and increasing harmonization of efforts in preventing the use of harmful drugs and adequately communicating the risks to health care practitioners, the public, and regulatory bodies in the interest of public health worldwide. We will look at this example with a view to consider the aspects of regulatory trials discussed in this chapter and finish with how to respond should a serious adverse event become apparent in one of your regulated clinical studies.

The details of the thalidomide tragedy are being recounted based on excerpts from Adriana Moro and Noela Invernizzi's article titled "The thalidomide tragedy: the struggle for victims' rights and improved pharmaceutical regulation." This article goes beyond discussing the regulatory and clinical history, but examines the role that the media, public, and public health advocates played in shaping history and pharmaceutical regulation and the current impacts being felt in the next generation of thalidomide victims in Brazil.[20]

Thalidomide was presented in the 1950s as a wonder drug, recognized worldwide as a treatment for insomnia after Herbert Keller of West Germany demonstrated its efficient use as a sedative and hypnotic in 1957. At that time, the tests

Table 23.1 Essential documents for a regulated clinical trial

Document	Purpose to document		
	Before the clinical trial starts	During the clinical trial	After the trial is completed or terminated
Investigator's Brochure	Relevant and current scientific information about the investigational product	That investigator is informed of relevant information as it becomes available	Filed in investigator's notebook
Signed protocol, amendments, sample clinical research forms (CRFs)	Investigator and sponsor agreement to the protocol/amendments and CRF	Revisions of these trial-related documents that take effect during trial	Filed in investigator's notebook
Information given to trial subjects	Informed consent obtained in accordance with GCP and subject recruitment is appropriate	Any revisions to information provided to subjects	Filed in investigator's notebook
Budgetary agreements	Financial agreement between the investigator/institution and the sponsor for the trial	Updated copy provided to investigator, if amended	Filed in investigator's notebook
Research Ethics Board (REB) communications	REB review and approval, including amendments	Amendment(s) and/or revision(s) have been subject to IRB/IEC review, were approved, and version number and dates recorded	Notifying REB of completion of trial
Regulatory authority authorization	Registration of trial protocol and authorization to complete the trial	Compliance with regulatory requirements	Notifying regulatory authority of completion of trial
CV, training logs, licenses	Qualifications to conduct trial and provide care	Updated as new members join the study team	Filed in investigator's notebook
Medical/laboratory/technical procedures	Normal values and/or ranges of the tests	Normal values and ranges that are revised during trial	X
Instructions for trials materials	Instructions to ensure proper storage, packaging, dispensing, and disposition of investigational product(s) and trial-related materials	Certification, accreditation, quality control, validation and that tests remain the same; shipment dates, batch numbers, method of shipment	X
Decoding procedures for blinded trials	How the identity of blinded product can be revealed, if needed	X	Any decoding that may have occurred and records of treatment allocation are returned to sponsor
Master randomization list	Method for randomization of trial population	X	Filed in investigator's notebook
Monitoring reports	Site is suitable for the trial and trial procedures were reviewed with site investigator and staff	Site visits and findings of monitor	That audit was performed and audit certificate received, if available

(Continued)

Table 23.1 (*Continued*) Essential documents for a regulated clinical trial

Document	Purpose to document		
Relevant communications with sponsor	Monitor visited site prior to the start date to prepare site	Administration, protocol deviations, serious adverse events, and other safety information	That all activities required for trial closeout are completed and copies of essential documents are held in the appropriate files
Source documents	X	Existence of subject and integrity of trial data	Kept on site in case of audit
Completed CRFs/ corrections	X	Investigator or authorized member of the investigator's staff confirms the observations recorded	All changes and corrections made after initial data collection
Subject screening log	X	Identify subjects who entered pretrial screening	Filed in investigator's notebook
Subject identification codes	X	Confidential list of all subjects allocated to trial numbers to allow identity to be revealed	Permission to identify all subjects enrolled in the trial in case follow-up is required
Signature sheet	All persons authorized to make CRF entries and corrections	All persons authorized to make CRF entries and corrections	Filed in investigator's notebook
Investigational product accountability	X	That investigational product(s) have been used according to the protocol	Investigational product(s) have been used according to the protocol, the final accounting of investigational product(s) received at the site, dispensed to subjects, returned by the subjects, returned to sponsor, and destruction of unused investigational product
Clinical study report	X	X	Results and interpretation of trial

Source: ICH 2016.[1]
Note: All documents addressed in this table may be subject to, and should be made available for, audit by the sponsor's auditor and inspection by regulatory authorities.

showed no toxicity, and a lethal dose was not established. Animal experimentation in science at that time was restricted to rats, and rarely birds, pigs, or mice. Teratological testing was limited and the literature of the era does not mention that the group of neuroleptic drugs, tranquilizers, sedatives, and antiemetics was tested.

The drug was launched on the market in 1956 as a cold and flu medication, under the trademark Grippex. Despite insufficient studies on its safety in humans, Grünenthal launched the drug Contergan as a sedative in October of 1957 and it

was one of the most widely sold medications in West Germany that year. Grünenthal launched an advertising campaign stating that the substance was innocuous and safe. Ads were planned for fifty top-line medical publications, in addition to two hundred thousand letters to physicians and fifty thousand to pharmacists around the world. Sales during the first year of production reached 90,000 units per month in twenty countries, and spread across the other continents. Thalidomide was marketed under at least 52 trade names worldwide. It was so successful that in 1958, the beverage distributor Distillers Biochemicals Ltd. (DBCL), which owned the Johnnie Walker label, became a distributor. Marketing efforts became so aggressive that advertisements in Brazil offered physicians literature and free samples for distribution. Ads also stated that the drug was well-tolerated by children and patients with liver damage. The United States was one of the few countries which did not allow this drug to be sold, on the recommendation of Frances Kelsey, a researcher at the Food and Drug Administration (FDA). Frances Kelsey's actions later formed the basis for transforming regulation in the United States and then across the world.

Adverse Events Reporting

In 1958, Grünenthal began to receive notifications from laypersons about peripheral neuropathies, represented by cramps, muscle weakness, and loss of motor coordination. In 1961, reports were made that the drug could cause constipation, dizziness, a hangover sensation, and memory loss. An initial study published in that same year in the *British Medical Journal* by James Murdoch advised against long-term use because no studies had been conducted on long-term effects. Lay reports about possible malformations had been made, but the first medical reports of cases of teratogenicity in children in Germany date back to 1959. These described a distinctive type of congenital malformation, caused by faulty development of the long bones in the arms and legs, as well as hands and feet which varied from rudimentary to normal. The first study that drew attention to the increasing incidence of extremity malformations was performed by Wiedemann in 1961.[30] In that same year, during the North Rhine-Westphalia Pediatric Meeting in Germany, Lenz[31] quoted another recent study and advocated removing the drug from the market until new studies were conducted, associating 34 cases of babies with congenital malformations of the extremities born to mothers who had used thalidomide during pregnancy. This hypothesis was confirmed by McBride in Australia (also in 1961), and by the presentation of other anomalies affecting various systems and organs which were described as teratogenic malformations.

The abnormalities caused by thalidomide include hearing loss, ocular alterations, deafness, facial paralysis, malformations in the larynx,

trachea, lungs, and heart, and mental retardation in 6.6% of affected individuals. The mortality rate among the victims ranged from 40 to 45%. Around the world, between 10,000 and 15,000 children were born with the characteristic abnormalities associated with thalidomide, and 40% died during the first year of life.[32] Thalidomide babies are still born today. Those who survive live with severe physical challenges.

Chemie Grünenthal withdrew the drug from the market through its distributor DBCL in December of 1961, after publication of the research that linked thalidomide to birth defects. Another distributor of the drug, Merrell Company, withdrew it in March of 1962.

How Regulation Was Transformed?

The thalidomide tragedy unfolded differently in two of the major western powers at that time, Germany and the United States, due to their different practices in the area of medicine and pharmaceutical regulation. Thanks to Frances Kelsey, a Canadian pharmacist employed by the FDA, the drug was not approved by the FDA for use in the United States, under the argument that the testing was insufficient. The cases of thalidomide-related teratogenicity recorded in the United States resulted from the use of the drug in pregnant women during clinical trials conducted by 1,200 physicians who received the medication directly from the company, since before this episode the government had no regulatory control over clinical trials. This has since changed, with the FDA transforming their role and establishing the Investigational New Drug Application procedure,[14] charged with monitoring the development of clinical trials that determine the safety and efficacy of new drugs.[33,10]

In Europe, the regulatory issue also took on transformative dimensions. In 1964, the World Medical Association published the Helsinki Declaration, which established standards for clinical research (see Chapter 10). Following this declaration, the then European Economic Community (EEC) recognized the need to regulate medications, and approved directive 65/65/EEC of January 26, 1965, which formed the basis of European pharmaceutical legislation. The Declaration of Helsinki, if you recall, laid the foundation for the International Conference on Harmonisation GCP guidelines, and ethical conduct of research involving human participants.

Think Practically

The history of thalidomide in Brazil was different from what occurred in other countries. Sales of the drug began in March 1958, almost 2 years after serious adverse events were identified in Germany. Notes on the withdrawal of thalidomide appeared in the Diário Oficial and O Estado de S. Paulo newspapers in August of 1962 and then later in 1965, 4 years after Germany. Even after the official withdrawal of thalidomide, it remained in some Brazilian drugstores for many years and continued to be sold by several laboratories because there was no regulation effectively banning its sale. In Brazil, 5,889,210 pills of thalidomide were distributed between 2005 and 2010.[32]

In 1965, after thalidomide was officially withdrawn from distribution, the drug was approved in Brazil for treatment of erythema nodosum leprosum, also known as leprosy. In 2013, between 30,000 and 33,000 "thalidomide baby" cases were registered in Brazil, demonstrating continuous use of thalidomide in the country. In 1961, the National Health Code (Código Nacional de Saúde) was approved, establishing general rules on the defense and protection of health, charging the Ministry of Health with adopting preventive measures and also instituting the Central Laboratory for Drug, Medication, and Food Control. Even though this action coincided with the initial phase of the reported events, it did not help impede the effects of thalidomide in the Brazilian population because the medication was only banned and recalled, legislation to support this work was not developed, and there were limited controls put in place to control other uses for the medication.

Since this time, many laws have been put in place in Brazil, where thalidomide is the only medication in the country to have its own law (Law 10.651). Several other standards have been established throughout Brazil, and there are efforts by multinational pharmaceutical corporations, international collaborative nonprofit originations, such as the ICH and WHO, and industry advocates to ensure public safety. As new uses for thalidomide continue to be researched, pharmacovigilance is still required to manage and prevent serious adverse events that take place.

What Is Your Role?

If you look at the differences between regulatory trials and conventional clinical trials, you will see that a number of characteristics of current regulatory trial design will impede future tragedies like the thalidomide disaster. The term "impede" is used because this was not the first such disaster in human health history,[34] and other disasters have taken place since this time.[27] By following GCP guidelines and considering responsibilities set forth by regulatory bodies, many actions are put in place to promote human health. Think about the following:

- In what ways do GCP guidelines protect you and your research team?
- You have a detailed protocol that you will follow. What other agencies have this protocol, knows that you will follow it, and supports you moving forward?
- Is your trial registered? If so, where, and how accessible is it?
- What type of adverse events qualifies for expedited reporting?
- Where is study documentation housed? Are you ready for an audit?
- Investigator qualifications and agreements are documented. Can you find the help or advice that you need?
- You see that your study is an extension of an earlier study. Where is that clinical study report?

Do You Know What to Do?

You are involved in a regulated trial. Recall that a serious adverse event (experience) or reaction is defined as any untoward medical occurrence that at any dose results in death, is life-threatening, requires inpatient hospitalization or prolongation of existing hospitalization, results in persistent or significant disability/incapacity, or is a congenital anomaly/birth defect.[28] You certainly were not expecting it, but a nurse from your clinical sites calls and accounts that a study participant had an ultrasound that appears abnormal. The long bones in the baby's arms seem short. Few details are given, but she will get back to you and hangs up. There are things that you can do to help.

Your site principal investigator must be notified by a telephone call, facsimile, or in person. Recall that the regulatory agency will need to be notified within 7 days or 15 days, depending on whether or not this is a life-threatening situation. This notification will come directly from the study sponsor. However, important information will need to be collected and you may play a big role in coordinating these efforts.[33] The study sponsor will need to be notified within 24 hours, to ensure that reporting timelines are met. Various study stakeholders have varying reporting responsibilities. You can begin by doing the following:

- Contacting your site principal investigator.
- Assembling contact/phone numbers for the study team, including the study sponsor, site principal investigator, clinician who initially contacted you, and IRB contact.
- Accessing and maintaining a means to collect pertinent information that needs to be reported, such as through the CIOMS-I.
- Reviewing the Trial Master File and ensuring the information is up-to-date and accessible, including the Investigator's Brochure and unblinding procedures.
- Do you have any additional information that might help the sponsor assess causality?

23.6 Conclusion

In this chapter, we discussed the key aspects of regulatory trials and how they differ from conventional clinical trials. We looked at what types of standards are in place that make regulatory trials expensive, labor intensive, time-consuming, and complicated, which are necessary to ensure impartial and effective oversight that is free of conflict of interest. Throughout this chapter, we discussed why these standards are in place, some of the key players involved in establishing these standards internationally, and how a research coordinator may put these standards into practice. Finally, we concluded by reviewing regulatory concepts presented in this chapter through the lens of the thalidomide tragedy and what responsibility a research coordinator has in contributing to promoting public health through good clinical conduct and timely safety reporting. We all have a role to play in ensuring that safe, effective, and high-quality medical interventions are developed, registered, and used in patient care. Research coordinators play a vital part in how patient care evidence is used and helps move innovation forward.

Definitions

- **Efficacy:** the performance of an intervention under ideal and controlled circumstances.

- **Harmonisation:** The process of creating common standards across the market, which governments can transpose into regulations for clinical trials involving human subjects.
- **Protocol:** A precise and detailed plan for the study of a medical or biomedical problem and/or plans for a medical intervention.
- **Serious adverse event:** Any untoward medical occurrence that at any dose results in death, is life-threatening, requires inpatient hospitalization or prolongation of existing hospitalization, results in persistent or significant disability/incapacity, or is a congenital anomaly/birth defect.
- **Trial registration:** The publication of an internationally agreed set of information about the design, conduct, and administration of clinical trials that are published on a publicly accessible website managed by a registry conforming to WHO standards.

References

[1] ICH Harmonised Tripartite Guideline: Guideline for Good Clinical Practice. 8. Essential Documents for the Conduct of a Clinical Trial. J Postgrad Med 2001;47:264

[2] Marsh J, Bryant D. Management Issues Unique to Regulatory Trials. J Long Term Eff Med Implants 2009;19(3):201–208

[3] Paine MF. Therapeutic Disasters that Hastened Safety Testing of New Drugs. Clin Pharmacol Ther 2017;101(4):430–434

[4] Vermeulen I. Regulatory Requirements. In: Shamley D, Wright B, eds. A Comprehensive and Practical Guide to Clinical Trials. London: Academic Press; 2017:27–42

[5] Abraham J. Bias in Science and Medical Knowledge: The Opren Controversy. Sociology 1994;28(3):717–736

[6] ICH. About ICH: History. Available from: https://www.ich.org/about/history.html. Accessed December 20, 2018

[7] Lourenco C, Orphanos N, Parker C. The International Council for Harmonisation: Positioning for the Future With its Recent Reform and Over 25 years of Harmonisation Work. Pharmaceuticals Policy and Law. 2016;18(1-4):79–89

[8] Health Canada. Health Canada's Clinical Trials Database (Web page). Available from: https://www.canada.ca/en/health-canada/services/drugs-health-products/drug-products/health-canada-clinical-trials-database.html. Accessed December 21, 2018

[9] Sprague S, Bhandari M. Organization and Planning. In: Gad SC, ed. Clinical Trials Handbook. New York, NY: Wiley; 2009:161–185

[10] US Food & Drug Administration. Available from: href="https://www.fda.gov/drugs/types-applications/investigational-new-drug-ind-application

[11] Arkin ML, Sondhi D, Worgall S, et al. Confronting the Issues of Therapeutic Misconception, Enrollment Decisions, and Personal Motives in Genetic Medicine-Based

Clinical Research Studies for Fatal Disorders. Hum Gene Ther 2005; 16(9):1028–1036

[12] World Medical Association. World Medical Association Declaration of Helsinki: Ethical Principles for Medical Research Involving Human Subjects. JAMA 2013;310(20):2191–2194

[13] European Commission. Directive 2001/20/EC of the European Parliament and of the Council of 4 April 2001 on the approximation of the laws, regulations and administrative provisions of the Member States relating to the implementation of good clinical practice in the conduct of clinical trials on medicinal products for human use. Official Journal of the European Communities 1.5.2001: L121/34–L121/44. www.eortc.be/services/doc/clinical-eu-directive-04-april-01.pdf

[14] U.S. Department of Health and Human Services; Food and Drug Administration; Center for Drug Evaluation and Research; Center for Biologics Evaluation and Research. Good Clinical Practice: Integrated Addendum to ICH E6(R1) Guidance for Industry E6(R2). Silver Spring, MD: Food and Drug Administration; 2018

[15] International Council for Harmonisation of Technical Requirements for Pharmaceuticals for Human Use. 1996. Available from: https://www.ich.org/fileadmin/Public_Web_Site/ICH_Products/Guidelines/Efficacy/E6/E6_R2__Step_4.pdf. Accessed August 8, 2018

[16] De Angelis C, Drazen JM, Frizelle FA, et al. International Committee of Medical Journal Editors. Clinical trial registration: a statement from the International Committee of Medical Journal Editors. CMAJ 2004;171(6):606–607

[17] Lemmens T, Vacaflor CH. Clinical Trial Transparency in the Americas: The Need to Coordinate Regulatory Spheres. BMJ 2018;362:k2493

[18] World Health Organization. International Standards for Clinical Trial Registries Version 3.0. Geneva: World Health Organization; 2018

[19] WHO. International Standards for Clinical Trial Registries. Geneva: World Health Organization; 2012

[20] Moro A, Invernizzi N. The Thalidomide Tragedy: The Struggle for Victims' Rights and Improved Pharmaceutical Regulation. Hist Cienc Saude Manguinhos 2017;24(3):603–622

[21] Moorthy VS, Karam G, Vannice KS, Kieny M-P. Rationale for WHO's New Position Calling for Prompt Reporting and Public Disclosure of Interventional Clinical Trial Results. PLoS Med 2015;12(4):e1001819

[22] Anderson ML, Chiswell K, Peterson ED, Tasneem A, Topping J, Califf RM. Compliance with Results Reporting at ClinicalTrials.gov. N Engl J Med 2015;372:1031–1039

[23] Prayle AP, Hurley MN, Smyth AR. Compliance with Mandatory Reporting of Clinical Trial Results on ClinicalTrials.gov: Cross Sectional Study. BMJ 2012;344:d7373

[24] Yao B, Zhu L, Jiang Q, Xia HA. Safety Monitoring in Clinical Trials. Pharmaceutics 2013;5(1):94–106

[25] CIOMS & WHO. International Ethical Guidelines for Biomedical Research Involving Human Subjects. Geneva: Who; 2002

[26] World Health Organization. The Importance of Pharmacovigilance. (Safety monitoring of Medicinal Products). Geneva: World Health Organization; 2002

[27] Ahmed SS, Schur PH, MacDonald NE, Steinman L. Narcolepsy, 2009 A(H1N1) Pandemic Influenza, and Pandemic Influenza Vaccinations: What is Known and Unknown About the Neurological Disorder, the Role for Autoimmunity, and Vaccine Adjuvants. J Autoimmun 2014;50:1–11

[28] International Council for Harmonisation of Technical Requirements for Pharmaceuticals for Human Use. Clinical Safety Data Management: Definitions and Standards for Expedited Reporting E2A. 1994. Available from: https://www.ich.org/fileadmin/Public_Web_Site/ICH_Products/Guidelines/Efficacy/E2A/Step4/E2A_Guideline.pdf. Accessed August 8, 2018

[29] ICH. ICH Harmonised Tripartite Guideline: Structure and Content of Clinical Study Reports E3. Geneva: ICH; 1995

[30] Oliveira MA, Bermudez JA, Souza AC. Thalidomide in Brazil: Monitoring with Shared Responsibility? Cad Saude Publica 1999;15(1):99–112

[31] Lenz W. A Short History of Thalidomide Embryopathy. Teratology 1988;38(3):203–215

[32] Sales Luiz Vianna F, Kowalski TW, Fraga LR, Sanseverino MT, Schuler-Faccini L. The Impact of Thalidomide Use in Birth Defects in Brazil. Eur J Med Genet 2017;60(1):12–15

[33] Crépin S, Villeneuve C, Merle L. Quality of Serious Adverse Events Reporting to Academic Sponsors of Clinical Trials: Far from Optimal. Pharmacoepidemiol Drug Saf 2016;25(6):719–724

[34] Rahalkar H. Historical Overview of Pharmaceutical Industry and Drug Regulatory Affairs. Pharm Regul Aff 2012;11:2

Further Readings

International Clinical Trials Registry Platform. International standards for Clinical Trial Registries. Geneva: World Health Organization; 2012

International Conference on Harmonisation (ICH) Guideline for Good Clinical Practice E6(R1). 1996. Available from: http://www.ich.org/fileadmin/Public_Web_Site/ICH_Products/Guidelines/Efficacy/E6_R1/Step4/E6_R1__Guideline.pdf. Accessed October 8, 2010

REGULATION (EU) No 536/2014 OF THE EUROPEAN PARLIAMENT AND OF THE COUNCIL of 16 April 2014 on clinical trials on medicinal products for human use, and repealing Directive 2001/20/EC

24 How to Survive a Site Audit

Annemieke I.J.M. Schellevis-Mintiens, Esther M.M. Van Lieshout

Abstract

In this chapter, we explain how to handle a site audit at a practical level. Good preparation of team and documentation, professional behavior during the audit, and extensive attention for the report and corrective actions are key. First, the difference between monitoring and auditing is explained more theoretically using the three lines of defense model.

Keywords: audit, compliance, documentation, quality control, responsibilities

24.1 Introduction

When you are part of a team conducting clinical research, you may dread the announcement that your study will be audited. However, surviving an audit is pretty straightforward, and a successful audit creates a moment to celebrate what went well as well as an opportunity to learn and improve where needed. In this chapter, we will give practical advice on how to act upon the announcement of an audit: how to prepare for it, how to act during the audit, and how to reply upon arrival of the report. Before getting to the tips and tricks on how to survive a site audit, we will explain the difference between monitoring and auditing, relating these processes to the three lines of defense model.

24.2 The Difference between Monitoring and Auditing

At first glance, the difference between monitoring and auditing may not seem obvious; monitors and auditors both check the study documents and conduct of the study. However, these are two distinct processes. Monitoring is meant to check and correct the execution of the study and is therefore always performed during the study. Preferably, monitoring starts early in the study so mistakes can be corrected and repetition of the same mistake can be avoided. For example, the monitor checks the informed consent process after inclusion of the first three participants and finds that the wrong versions of the information sheet and consent form have been used. This will

be stated in the monitoring report including the subject ID numbers. Upon receipt of the monitoring report, the principal investigator (PI) will take three actions: (1) they will make sure the subjects are re-consented as soon as possible, (2) they will make sure the re-consent process is adequately documented in the study file, and (3) they will make sure the correct version of the consent documents is being used from that point onward subject by instructing the study staff and making sure only the approved versions of the consent documents are accessible. As a rule of thumb, the intensity of monitoring is risk based; the greater the risk, the more items checked.

Auditors also check the study, but they do this on the level of the study processes so they can assess proper organization and execution of the study including monitoring. One of the aspects they verify is indeed monitoring. Auditors ask whether the study is monitored by a qualified monitor who is not otherwise involved in the study. They check whether reports are being made and whether appropriate actions are taken by those responsible for the study. Other processes checked by auditors include the informed consent process, the serious adverse event (SAE) reporting and handling process, and privacy of subjects. Apart from obvious compliance aspects, auditors may also focus on proper delegation of responsibilities. Audits may focus on one study but may also look at the performance of a department or institution. Audits may be performed during or after a study.

Monitoring and auditing are both about quality and compliance. The relation and differences between monitoring and auditing has been made clearer by the "three lines of defense" model that originates from financial auditing.

24.2.1 First Line of Defense: Procedures

To make sure a task is done properly, you need to have a set of standard operating procedures (SOPs). SOPs ensure that tasks are standardized and processes are formalized. Standardized procedures are your first line of defense against bad science. An example of the first line of defense is double data entry into the database, which is aimed at ensuring that the final database has no entry errors.

24.2.2 Second Line of Defense: Monitoring

Monitoring is defined as "the act of overseeing the progress of a clinical trial, and ensuring that it is conducted, recorded, and reported in accordance with the protocol, SOPs, Good Clinical Practice (GCP), and the applicable regulatory requirement(s)" (ICH 1.38).[1]

The aim of monitoring is to verify that:

- The rights and well-being of the study participants are protected.
- The reported study data are accurate, complete, and verifiable from source documents.
- The conduct of the study is in compliance with the approved protocol (or amendment), with GCP and with the applicable regulatory requirements.

Monitors are the main line of communication between the sponsor and the investigator. They are appointed by the sponsor. They need to be properly trained and should have sufficient scientific and clinical knowledge to monitor the study adequately. More specifically, they need to have detailed knowledge of the investigational product, the protocol, the informed consent form, the SOPs, GCP, and the regulatory requirements.

Examples of tasks performed by a monitor are to check (at least for the first few patients and then a random sample) the informed consent forms, eligibility criteria, source document verification (SDV), protocol compliance, adverse event (AE) reporting, and presence and completeness of the Trial Master File and Investigator File.

24.2.3 Third Line of Defense: Auditing

An audit is defined as "a systematic and independent examination of study-related activities and documents to determine whether the evaluated study-related activities were conducted, and the data were recorded, analyzed, and accurately reported according to the protocol, sponsor's SOPs, GCP, and the applicable regulatory requirement(s)" (ICH 1.6).[1] Audits are not done

continuously the way monitoring is performed during a study, but instead are compliance snapshots in time.

A fundamental difference with monitors is that authors are independent of a clinical study, data collection system, sponsor, contract research organization, or study site.

In general, research audits have three main functions:

1. To ensure participants' rights, well-being, and safety.
2. To ensure integrity of clinical and research data.
3. To allow sound decision-making regarding efficacy and safety of investigational (medicinal) product(s) or procedures.

Auditors assess this by thoroughly checking the study and clinical documentation to ensure compliance with GCP guidelines and regulations and to ensure that monitoring responsibilities have been undertaken to a satisfactory level. Auditors also check to ensure that data received by regulatory authorities can be verified through source data at each study site.

Research audits can be done by the institute's internal audit team, but also by health care inspectors or regulatory authorities. The latter may also be referred to as the fourth line of defense. The specifics of regulatory audits are beyond the scope of this chapter. For research coordinators, the workflow of internal and regulatory audits is basically the same.

The essential differences between monitoring and auditing are listed in ▶ Table 24.1.

Table 24.1 Essential differences between monitoring and auditing

Monitoring	Auditing
• Continuous process	• Done either during the study or after completion of the study
• Controls quality of the study	• Assures quality of the study
• Is done by a monitor who is part of the study	• Is done by independent personnel
• Monitor is appointed by the sponsor	• Auditor is appointed by the sponsor (sponsor audit) or by the hospital board (internal hospital audit)

24.3 What to Do When You Find Out You Will Be Audited

It may seem like a catastrophe or at least an enormous mountain of work: your schedule was more than full as it was, and now auditors will come and check every detail of the study within a matter of weeks! Actually, all you need is to keep calm and beware of six points. These points are explained below, along with some specific dos and don'ts.

1. Content of the study: the big picture.
2. Documentation.
3. Meeting and interviews with auditors.
4. Role of the PI, research coordinator, and team.
5. Practical aspects: travel, space, food, and drinks.
6. Report and corrective action/preventive action (CAPA) plan.

24.4 Content of the Study: The Big Picture

What exactly is the study about? What is the research question? How many patients will be recruited? Which drug/device/intervention is being studied and what is the comparator? When will the results of the study be implemented on daily practice? What is the status of the study today? Who is doing what in the study? These are some questions that may be asked at the beginning of or during an audit interview, and they may take you—or

the PI!—off guard when you are fully focused on details like version dates and delegation logs.

DO: Make sure everyone involved is aware of the study. Prepare a short text (one page) on the study and share it with the team as soon as possible. Update the document with the current situation/progress 1 day before they audit and email it to the team.

24.5 Documentation

As we say in the audit world, *if it hasn't been documented, it hasn't happened.* So, you will be required to provide written proof of just about everything in your study. But how will you check the status of your documentation weeks before the audit? A first check of the documentation should have been done by the monitor visiting your site. Therefore, monitoring reports may be a good place to start checking site file status. Checking the monitor's report may not be sufficient, especially when a clinical study has been ongoing for quite a while, or even if the study has been stopped some time ago, you will need to step back and see what has been done, and what has happened in your study from the very start until today.

DO: Take about 1 hour and make a timeline of the study. You may wish to start with ethics committee approval, or with the first patient enrolled at your site. Make a six-column table (see ▶Table 24.2). Note the event in column 1 and the date in column 2. In columns 3 and 4, note the document that

Table 24.2 Study timeline example (layout can be adapted)

Event	Date	Document	Document version	Consequence	Remarks
Ethics approval	May 3, 2016	Positive opinion/approved	Letter on date of event	All consents should be no sooner than May 3, 2016	Protocol approved on May 3 included amendment 1
First patient enrolled	June 16, 2016	Letter to the ethics committee to confirm that the study has started[a]	June 20, 2016		
Amend 2 submitted to ethics committee	December 12, 2016	Amend 2: amended protocol includes amends 1 and 2	Amend 2 version date: December 9, 2016	Awaiting approval	No consequence for subjects/consent procedure
...	...	...	...	...	...

[a]Not required in all jurisdictions.

describes or proves the event and the date it was issued. In the remaining columns 5 and 6, consequences and remarks can be noted. Starting from the ethics committee approval, work your way back to the very beginning and forward until today.

Remember the acronym "KISS": Keep It Short and Simple. There is no need to go into every detail of the study. It is all about milestones, for example, when the study was approved by the ethics committee, first patient enrolled, when an amendment was needed, and when items were submitted, approved, and implemented. It is also important to note any SAEs with major consequences for the study. Ensure that all versions of the protocol have been approved by the ethics committee, and note which versions of the protocol each participant was recruited under. Note key monitoring dates like when the PI received the monitoring report *and* resolved the issues described in the report.

DO NOT drown in the hundreds of minor details. For example, there is no need to enter every letter to the ethics committee in this table, only submissions and approvals. Do not make a list of all sorts of correspondence. Do not enter cancelled monitoring visits or emails to monitors unless they document a vital aspect of the study.

DO: Discuss the table briefly with the PI, so they have a general knowledge of the content. No auditor will require you or the PI to know all approval dates by heart. They will, however, appreciate if you can swiftly and correctly answer such questions and that you have the paperwork to corroborate your answer.

DO: Check the Trial Master File. It needs to document every aspect of the study. Make sure the master file is complete according to GCP (see Chapter 10 for a list of required documentation before the start of the study, during the study, and after completion of the study). GCP also offers clear information on the location of each document (e.g., at the sponsor's site or at the investigator's site). Print the GCP list and work your way through it checking what is missing, old, incomplete, or unclear. Then work your way through the file once more, checking what is in there that is not on the GCP list. Check all monitoring reports for findings on the file and make sure these were properly addressed by the PI. The next action is to organize the file in a clear way and to make sure the table of contents matches the actual content. You may want to add a note explaining how consents were organized. For example, were they organized by enrollment date (screen failures separately) or by subgroup or even alphabetically by patient name? Make sure the auditor can see this immediately, thus avoiding puzzles for the audit team.

DO NOT date documents in the past to make it seem you have had them since the beginning of the study. It is fraud, it is wrong, and it is obvious to the auditors. If a document is missing or in any other way inadequate, make a note to file explaining what is wrong, when you found out, and how did you (attempt) to correct it. It may still be an audit finding, but depending on the document missing it may be a minor finding if you tried to correct it.

24.6 Meetings and Interviews with Auditors

24.6.1 Introduction or Start–Up Meeting

Auditors may ask the site to organize an introduction or start-up meeting just before the actual start of the audit. During this meeting, the auditors will introduce themselves, elaborate on the aim of the audit, and answer questions on the audit process. Apart from this, they may ask the team to introduce themselves and they may ask for a summary of the study, which will normally be presented by the PI. What auditors will also do during this meeting is observe the team and get a feel of the atmosphere at the site.

DO: make sure the meeting is well prepared and all required personnel are present and punctual. Keep introductions brief and to the point.

DO NOT: volunteer to mention any study problems discovered during audit preparation during this meeting. You will get the opportunity to discuss this during the interviews.

24.6.2 Audit Interviews

Several team members are typically invited for an audit interview as a group or separately. This may be exciting or scary, but there is no need to worry. You will be asked a number of questions about your study, your daily practice, and your field of expertise.

DO: Keep it simple, be honest, keep calm, and be polite. Auditors may ask questions that seem obvious, but they may just be testing your knowledge or double-checking an answer from another interview. They also may ask off-topic questions.

As long as these are not intrusive or inappropriate, just answer briefly, politely, and to the point. If you do not know the answer to a question, admit to it. Good responses in this situation are "I don't know, but I will make sure to look up the answer in our documentation and I will respond just after lunch. Will that be ok?" or "I don't know. I will discuss this question with the PI and have him/her reply to you."

DO NOT: volunteer extra information; just answer the question. Do not make up elaborate answers to hide the fact you do not know what you are talking about. Do not overemphasize your role in the study by beginning every reply with "I made sure" or "I arranged." Every study is a team effort and even if you pay the largest role in the process, make sure everyone's contribution is clearly illustrated. Last but not least, do not gossip and do not complain about colleagues, the company you work for, vendors you work with, or whomever. Gossip and complaining is always considered lack of taking responsibility.

24.6.3 Daily Briefings

When an audit is planned over several days, usually auditors will brief the team daily on progress and outstanding issues.

DO: Make sure these meetings are well organized and are attended by at least the PI and one or two team members. Issues addressed during these meetings will require follow-up, so make sure someone makes a list of issues and remarks and follow up during the audit. Make sure the PI takes action or delegates appropriately.

24.6.4 Informal Conversations in between Audit Events

Auditors may ask you or your colleagues informal questions during coffee breaks, lunch, or as you show them to their hotel. Conversations may include things like the following: "It must be hard for you to combine this function with your family life" or "Dr. X is very lucky to have a research office to which he/she can delegate most of the study work." Please be aware every conversation you have with them is actually an interview. The audit is not over until the auditor has left the premises.

24.6.5 Final Audit Meeting

At the end of the audit, the audit team usually will want to meet with the team and discuss what has been done and will share some of the positive and negative findings. Also, a timeline for the report and CAPA plan (Corrective Action, Preventive Action plan) will be discussed.

DO: Make sure the meeting is well organized and well attended. Have someone take notes. Be aware that the audit is not finished and statements made during this meeting will be part of the audit report. Ask the team members not to engage in discussions at this meeting unless the auditor explicitly asks to discuss a finding.

DO NOT: It is usually not a good idea to defend yourself with regard to negative findings at this point. The audit is nearly finished; everybody, including the auditors, is tired and wants to conclude the audit. It is better to have an open mind and realize that you and your team will learn from all findings and that you will take appropriate action after the audit. Thank the audit team and escort them to the exit of your department, building, or facility.

24.7 Role of the PI, Research Coordinator, and Team

Who is doing what in the study and who was doing what last month? Auditors are interested in which decisions were taken by whom and whether this person is actually qualified to do so at that time. It is vital that the PI of your site knows exactly who is doing what, why, and when. This brings us to the most important piece of advice about dealing with an audit.

DO: *Make sure the PI owns their responsibility.* The PI—not the research coordinator—is responsible for what has been done and for what is going on in the study. Make sure they do not hide, make excuses, or show up late for the audit. Make the PI aware of the importance of the audit. Make sure the PI realizes that during the audit it is all about the study. The worst excuse an auditor will ever hear is "I am too busy," whether they mean that they are too busy for this audit, to document every AE, or to be compliant to all these rules and regulations. As soon as the audit is announced, take a look at the schedule of the PI and other key team members to see when their presence is required. Other activities and appointments may need to be rescheduled.

After discussing all this advice with the PI, step back! Be aware of where the research coordinator's responsibilities start and where they end. Research coordinators may be asked to arrange many aspects of the audit, but it is first and foremost the PI's audit, not the coordinator's. Help and arrange wherever you can, but do not overdo it.

24.8 Practical Aspects: Travel, Space, Food and Drinks

Whether the auditor is flying in from across the globe or walking in form across the building, practical aspects are important.

DO: Make sure any applicable travel arrangements are well communicated, and the auditors will be met as agreed, so you will be off to a good start.

As soon as the audit is announced, make sure you book two meeting rooms or separate working spaces: one for the auditors to work in and a separate room, not too close to the audit room, for the study team to use, prepare, and discuss what is going on. Make sure refreshments are present in the audit room: coffee, tea, water, juice, fruit. Occasional cake, cookies, or chocolate may be nice, but do not overdo it. There is no need for a nauseated auditor, nor one that feels overly pampered. Find the balance.

It may be a good idea to provide lunch arrangements; it will however be exhausting to spend the entire audit day(s) including lunch(es) with the auditors. For example, you could arrange for the PI to have lunch with them on day 1, have a lunch delivered for them on day 2, and suggest you may have lunch with them on day 3. Make sure you have real breaks in between audit activities. Take breaks with some fresh air, a drink, and no conversations about the study or the audit(or).

Make sure the PI is aware of all arrangements including your availability and the limitations thereof during the audit days. Include the PI's administrative assistant (if applicable) in all practical arrangements.

24.9 Report and Corrective Action/Preventive Action Plan

24.9.1 Audit Report

During the audit, the auditor will announce when you will receive the draft report. Upon getting the report, take some time to read it calmly.

Audit finding may be classified in several ways:
- *Critical, major, minor.* Usually this is risk based: critical findings will be those that

entail a risk for the participant and/or the integrity of the study date and need immediate action. Major findings may cause harm to the participant and entail a risk to the integrity of the study data. Minor findings are smaller findings that will still need action but are not urgent.
- Another way of classifying findings is urgent–not urgent, which is self-explanatory. Make sure you check when action is required for every finding.

In any case, the audit report will include an overview of the classification of the findings, their possible consequences, and required timeline of action. Make sure to read the explanation and to include every finding in the CAPA plan even the minor or nonurgent ones.

DO: It is vital to send the auditor a polite, correct, complete, and timely answer. Normally, you will be asked to check the report for errors. Check the findings you are not sure of and have them double-checked by the PI. If there is actually an error in the report, state this in a concise, neutral way, adding documentation if needed.

DO NOT react immediately, emotionally, and/or defensively. Do not take the opportunity to explain findings that have been stated correctly in the report, nor defend yourself in the reaction to the draft report.

24.9.2 Corrective Action/ Preventive Action (CAPA) Plan

After responding to the draft report, you will receive a definitive report and a request to make a CAPA plan. This is a plan describing how the research team will improve compliance, addressing all action items from the audit. For every finding, you need to describe how you will correct the issue, how you will document it, and—most importantly—how you will prevent the issue from happening again.

DO: Be concise. Include how issues will be solved by whom and when. Make sure the PI has, for example, weekly or monthly checks to monitor the status of the CAPA plan. Document the actions taken and file it in the study file.

DO NOT: make promises you cannot keep in terms of actions, timelines, or otherwise. You will be asked to update the CAPA plan at some point in the future.

24.9.3 Life after the Audit

After you have survived the audit, you may want to share the experience with the rest of your department. Researchers and other colleagues may learn how to handle things in case of another audit, and they may pick up some tips and pointers on how to organize, perform, and document their studies even better. You may want to consider writing an audit SOP for your company.

DO: celebrate the end of the audit, or even better, the completion of actions on the CAPA plan by having a get-together with the team. Make sure all contributions to the successful audit experience are acknowledged appropriately.

DO NOT: throw the audit report in a drawer, ignore the CAPA plan actions, and never speak of the audit again unless to explain what a horrible experience it was.

24.10 Practical Application

The tips and tricks discussed earlier are meant to be used as soon as an audit is announced. Obviously, organizing a study and keeping records in compliance with laws and regulations from day 1 is the best way to minimize the need for extensive audit preparations.

Definitions

- An audit may be a lot of work. Keeping cool and organizing is the best way forward. **Preparations** include not only the site and the files but also clear instructions to team members and the PI. Practical aspects like audit venue need to be arranged timely.
- **During the audit**, it is key that all those involved are honest, to the point, and polite; they should show up on time and act professionally at all times.
- **The follow-up** of the audit includes reacting correctly to the audit report and making and executing a CAPA plan. Celebrate what went well and learn from your mistakes. Sharing audit results and experiences with other departments will increase the learning experience for your organization.

Reference

[1] International Council for Harmonisation of Technical Requirements for Pharmaceuticals for Human Use (ICH). ICH Harmonised Guideline Integrated Addendum to ICH E6(R1): Guideline for Good Clinical Practice E6(R2). Current Step 4 version. November 9, 2016. Available at: https://www.ich.org/fileadmin/Public_Web_Site/ICH_Products/Guidelines/Efficacy/E6/E6_R2__Step_4_2016_1109.pdf

25 Monitoring in a Clinical Study: Why and How?

David Pogorzelski

Abstract

Monitoring is an essential requirement of clinical studies involving human subjects. The purpose of monitoring is well defined, but there is no set approach to monitoring that works best for all studies. This chapter will describe how and why monitoring is performed, who performs study monitoring, and the various approaches that are used.

Keywords: monitor, source data verification, site selection visit, site initiation visit, routine monitoring visit, closeout visit, data safety monitoring committee

25.1 Introduction

The International Conference on Harmonisation of Technical Requirements for Registration of Pharmaceuticals for Human Use Good Clinical Practice (ICH-GCP) is the set of standards that govern clinical studies involving humans.[1] ICH-GCP requires sponsors of clinical research to ensure that the study involving human subjects is adequately monitored.[1] Given this essential requirement, the sponsor must implement a monitoring plan for every study. In this chapter, we will describe who is responsible for monitoring, the purpose and requirements of monitoring, why monitoring is necessary, and the various approaches that are used.

25.2 Purpose of Monitoring

The purposes of monitoring are to ensure the following[1]:

- The rights and well-being of human subjects are protected.
- The reported study data are accurate, complete, and verifiable from source documents.
- The conduct of the study is in compliance with the currently approved protocol/amendment(s), with GCP and with the applicable regulatory requirements.

Monitoring provides assurance for users to feel comfortable in using the medications and devices after they are approved for use.

25.3 Responsibilities, Extent, and Nature of Monitoring

The responsibilities of a monitor are outlined in ICH-GCP Section 5.18.4.[1] Conducting a study in compliance with ICH-GCP should ensure the safety of the study subjects and reliability of the study results. Since every study is different, the risks to safety of the subjects and reliability of the results are not equal in every study. As a result, the amount of monitoring should be proportional to the amount of risk associated with the study. To determine the amount of risk, factors such as the objective, design, purpose, size, complexity, sites, data collection, and endpoints of the study should be considered. Not surprisingly, studies with minimal risk such as those with little data collection using extensively studied drugs with few known adverse events (AEs; e.g., phase IV trials) should not require as much monitoring as complex trials in vulnerable subjects with little human exposure and lots of known AEs associated with its use. Regardless of how much monitoring is required, studies should have a monitoring plan that clearly describes the monitoring that will be performed in the study and it should be reflective of the risk associated with the study.

25.4 Monitor Qualifications

The sponsor must appoint a monitor who is capable of performing the responsibilities listed earlier.[1] In order to do so, monitors, also known as clinical research associates (CRAs), should have a strong knowledge of study investigational products, be appropriately trained, and have the scientific understanding of the protocol to be able to monitor the study according to the sponsor's standard operating procedures (SOPs), ICH-GCP, and the applicable regulatory requirements.

Larger studies with many sites will often require multiple monitors to monitor the study. In smaller studies, monitors may have additional responsibilities such as creating study documents, planning investigator meetings, and preparing reports. Regardless of who is monitoring the study, the person must have the resources and qualifications necessary for the job and a copy of their qualifications and training should be kept on file in case of a study audit (see Chapter 24).

Although we listed the general set of responsibilities of a monitor, applicability of these responsibilities will vary based on many factors. For example, vaccine studies may have more emphasis on handling and storage given their narrow temperature storage conditions permitted and low tolerance for temperature deviations.[2] Blinded studies will require monitoring for assurance that blinding is maintained. Monitoring early in the study may focus more on site training, whereas monitoring later in the study will focus more on data verification. Monitors should be aware of what aspects are critical for monitoring and focus their attention accordingly.

For multicenter studies, monitoring often involves traveling to be able to perform the necessary responsibilities. If sites are spread far apart, traveling can occupy a large proportion of a monitor's time. In these situations, monitors may spend much of their time in hotels and airports traveling between sites. Other studies may have sites closer together in a specific region, which often requires less traveling. In some cases, a sponsor may have a number of sites in a specific region but across multiple studies. In these cases, a monitor may oversee all of these sites in a region and therefore may be involved in multiple studies.

25.5 Monitoring Visits

Performing on-site monitoring visits are the traditional approach toward monitoring a study. After all, being on site leaves almost no limitations to what can be monitored. The monitor should meet with the personnel responsible for the various aspects of the trial that they are monitoring. A wrap-up session should be scheduled with the principal investigator (PI) if they are unavailable during the visit. The requirements of monitoring visits will be different depending on how far along a study is at a site and are typically broken down into four types of visits.

25.6 Site Selection Visit

All studies must have assurance of the quality of every aspect of a study.[1] One way to ensure quality is by selecting good sites to conduct the study. In the early stages of a study, sponsors will typically have an idea of how many sites they would like to participate in the study and will reach out to sites regarding participation. They will usually provide relevant information related to the study such as the protocol and investigator's brochure and collect information regarding their ability to conduct the study. Once all of the information is collected from each of the prospective sites, the sponsor will narrow down the list of sites to the most qualified ones to participate. This selection process often involves a visit to the site to assess the site's qualifications. Monitors often perform this visit and meet with the local PI and research coordinator. Other site personnel including allied health professionals that may be involved in the study may also attend for their input on certain aspects of the study.

The main purpose of the site selection visit (SSV) is to determine if the site is able to conduct the study. Oftentimes, the most important factor to assess is the site's ability to enroll subjects. There is very little point to including a site that cannot enroll the study subjects of interest. Other factors that require assessment are the PI's and research coordinator's qualifications and experience, equipment, drug storage location, availability of space, and time to devote to the study. In many cases, the budget will also be a big factor as to whether the sites can perform the study.

In some cases, the sponsor may already have a long-standing relationship with a particular site and therefore may already be aware of the site's capability of conducting the study. This is often the case when an investigator has been involved in the earlier phases of the development of a product. In these cases, the selection process may not be as thorough. For new sites, the evaluation of a site should be thorough and may entail discussions with the PI and visits to all the areas where study activities may take place. A monitor sometimes has to rely on their judgment as to whether the site should be included in the study. For example, an investigator may appear interested in participating in the study and have all the resources to conduct the study but may have too many other obligations to provide sufficient oversight or to perform study requirements in a timely fashion.

Conversely, a site may be very interested and eager to participate but may be missing a key requirement. In some cases, the sponsor or site may be able to come up with a solution for the missing requirement. For example, an MRI can sometimes be outsourced to a third party or a refrigerator, ECG machine, or temperature-monitoring equipment can be provided by the sponsor or vendor. Sponsors should consider trying to find a solution if suitable sites are hard to find or the site would otherwise be a strong site. Ultimately, the monitor should gather enough information to make an educated decision as to whether to include the site in the study. After all, highly capable sites are required for a successful study.

In order to identify the most suitable sites, a typical agenda for an SSV may include the following:
- Background and discussion of the investigational product.
- Review the protocol.
- Recruitment ability.
- Roles within the study team.
- Availability of equipment.
- Ethics committee.
- Regulatory requirements.
- Documents (including CVs).
- Budget and publication policies.
- Assessment of facilities.
- Timelines for initiation.

25.7 Site Initiation Visit

After a site has been selected to participate in a study, a number of requirements need to be fulfilled before a site is ready to begin enrollment. Ethics approvals are required and an agreement between the sponsor and site needs to be in place. Sites should have a Trial Master File (TMF) or Investigator Site File (ISF) in place that contains all the essential documents for the study (see Chapter 13). If all of the requirements are in place, a site initiation visit (SIV) is usually conducted.

The purpose of the SIV is to ensure that the site is in fact ready to begin enrollment. This will entail training on the study procedures, going over roles, responsibilities, regulatory obligations, case record form (CRF) completion, record management, drug handling and storage, enrollment, and serious adverse event (SAE) reporting. Although training is required, the amount of training at these visits depends on a few factors. Highly experienced sites may not require as much training on certain aspects such as regulatory obligations and SAE reporting as new sites. Sites that are familiar with the product under investigation may not require as much information about it. Many studies will have an investigator's meeting around the time

of the SIV. The purpose of this meeting is to train investigators and their lead staff on the study-related procedures. If the site recently attended the investigator's meeting, less training during the SIV will be needed. It is important that all training and qualifications of the site personnel are documented and available for audit.

During the SIV, the monitor will usually spend most of their time with the research coordinator but should meet with the investigator for a review of the visit, perform any necessary training, and answer any questions. During the visit, monitors should physically review the TMF, verify the drug is being stored properly, and check that all supplies and equipment are ready for use. If there are any outstanding issues, enrollment should not proceed until the issues are resolved. Once all requirements are met, the site can be notified to begin enrollment.

25.8 Routine Monitoring Visits

Once subject enrollment and data collection is under way, a routine monitoring visit is usually scheduled. This visit will often occur multiple times during enrollment and follow-up. The main purpose of the routine monitoring visit is to ensure all aspects of the study are being conducted properly. This includes verification that the conduct of the study is in compliance with all regulations, the data are being reported accurately, the safety of the subjects is being maintained, the investigational product is being stored, dispensed, and maintained properly, and that the site has all the resources to perform the study.

The TMF should be reviewed again. A comprehensive review may not be necessary if it was in order during the previous visit and not much time has elapsed. Monitors should be aware of any changes that have occurred and verify if they are reflected in the TMF. For example, if it has been over a year since the site's ethics approval, the monitor should verify whether a renewal has been obtained given that ethics approvals are only granted for a period of up to 1 year in most jurisdictions.[3] They should verify that any protocol amendments and deviations have been approved by the ethics committee and that any new personnel have had their responsibilities delegated.

The rights and well-being of the subjects in a study has to be protected. The monitor must ensure all safety issues have been identified and reported (if required), and the subject has received the proper medical attention. Any untoward medical occurrence in a subject administered a pharmaceutical product is an AE. If the AE is related to the drug, it is called an adverse drug reaction. If the AE is related to a medical device, it is called an adverse device effect. These events are considered serious if they:

- Result in death.
- Resulted in life-threatening illness or injury.
- Resulted in permanent impairment of body structure or body function.
- Required hospitalization or prolongation of existing hospitalization.
- Resulted in medical or surgical treatment to prevent the above.

AEs are usually classified as either related or unrelated and expected or unexpected. These determinations can be made by reviewing the Investigator's Brochure if the product is investigational or the product's label if it has been approved for use. All monitors must be aware of the AEs and keep an eye out for any untoward medical occurrence meeting these definitions.

The most time-consuming part of this visit is usually verifying that the data are entered correctly. To do this, monitors will go through each subject's CRFs and compare it with source documentation. Any discrepancies will be identified and should be discussed with the research coordinator so that they can be resolved. Source documents are where the data required for the study are first recorded and frequently refer to the subject's medical records. As a result, monitors will require access to subject's medical records in order to verify the data. If subjects are provided questionnaires, diaries, or logs to complete, they can be considered source documents and used for verification purposes. If subjects are asked questions in person or over the phone, the form where the data are initially recorded will be the source document. If a subject responds to a question over email, then the email would be considered the source document.

Technology is becoming more widely adopted in clinical studies, particularly in the collection of subject data. Wearable technology that tracks activity level and heart rate can be used as source data. Text messages and blood glucose monitors can also be used as sources of data. Printouts of various monitoring equipment often seen in intensive care unit settings can also be source documents. Regardless of what the source is, it must be available for verification of the study data during the visit. Clinical research has long abided by the old saying "if it's not documented, then it didn't happen."

25.9 Closeout Visit

Once the study is completed at a site, a closeout visit (COV) is often performed. COVs occur when the final subject has completed their last visit, all data have been entered, and all queries have been resolved. The COV is an important part of the quality control of a study.

The COV usually requires a final check of the study database to ensure there is no outstanding information and all queries are resolved. Once this is completed at all sites, the database is usually locked and ready for analysis by the sponsor or its delegate. During the visit, the monitor should arrange for the return of all study equipment and supplies if they have not been returned at the time of the visit. All unused investigational product must be accounted for and returned to the sponsor. Sites will often be permitted to destroy the unused product if the site has an SOP to do so. Proper documentation regarding destruction must be maintained to ensure accountability of all investigational products. The monitor should review that all SAEs have been reported and a final report has been submitted to the ethics committee. The monitor should review the site's TMF and ensure that it is in perfect order and signed off by the investigator where applicable. If everything is in good order, archiving all research records is required. At a minimum, records must be kept for 2 years following the approval of the last marketing application.[1] Depending on the applicable regulatory agencies, the length of time may be considerably longer. All research records must remain accessible during this period of time. If a regulatory agency or the sponsor were to revisit the site following the study closeout, they should be able to identify what has occurred and when and should be able to access any document or record to verify proper execution of the study.

The ideal closeout scenario follows the completion of a successful clinical study after all subjects have been enrolled; however, COVs can occur for other reasons. Studies can fall behind on enrollment, can go over budget, or the safety risk can become too high, all of which can prompt early termination. Slow enrollment, noncompliance, or safety issues may prompt the sponsor to close out a site prematurely. A site may wish to terminate their involvement in a study for financial reasons or a lack of resources to be able to conduct the study properly. Many times, key personnel such as the investigator, coinvestigator, or research coordinator may relocate to another institution with no suitable replacement available. In any of these circumstances, a final COV should be performed by the study monitor even if study activity is ongoing at other sites.

25.10 Monitoring Reports

Every site visit requires a monitoring report to be completed. This is essential to demonstrating proper oversight of a clinical study.[1] It is typically issued by the monitor shortly after the monitoring visit and usually no later than 5 days after the visit. The report should include the date, site, name of the monitor, and name of the site attendees. This report summarizes what was reviewed during the visit and any findings the monitor observed during this visit. The report also provides a list of action items that must be completed. Many sponsors or CROs (contract research organizations) have a template for the report. Please see ▶ Fig. 25.1 for an example of what a monitoring report may look like. Following the issuance of a report, monitors should follow up on the report and research coordinators should prioritize ensuring that all outstanding items are addressed. Many monitors will verify that all action items from the previous visit have been address at the start of their next visit.

Key tips to writing a good monitoring report are as follows:

- Review all aspects of the study during the visit and use time wisely.
- Be observant and take good notes during the visit.
- Complete the report as soon as possible after the visit.
- Review the report carefully.
- Only include relevant information pertaining to the visit.

25.11 Centralized Monitoring

Traditionally, study monitoring has been performed through frequent on-site visits. One of the drawbacks of frequent visits is the high cost, which can be up to 30% of a study's budget.[4] Not surprisingly, centralized monitoring is increasingly been adopted to monitor clinical studies to help keep costs low.[5]

Centralized monitoring is the evaluation of a site from a remote location. To do this, sites conduct the study as they normally would but also send source documents electronically to the monitor for verification. Most electronic data capture (EDC) systems have capabilities to attach source documents within them so monitors can compare the data entered into the EDC system to the source documents for discrepancies. For example, to verify that a lab value entered into the EDC system is accurate, research coordinators will also attach a copy of the lab report so it can be verified for accuracy by a central monitor. Central monitoring is not just limited to data verification. Sites can send screening logs and various documents from the TMF for central monitoring. The most common modes of transmission typically involve email, fax, or directly through a secure file hosting service or the EDC system. Review of data through a centralized approach can allow for the comparison of data across sites, which is not as easily done via on-site monitoring. This is useful if the sponsor wishes to identify trends or inconsistencies in the reporting of data. Sites must be careful to remain in compliance with all privacy regulations when submitting source documents electronically for verification.

Most EDC systems are also capable of checking for incorrect or unrealistic values instantly. For example, an EDC system can be set up initially to not accept birth dates that would make a subject ineligible based on age, or to recognize and query unrealistic heights or weights. This monitoring approach provides the benefit of identifying queries immediately and allows monitors to allocate resources to other functions that cannot be performed centrally. It can reduce the amount of on-site visits, which can in turn reduce the travel costs associated with monitoring.

Critics of central monitoring point out the increased burden of uploading source documents by site research coordinators, the increased possibility of a privacy breach, and the upfront investment associated with programming the EDC system to identify incorrect or unrealistic data. Despite the criticism, regulators are encouraging the adoption of a range of monitoring approaches, and growing evidence is suggestive that that centralized monitoring does reduce costs and can be a very effective strategy for trial monitoring.[6,7,8]

Monitoring visit report form

Visit details	
Sponsor:	Protocol number:
PI:	Monitor:
Visit date:	Previous visit:
Site Name:	
Site number:	

Visit attendees

Study status	
Study start date:	Subjects screened:
Date of last visit	Subjects enrolled:
Number of SAEs	Subjects completed:
Number of protocol deviations	Subjects withdrawn:

Regulatory binder review	Acceptable?	Comment

IP accountability and storage	Acceptable?	Comment

Source document verification	Acceptable?	Comment

Fig. 25.1 Sample monitoring report.

25.12 Risk-Based Monitoring

Most studies have a monitoring plan or a source document verification (SDV) plan that will indicate the amount of SDV required for the study. The traditional approach to monitoring relies on 100% SDV for all subjects as the most reliable way to ensure correct data.[9] Recent findings have shown that 100% SDV is not necessarily more effective than a targeted or risk-based SDV approach[10] and the recent introduction of Food and Drug Administration (FDA) and European Medicines Agency (EMA) guidelines encouraging alternative approaches to monitoring has sped up the adoption of risk-based monitoring.[9] Risk-based monitoring targets resources where data and safety are more likely to be compromised. ▶ Fig. 25.2 illustrates an example

of a risk-based monitoring approach. In this example, risk assessment is performed at the onset of a study and a monitoring plan is developed proportionate to the level of risk. When on-site monitoring is performed, the findings from the monitoring visit will determine the subsequent level of monitoring that will be performed and any additional steps that may be required. This approach often requires a threshold level to be in place to trigger subsequent steps. For example, sites that pass a threshold number of SAEs may require additional monitoring visits and sites below a threshold number of SAEs may require retraining on SAE reporting. Similarly, sites that pass a threshold of data discrepancies may require additional visits and training, while sites below a threshold of discrepancies may require fewer visits.

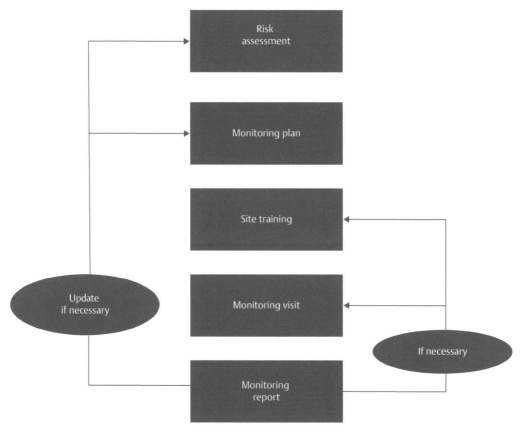

Fig. 25.2 Risk-based monitoring approach.

25.13 Data and Safety Monitoring Committee

Another type of monitoring is performed by a Data Safety Monitoring Committee (DSMC), also known as a Data Safety Monitoring Board (DSMB). DSMCs provide ongoing data and safety monitoring during the course of a study. The main responsibility of the DSMC is to evaluate the safety information of the study and advise on stopping or continuing the study based on the safety information that becomes available during the study. The DSMC is typically composed of three to five clinicians knowledgeable in the subject area and at least one statistician, all of whom are independent of the study's steering committee and sponsor. Independence is a crucial factor, as independence allows for their unbiased interpretation and reporting. The DSMC reviews incoming safety data during the study and they meet at various times during a study to evaluate all safety information to advise on continuation/termination of the study.[11] The exact scope of their responsibilities, meeting frequency, and stopping criteria is typically described in a DSMC charter that is prepared and signed off by all parties at the start of a study.

All clinical studies require safety monitoring; however, a formal committee is not always necessary. Studies that pose minimal safety risks to subjects like behavioral or nutritional studies, ones without mortality or other serious outcomes, as well as single-center and phase I and II trials are often exempt from having a formal DSMC.

25.14 Practical Application: Ensuring an AWESOME Site Visit

There are a number of things a research coordinator can do to ensure their site visit goes well. The various stages associated with a site visit are discussed in the following sections.

25.15 Scheduling

The study monitor is often the person who will initiate a site visit, and in many cases they will make the arrangements with the research coordinator. This visit will usually be scheduled weeks in advance and an agenda will be provided by the monitor. The research coordinator should review the agenda and ensure that there will be no issues with any of the items on the agenda. Before finalizing the date and time, the research coordinator should ensure the availability of everyone who needs to attend and give enough time to review the material and prepare for the visit. The research coordinator should book a room that is quiet with ample space for the visit. If the monitor would like to visit any of the areas where study-related activities will be performed, the research coordinator should make arrangements for this to be done if necessary. For routine monitoring visits, enough time should be given to enter any outstanding data into the study database, resolve all queries, and retrieve source documents for verification. The timing of the visit should also be appropriate for the visit being scheduled. For example, sites should almost be ready for enrollment on the date of the SIV. All data should be entered into the EDC system, all queries should be resolved, and the TMF and other study documents should be in good order and ready for archiving at the COV.

25.16 Preparation

Upon confirmation of the visit, the research coordinator should do a thorough review of the agenda and any material provided for the visit. They should identify any questions they may have and have them ready for the visit. The TMF should be up-to-date and should contain all the essential documents for the trial. All data should be entered into the study database and be query free. The investigational product should be stored properly and all records should be properly maintained and be ready for review. There should be no outstanding items with the ethics committee or regulatory agencies prior to any site visit.

25.17 Previous Monitoring Reports

If there has been a previous study visit, the research coordinator should review the monitoring report and ensure every recommendation/action item has been addressed. If there are any items that remain unaddressed, the research coordinator should prioritize addressing them before addressing any other items that might be relevant for the visit.

25.18 During the Visit

The research coordinator and monitor will typically arrange to meet at a certain time and place. The research coordinator should be available for all monitoring visits and the investigator should be available for at least part of the visit to provide any feedback and ask any questions. Any new members of the study team should receive training. If the research coordinator is not available for the whole visit, they should be easily accessible if needed or have another member of the study team available. Research coordinators should also ask questions and not be hesitant to ask for advice during a visit. This is a key to building a good relationship. After all, monitors and research coordinators share the same goals of ensuring the study is a success. Strong communication can help achieve this goal.

25.19 After the Visit

Ensuring a strong monitoring visit does not end at the completion of the visit. Strong communication is required between visits as well. Study monitors should provide a monitoring report after each visit. If the research coordinator has not received the report after a couple of days, they should follow up with the monitor. This can help leave a positive impression that the site is serious about the study and on top of their responsibilities. Once the monitoring report is received, the research coordinator should review it and get started immediately on addressing any items it contains. Sites should aim to have all items addressed within a few weeks of the visits and should be communicating their progress along the way and asking for help or for any questions that arise.

25.20 Managing Expectations

A key skill of a good research coordinator is their ability to manage the expectations of the monitors. Many sites provide enrollment projections that are far below their actual capabilities. Investigators and research coordinators should carefully review the eligibility criteria of a study before providing projections on enrollment. If it is not entirely clear,

it might be helpful to provide a range. Research coordinators should provide adequate space to perform any monitoring responsibilities. Finally, research coordinators should provide advance notice regarding availability of any site personnel or requirements during the visit. Monitors often come from a long distance away and last minute changes can disrupt a monitor's schedule and wind up being costly if an additional visit is required and/or flights and accommodations have to be changed.

References

[1] International Conference on Harmonisation of Technical Requirements for Registration of Pharmaceuticals for Human Use. Guideline for Good Clinical Practice E6. 1996. Available from: http://www.ich.org/fileadmin/Public_Web_Site/ICH_Products/Guidelines/Efficacy/E6/E6_R1_Guideline.pdf. Accessed June 17, 2018

[2] Centers for Disease Control and Prevention. Epidemiology and Prevention of Vaccine-Preventable Diseases. Washington, DC: Public Health Foundation; 2015

[3] Department of Health and Human Services. IRB review of research, 45 C.F.R 46.109. 2009. Available from: https://www.hhs.gov/ohrp/regulations-and-policy/regulations/45-cfr-46/index.html#46.109. Accessed June 23, 2018

[4] De S. Hybrid Approaches to Clinical Trial Monitoring: Practical Alternatives to 100% Source Data Verification. Perspect Clin Res 2011;2(3):100–104

[5] Hind D, Reeves BC, Bathers S, et al. Comparative Costs and Activity from a Sample of UK Clinical Trials Units. Trials 2017;18(1):203

[6] Macefield RC, Beswick AD, Blazeby JM, Lane JA. A Systematic Review of On-Site Monitoring Methods for Health-Care Randomised Controlled Trials. Clin Trials 2013;10(1):104–124

[7] Baigent C, Harrell FE, Buyse M, Emberson JR, Altman DG. Ensuring Trial Validity by Data Quality Assurance and Diversification of Monitoring Methods. Clin Trials 2008;5(1):49–55

[8] Bakobaki JM, Rauchenberger M, Joffe N, McCormack S, Stenning S, Meredith S. The Potential for Central Monitoring Techniques to Replace On-Site Monitoring: Findings from an International Multi-Centre Clinical Trial. Clin Trials 2012;9(2):257–264

[9] Gupta A. Taking the "Risk" out of Risk-Based Monitoring. Perspect Clin Res 2013;4(4):193–195

[10] Olsen R, Bihlet AR, Kalakou F, Andersen JR. The Impact of Clinical Trial Monitoring Approaches on Data Integrity and Cost: A Review of Current Literature. Eur J Clin Pharmacol 2016;72(4):399–412

[11] Wilhelmsen L. Role of the Data and Safety Monitoring Committee (DSMC). 2002:2823–2829

26 Managing Large Studies: Organization and Committees

Stephanie L. Tanner

Abstract

Large studies require formal structure and organization to reach successful completion. The size and complexity of each study will affect the overall infrastructure required. Most large studies will require a study team to assist the Study Principal Investigator including at minimum a Study Manager. Additional Study Management Committee members are often required. Study oversight is also improved with the addition of a Steering Committee to guide the overall study management. A Data Safety Monitoring Committee may be required to provide additional safety oversight for the study participants. Outcome Adjudication Committees can improve the accuracy of subjective outcome evaluation.

Keywords: study management, study committees, methods center, steering committee, data safety monitoring, large studies

26.1 Introduction

Clinical studies come in different sizes and complexities. Small clinical studies can sometimes be completed with a small number of dedicated individuals. However, for large clinical studies to be successful, they often require teams of individuals. When working with these often sizable teams, it is imperative to develop a clear organizational structure at the start of the study for more streamlined study execution.

This chapter will describe common organization and committee structures for managing large clinical studies. It will present the purpose of the Study Management Committee and describe the roles and responsibilities of members of the Study Management Committee. Additionally, the chapter will identify and describe the roles and functions of common clinical study committees, primarily the Steering Committee, Data Safety Monitoring Board (DSMB), and the Adjudication Committee. This chapter does not describe roles and functions of individual clinical study site investigators and staff, as these are described in detail in previous chapters.

26.2 Study Management Committee

The intricacies of a particular study will often determine the composition of an individual study team. All large studies require a Study Management Committee (also known as a Study Management Group, Study Management Team, or Methods Center) to ensure the success of the study. This overarching committee is responsible for all day-to-day elements of the study from study design and protocol development through final data dissemination. Study Management Committees are responsible for creating the study protocol, data collection forms/systems, developing and maintaining study randomization, and creating study manuals and other study resources. The Study Management Committee is also responsible for budgeting and securing grant (or other) funding to conduct the study. Additionally, the Study Management Committee is responsible for the ongoing data validation, query management, and problem-solving. The Study Management Committee also manages all study communication including study newsletters, site initiation/monitoring/closeout visits, Investigator/Coordinator Meetings, teleconferencing, and individual study site communication. Interim data reports, grant reporting, final data analysis, reporting, and data dissemination through presentations and submitted manuscripts are also managed by the Study Management Committee.

The duties of individual Study Management Committee members are outlined below. However, in many studies, the individual duties maybe combined depending on the size and complexity of the clinical study. ▶ Table 26.1 summarizes individual Study Management Committee member responsibilities.

26.2.1 Study Principal Investigator

All clinical studies must have a Study Principal Investigator or Chief Investigator. The Study

Table 26.1 Primary roles of members of the Study Management Committee

Study Principal Investigator	Overall responsibility for the design and conduct of the clinical study
Co-investigators	Highly involved and make significant contributions to the clinical study; however, they do not share in the overall responsibility for the study.
Study Manager	Responsible for the day-to-day management of the clinical study. Administrator over all aspects of the clinical study, from protocol management, site recruitment, contracts, budgets and finance, data collection, and study development.
Database Managers	Responsible for creating, managing, and maintaining study-specific databases. Also responsible for ongoing data validation, data cleaning, and data query management.
Financial Analysts/Business Analysts	Manages the study budget, prepare financial reports, and create and monitor study budget projections. Responsible for study contracts and ensuing that study invoices are prepared and paid in a timely manner.
Research Assistants	Duties vary depending on study team needs. Often responsible for assembling and distributing case report forms and study binders to research sites. Assist with data validation and data query resolutions, remind sites of overdue study visits, prepare adjudication materials, prepare study newsletters, and other duties as delegated.
Study Statistician	Provides statistical input in the study design and monitoring. Performs interim analysis and final data analysis.
Study Monitors	Reviews regulatory documentation at individual sites to ensure compliance. Monitors sites for protocol adherence, event reporting, quality control, and accurate data entry.

Principal Investigator, who is generally a clinician in traditional clinical studies, is the leader of the overall study. They have the overall responsibility for the design and conduct of the clinical study. The Study Principal Investigator should be knowledgeable of both the specific study and research best practices in order to handle clinical and scientific issues that may arise during the study. Study Principal Investigators should have experience in conducting clinical research as a site investigator and as part of the design and management of a large clinical study. If the Study Principal Investigator does not have experience in managing large studies, it is vital to the study that other study team members have this experience.

Two often overlooked, however vitally important, requirements of a Study Principal Investigator are that they should be committed to the study and be available to conduct the study. They must be committed to the proper and ethical execution and completion of the study. Clinical studies may take years to complete, and the Study Principal Investigator must remain interested and invested throughout the study for the successful completion of the study. It is also important that the Study Principal Investigator be available by having time dedicated to the oversight and conduct of the clinical study. If a clinician does not have protected time from a busy clinical practice, then their study responsibilities often get ignored, delayed, or delegated. However, it is important for the Study Principal Investigator to remember that they generally hold the primary responsibilities of the successful conduct and completion of the study.

In some clinical studies, there may be Study Co-Principal Investigators. This occurs when more than one individual has equal responsibility for the conduct of a study. Co-Principal Investigators are often used in multinational studies, where the individual Principal Investigators will have the responsibility for the study conduct in their country of practice.

26.2.2 Co-investigators

Very few studies can be conducted with only one investigator. Co-Investigators are highly involved in clinical studies and make significant contributions. However, they do not share in the overall responsibility for the study. Co-Investigators are able to provide additional insight into the clinical problem, help troubleshoot possible roadblocks for the completion of a study, and can provide assistance in enrolling patients in order to meet the sample size needed. Co-Investigators are involved in all aspects of the study from study design, implementation, and dissemination of study findings.

26.2.3 Study Manager

A Study Manager is a key element of successful clinical studies.[1] This individual may have different titles depending on the individual study (study manager/trial manager/study coordinator/trial coordinator, etc.). However, this is the individual charged with the day-to-day management of the clinical study. This individual is often the administrator over all aspects of the clinical study, from protocol management, site recruitment, contracts, and budgets and finance to data collection and study development. Ideally, a study manager will be involved from the initial study design through study completion. While having a study manager on board in the beginning stages of the study design is often difficult due to budgetary constraints, the Study Manager should be brought into the study team as soon as possible.

In additional to protocol and funding management, the Study Manager is also responsible for creating any study specific manual of operations, standard operating practices, and data collection forms. In large studies, the Study Manager will often also manage additional research staff including data analysts, database managers, research assistants, etc.

A Study Manager should have significant experience in conducting clinical studies prior to managing a clinical study. Experience on a Primary Study Team or at minimum experience as site study coordinator for multiple studies provides the foundation of skills required to be a successful Study Manager. Education in clinical research methodology or biostatistics provides additional tools that are beneficial to a Study Manager. A solid understanding of budgeting and resource management is also required for Study Managers in most settings. Finally, a Study Manager must work closely with the Study Principal Investigator for the study to be successful. A successful Study Manager and Study Principal Investigator team has a foundation in trust, mutual respect, and open communication.

In addition to the above-stated experience, there are a number of skills required of a successful Study Manager. These include a strong skill set in communication, organization, operational management, and budget management. Additionally, a successful study manager will exhibit enthusiasm, leadership, independent thinking, and problem-solving skills.

26.2.4 Database Managers

In large clinical studies, there is a large amount of data that need to get into the data collection system and need to be processed appropriately. Database managers are often charged with creating and managing study participant randomizations, and any systems that assist with the randomization process. Database managers should work closely with the Study Manager to develop case report forms (CRFs) to ensure that all data required for the study are able to be collected and managed in the most efficient way to achieve high-quality data. The Database Manager is also responsible for the programing and maintaining the study-specific database.

Database Managers may also be responsible for ongoing data validation. Study data need to be reviewed in a timely manner to monitor for any clinical problems or data collection problems with the study. Data managers are often responsible for developing the processes to obtain this clinical study data, along with data cleaning, data query management, and data verification. In small clinical studies, the Study Manager may also perform the duties of the Database Managers. While in larger studies, some of these tasks, such as data cleaning and query management, may be delegated to Research Assistants.

26.2.5 Financial Analysts/Business Analysts

Financial or Business Analysts may also play a large role in the conduct of clinical studies. The Financial Analysts will work with the Study Manager to develop and manage the study budget, prepare financial reports, and create and monitor study budget projections. This individual will also be responsible for ensuring appropriate contracting between the funding agency, methods center, and study sites. They will ensure that invoices are appropriate and substantiated, and that all payments or fund transfers occur in an appropriate manner. In larger research groups, an individual financial analyst may manage the study finances of a number of different studies. While in small clinical studies, the duties of the financial analyst may be assigned to the Study Manager.[2]

26.2.6 Research Assistants

Research Assistants may also be an invaluable asset to a study team. The roles of a Research Assistant can vary depending on the needs of an individual study team. In some research teams, Research Assistants may be responsible for assembling and distributing CRFs and study binders to research sites. They may assist with data validation and data query resolutions, remind sites of overdue study visits, prepare adjudication materials, or prepare study newsletters and other site communications under the supervision of the Study Manager.

26.2.7 Study Statistician

Large studies require an individual with advanced statistical training to provide statistical input in the study design, monitoring, interim analysis, and final data analysis. This individual may be employed by an individual study team (generally working on multiple projects) or contracted to analyze certain portions of the research data.

26.2.8 Study Monitors

On-site monitoring of study data is generally conducted by Study Monitors. In purely academic studies, study monitoring may be conducted by the data coordinators, or the Study Manager. However, industry-sponsored clinical studies either provide study monitors themselves or use a contract research organization (CRO) to help assure that the regulatory requirements are met.

Study Monitors review regulatory documentation at individual sites to ensure that all regulatory requirements have been met, are up-to-date, and on file at each institution. Additionally, Study Monitors compare reported data elements to source documentation to monitor for protocol adherence, event reporting, quality control, and accurate data entry.

26.2.9 Additional Team Members

Depending on the size and complexity of a given study, additional team members may be included. For example, Adjudication Coordinators, Administrative Assistants, and Regulatory Coordinators may be valuable members to a Study Management Committee.

For studies that require extensive outcomes adjudication, an Adjudication Coordinator may be required to gather, prepare, and disseminate information needed for outcomes adjudication. This individual is responsible for ensuring that all supporting information including blinded clinic notes, imaging, and test results are available for review by the Adjudication Committee. The Adjudication Coordinator may also record and manage the integrity of the adjudicated data.

Administrative Assistants can assist in preparation of study documents, shipping, and management of study supplies to study sites, and assist in dissemination of study documents. In some studies, Administrative Assistants may be responsible for maintaining updated contracts, invoicing, and site payments. Administrative Assistants may also be responsible for scheduling Study Management staff travel to study sites.

In large multicenter studies, a Regulatory or Ethics Review Coordinator is beneficial to ensure that all study sites have appropriate regulatory, Ethics, or Institutional Review Board approval and up-to-date regulatory submissions across all study sites. Multisite regulatory compliance can be especially tricky if the study is being conducted in multiple countries with different regulatory requirements or if the study requires additional regulatory review such as approval from the Food and Drug Administration or from a governmental granting agency.

26.3 Additional Study Oversight Committees

In addition to the Study Management Committee, large studies also rely on a number of committees to help make the studies successful. The duties of these committees may vary in scope depending on the individual study needs.

There are some guidelines that are helpful for all study committees. All study committees should have clear communication with the Study Principal Investigator. The written charter for each committee should define the roles and responsibilities of the committee clearly defined. Additionally, the charter should guide the actions and decision of the committees throughout the study.

In general, study committees should involve an odd number of committee members to help assure a majority rule. Each committee should also have a designated chairperson with prior expertise in the committee functions. Committee member personalities should also be carefully considered. When one member has a more dominant personality, committee decisions can be biased by the dominant personality's opinion. Conversely, more timid personalities may be less likely to voice and stick to their opinions and concerns. The designated chairperson must make sure that all committee members' thought and opinions are able to be freely shared and discussed.[3] Finally, committee members should be able to commit the time needed to meet the expectations and responsibilities of the committee throughout the length of the study.

This chapter will focus on three additional study oversight committees: Steering Committees, DSMBs, and Outcomes Adjudication Committees.

26.3.1 Steering Committee

A number of different models have been proposed for Steering Committees. However, most Steering Committees are a group of individuals with expertise in the clinical topic being investigated and/or clinical study management who are responsible for decision-making and the highest level of oversight of a study. It is generally preferable that the Steering Committee is made up of individuals from different stakeholders and backgrounds. Steering Committee members have been described as a "critical friend." They are individuals who are invested in the study, but able to ask the big questions since they are not as close to the study as the Principal Investigator.[4]

Steering Committees generally consist of the Study Principal Investigator, one to three clinicians, and a statistician and/or study methodologists. The clinicians may or may not participate as site investigators in the study. Sponsored or funded studies will often have a delegate on the Steering Committee from the sponsor or funding agency. A multidisciplinary team of clinicians is very beneficial, especially if the clinical outcomes cover multiple specialties. For example, a study involving the effect of diabetes on infection rates following total joint replacement surgery may be led by an orthopaedic surgeon as the PI. However, having an endocrinologist and an infectious disease expert on the Steering Committee can add new points of view and expertise to the study.

More recently, there has been a huge push internationally for more patient-centered research and more patient and public involvement in clinical research. Including a patient advocate into the Steering Committee can help ensure that the study is adequately evaluating what outcomes are important to patients and thus is more likely to change current practice.[5,6]

Steering Committees review and approve the main study protocol and any study amendments. They recommend changes to the protocol as needed. They also monitor and supervise the overall conduct of the study. They maintain regular contact with the other study committees such as the Data Monitoring Committee, Adjudication Committee, and the Primary Study team. At study completion, the Steering Committee is responsible for the final data analysis, dissemination of findings, and manuscript preparation.[2]

26.3.2 Data Safety Monitoring Committee/Data Safety Monitoring Boards

A Data Safety Monitoring Committee (DSMC), also known as an Independent Data Monitoring Committee (IDMC) or Data Safety Monitoring Board (DSMB), is established "to assess at intervals the progress of a clinical study, the safety data, and the critical efficacy endpoints, and to recommend to the sponsor whether to continue, modify, or stop a trial."[7]

DSMCs are charged with monitoring study data to evaluate the safety and effectiveness of the interventions being tested, along with monitoring study compliance and conduct. Specifically, DSMCs will review all adverse events, unanticipated events, and study outcomes to ensure that the participants are not undergoing undue harm due to study participation. They should also have the ability to recommend changes to the protocol, such as changing study inclusion criteria, dosage, or require additional screening tests or outcome measures to evaluate of the safety and efficacy of the intervention. DSMCs may also recommend terminating a study in the event of related serious adverse events. Many DSMCs review study protocol compliance, including protocol deviations, screen failures, missed evaluations, and improper treatment allocations/randomizations. They also evaluate for any issues with recruitment or participant retention. However, other DSMC models only evaluate for adverse events and unanticipated problems.

DSMCs should also be aware of any data from outside of the study that may have an effect on the safety of the study. For example, new publications reporting on unanticipated side effects of the drug or drug class being evaluated. However, to minimize bias, it is important that the DSMC only recommend protocol changes that directly relate to the safety of the studies. Other changes should be initiated by the Principal Investigator or the Steering Committee.

While a DSMC is not required for every study, they are often required for industry-supported clinical studies and studies funded by federal agencies to monitor patient safety and study progress. The U.S. Food and Drug Administration has recommended that sponsors and investigators consider a number of characteristics to decide if DSMC is needed.[8] When one or more of the characteristics included in ▶ Table 26.2 are met, the inclusion of an independent DSMC is recommended. Additional authors have recommended that DSMCs should be utilized if the risks are unknown, when a pharmaceutical or device company is involved, or where a company's or institution's standard operating practices may not be followed.[9,10] However, short-term studies, studies where events would accrue before the DSMC could review, studies with minor risks from the treatment, and studies evaluating symptom relief may not require a DSMC.[8,9]

Many different examples of DSMC structures have been proposed. Different models may work in different clinical study scenarios and the safety concerns related to each study. In general, DSMCs should have a minimum of three members, who should be carefully chosen by the Steering Committee to ensure that the members have the appropriate experience and expertise to participate. In general, DSMCs consist of clinicians with expertise in the condition being studied; however, they must also be independent of all other aspects of the study and without any serious conflict of interest. DSMC members should not have any financial, intellectual, or personal relationships with members of the Primary Study Team, Steering Committee, or sponsoring organization. Each DSMC should also contain at least one biostatistician who is also independent of the clinical study. Some studies may require more specialized individuals to participate in the DSMC. These may consist of medical ethicists, pharmacists, epidemiologists, etc. Nonscientists are also often participating in DSMCs to provide the perspective of the population being studied.[8]

It is also important that DSMC members have appropriate training, experience, and expertise in participating on DSMCs. However, currently there is a lack of standardized processes and trainings for DSMCs. DSMC members should have clinical expertise in the condition being studied, and understanding of applicable regulations, clinical study design, and data analysis. At minimum, the Chair of the DSMC, whether a clinician or a biostatistician, should have experience participating in DSMC committees.

It is vitally important to clinical studies that the data reviewed by the DSMC remain strictly confidential. Early release of incomplete study data may lead to prejudgments about the efficacy of an investigational product or procedure, which

Table 26.2 Characteristics of studies that will benefit from the establishment of a Data Monitoring Committee

A highly favorable or unfavorable study endpoint, or even a finding of futility, at an interim analysis might ethically require termination of the study before its planned completion.

Known reasons, a priori, for a particular safety concern, as, for example, if the procedure for administering the treatment is particularly invasive.

Prior information suggesting the possibility of serious toxicity with the study treatment.

The study population is potentially fragile (such as children, pregnant women, or the very elderly), or other vulnerable (terminally ill or of diminished mental capacity).

The study population has an elevated risk of death or other serious outcomes, even when the study objective addresses a lesser endpoint.

The study is large, of long duration, and multicenter.

The study intervention is complex, which may increase the overall risk to the participants.

Source: Adapted from FDA Guidance 2006 and 2012.

may affect the ability to complete the study or undermine the ability of the study to provide clear answers to the study question. Study management staff and sponsor representatives should not be involved in the closed sessions of the DSMC where unblinded data are discussed. Often DSMC members are required to sign confidentiality agreements for the time of the study and for some time following the study closeout.

DSMCs should be governed by DSMC charters and standard operating procedures (SOPs). These should be developed early in the study prior to interim data analysis. These charters and SOPs should be reviewed and approved by all members of the DSMC. DSMC charters should include the meeting format, frequency of meetings, guidelines for reports, minutes and other communication, statistical guidelines for interim analyses, as well as procedures for maintaining confidentiality, and managing any potential conflicts of interest the DSMC members may have or develop.

Detailed minutes should be maintained for all DMSC meetings. These minutes are generally kept in two distinct sections. One section should contain the overall recommendations to the DSMC. This section should not report any unblinded data, but should only report blinded, aggregate data. This section can then be shared with the sponsor and study sites as documentation of the completed DSMC meeting. If the minutes are to contain any unblended data and analysis, this information should be kept separate and not distributed to anyone outside of the DSMC during the conduct of the clinical study.

26.3.3 Adjudication Committee

Adjudication Committees, also known as Endpoint Assessment Committees or Outcomes Adjudication Committees, are used in some studies to evaluate important outcomes or participant eligibility to determine if the data reported by the Site Investigators meet the protocol-specific criteria.

Similar to DSMCs, not every study will require an Adjudication Committee. The primary outcome and resource availability are the two driving points behind the need for an Adjudication Committee. These committees are especially beneficial when the outcomes are subjective or when the study intervention is not blinded to the treating investigators. Adjudicating these outcomes will reduce the effects of any bias introduced by the

subjective nature of the outcome. However, in studies where the primary outcomes are laboratory values, all-cause readmissions, or all-cause mortality, the need for outcome adjudication is greatly reduced. Additionally, unfunded or significantly underfunded studies will often not have the resources available to adequately prepare, distribute, and process adjudication committee materials and decisions.

Adjudication committee members are blinded to the treatment allocation of an individual subject when adjudicating whether the outcome meets the protocol-specific criteria. They review the clinical supporting data (whether blinded copies of clinical notes or imaging studies) to determine if the participant meets study eligibility, or if a study outcome event has occurred.

An Adjudication Charter must be created to outline the responsibilities of the Adjudication Committee members, describe which items will be adjudicated, provide decision rules, and indicate when outcomes will be adjudicated. The adjudication charter should also clearly define the level of agreement required for the committee. Ideally, complete consensus is used in most clinical studies; however, with larger committees and subjective outcomes this may be difficult to obtain; thus, a majority consensus may be used if described in the Adjudication Committee Charter.[11]

The Adjudication Coordinator, or other members of the Study Management Committee, is generally responsible for preparing materials for adjudication. The Adjudication Coordinator gathers all clinical notes, imaging files, laboratory data, etc., from the local sites and ensures that the materials are all blinded in regard to the patient and site. These tasks take a significant amount of time. Additionally, the Adjudication Coordinator and members of the Study Management Committee schedule and attend the adjudication meetings. The Adjudication Coordinator is generally responsible for getting the adjudicated data to the biostatisticians for data analyses and reporting.

Outcomes adjudication should begin once study-specific outcomes begin being reported to the methods center. These committees should meet at frequent intervals to stay as up-to-date as possible with the outcomes adjudication. While it may seem more budget friendly to conduct adjudication at the end of the study, it is important to have adjudication meetings throughout the study. This provides the opportunity to identify early on if additional information is needed for the committee to make their assessments, identify common errors in data collection, and identify issues relating to the safety of participants. This also allows for the adjudicated data to be used in any interim reports or DSMC meeting to help assure that the data are free of bias.[8,11]

26.4 Other Study Committees

26.4.1 Writing Committee/Data Dissemination Committee

In large clinical studies, a Writing Committee or Data Dissemination Committee may be tasked with the writing of any manuscript for the study team. This committee generally consists of the Study Principal Investigation, Study Manager, Biostatistician, and other interested investigators or study team members. This committee takes on the responsibility for the primary study manuscript preparation along with submissions to any scientific conference for presentation, or to regulatory bodies as needed. Additionally, this committee may prepare secondary manuscripts from the initial study data as appropriate.

26.4.2 Audit/Monitoring Committee

In some large studies, the site audit or monitoring responsibilities may necessitate the creation of an Audit or Monitoring Committee outside of the Study Management Committee. This committee is then responsible for auditing/monitoring of data collected from study sites. Common monitoring checklists and procedures are developed to ensure accurate and consistent review of study data.

26.5 Practical Application

In a large multicenter trial evaluating a new insulin and blood glucose management system for individuals with Type I diabetes, the Study Principal Investigator, an endocrinologist with a specific interest in Type I diabetes, consulted with colleagues on a possible investigation of a new insulin and glucose management system. Following positive feedback from colleagues, the Study Principal Investigator consulted with an individual with experience as a Study Manager in conducting clinical trials in patients with Type I diabetes. The team was successful in obtaining funding for their research. The Study Manager was able to hire an experienced database manager and a research assistant to work as part of the Study Management Committee. An experienced biostatistician was contracted to assist with the data analysis for the study. The Study Manager, who had previous experience in grant management, took on the duties of the financial analyst. All other Study Management Committee duties were split between the Study Manager, Database Manager, and Research Assistant.

The Study Principal Investigator was able to recruit two of the three colleagues (one endocrinologist and one Certified Diabetes Educator) that they initially contacted about the study idea to participate in the Study Steering Committee. In addition to the biostatistician, the Study Principal Investigator consulted with a local Type I diabetes support group and was able to identify an individual who was diagnosed with Type I diabetes 15 years prior. This individual was recruited to participate as a Steering Committee member to provide input into outcomes of interest and barriers to protocol compliance faced by individuals with Type I diabetes.

Since a malfunction in the insulin and glucose management system could cause significant adverse events to the study participants, and the population is already at risk for complications, it was decided to have a DSMC as additional safety oversight. An endocrinologist who was an experienced DSMC member, without a potential conflict of interest, was recruited to be the chair of the DSMC. An additional endocrinologists and an independent biostatistician were also recruited to participate in the DSMC.

The primary outcomes were determined to be the change in hemoglobin A1C from baseline to 6 months and the number of episodes of hypoglycemia as reported by the study participants. These outcomes were determined to be objective and therefore the decision was made to not have an Outcome Adjudication Committee.

26.6 Conclusion

Successful large clinical studies require study management infrastructure and committees to complete. This team of individuals required for a successful study varies depending on the needs of a study and the resources available. At minimum, clinical studies require a knowledgeable, committed, and available Study Principal Investigator, and a dedicated and organized Study Manager. Additional team members are needed for larger and more complex studies to ensure protocol optimization, protocol adherence, and accurate data collection that can lead to clear study conclusions. Steering Committees, Data Monitoring Committees, and Outcome Adjudication Committees, while not always required, often add additional levels of study oversight to enhance the overall study, protect the safety of the patients, and minimize bias.

Definitions

- **Adjudication:** The process of making a formal decision or judgment. In clinical studies, subjective outcomes are often adjudicated by a committee of experts who review all supporting documentation to make a formal decision on the outcome in question.
- **Dissemination:** The process of spreading and sharing information. In clinical studies, dissemination of results usually refers to the publication and presentation of study outcomes and conclusions.

References

[1] Farrell B, Kenyon S, Shakur H. Managing Clinical Trials. Trials 2010;11:78

[2] Bhandari M, Jönsson A, Eds. Clinical Research for Surgeons. 1st ed. New York, NY: Thieme; 2008

[3] Simunovic N, Walter S, Devereaux PJ, et al. SPRINT Investigators. Outcomes Assessment in the SPRINT Multicenter Tibial Fracture Trial: Adjudication Committee Size has Trivial Effect on Trial Results. J Clin Epidemiol 2011;64(9):1023–1033

[4] Harman NL, Conroy EJ, Lewis SC, et al. Exploring the Role and Function of Trial Steering Committees: Results of an Expert Panel Meeting. Trials 2015;16:597

[5] Bagley HJ, Short H, Harman NL, et al. A Patient and Public Involvement (PPI) Toolkit for Meaningful and Flexible Involvement in Clinical Trials - A Work in Progress. Res Involv Engagem 2016;2:15

[6] South A, Hanley B, Gafos M, et al. Models and Impact of Patient and Public Involvement in Studies Carried out by the Medical Research Council Clinical Trials Unit at University College London: Findings from Ten Case Studies. Trials 2016;17:376

[7] International Council for Harmonisation of Technical Requirements for Pharmaceuticals for Human Use. Integrated Addendum to ICH E6(R1): Guideline for Good Clinical Practice E6(R2). 2016. Available from: https://www.ich.org/fileadmin/Public_Web_Site/ICH_Products/Guidelines/Efficacy/E6/E6_R2__Step_4_2016_1109.pdf. Accessed October 23, 2018

[8] United States Food and Drug Administration. Guidance for Clinical Trial Sponsors: Establishment and Operation of Clinical Trial Data Monitoring Committees. 2006. Available from: https://www.fda.gov/downloads/RegulatoryInformation/Guidances/ucm127073.pdf. Accessed October 24, 2018

[9] Sydes MR, Spiegelhalter DJ, Altman DG, Babiker AB, Parmar MK; DAMOCLES Group. Systematic Qualitative Review of the Literature on Data Monitoring Committees for Randomized Controlled Trials. Clin Trials 2004;1(1):60–79

[10] Calis KA, Archdeacon P, Bain RP, Forrest A, Perlmutter J, DeMets DL. Understanding the Functions and Operations of Data Monitoring Committees: Survey and Focus Group Findings. Clin Trials 2017;14(1):59–66

[11] Vannabouathong C, Saccone M, Sprague S, Schemitsch EH, Bhandari M. Adjudicating Outcomes: Fundamentals. J Bone Joint Surg Am 2012;94(Suppl 1):70–74

27 International Research: Challenges and Successes

Chuan Silvia Li, Mandeep S. Dhillon

Abstract

The importance of conducting medical research on a global or international platform cannot be overemphasized in current times. Establishment of international research is indispensable to the advancement of science and the improvement of patient outcomes on a global scale. In this chapter, we describe the common challenges faced when conducting international research, especially in low- and middle-income countries (LMICs), and provide a successful example of coordinating an international multicenter research study in LMICs: the International Orthopaedic Multicenter Study in Fracture Care (IMORMUS) study.

Keywords: international research, international collaboration, low- and middle-income countries

27.1 Introduction

Traditionally, the medical literature has been dominated by small studies that were largely single-center initiatives. In recent years, there has been a paradigm shift toward larger, multicenter, international collaborative research studies, as the medical community embraced the concepts of evidence-based medicine and the need for high-quality research to guide clinical practice.[1] The importance of conducting medical research on a global or international platform cannot be overemphasized in current times.[2] With one-fifth of the world's scientific papers coauthored internationally, there is a sustained move on the part of researchers throughout the world to engage collaboratively in the production of knowledge and innovation.[3] In 2013, the WHO stated that unless low- and middle-income countries (LMICs) become producers of research, health goals would be hard to achieve. The ability to conduct clinical studies is important for institutions in LMICs.[4] There is a need and growing interest for executing clinical studies in LMICs.[5] Conducting international clinical studies increases access to potentially eligible study subjects and reduces overall recruitment and enrollment time, leading to more rapid advancement in science and conservation of research-specific resources. Rapid advancement in science can reduce the burden of disease, promote

health, and extend longevity for all people. In addition, generalizability will increase when recruiting patients from multiple countries and multiple ethnicities.[2] Establishment of international research is indispensable to the advancement of science and the improvement of patient outcomes on a global scale.

Numerous barriers exist preventing both clinical study design and execution while implementing an international clinical study, especially in resource-limited countries. Common challenges faced include lack of infrastructure, heterogeneity of resource availability among countries, unfamiliarity with clinical study regulations, cultural and ethical issues, and other legal issues. In this chapter, we describe the challenges associated with initiating and conducting clinical studies in LMICs and provide successful examples of coordinating an international multicenter research study in LMICs—the International Orthopaedic Multicenter Study in Fracture Care (INORMUS) study.[6,7]

27.2 Study Planning Phase

The planning of a study should begin years before the start of patient enrollment. It is beneficial to involve site investigators and encourage active contribution to the study design and protocol. This can be done through multiple investigator meetings (in-person and/or teleconference). This may lead to frequent changes to study protocol. When planning for a multinational study, one must take into account potential differences in the standard-of-care and cultural practices that could impact implementation of the protocol.[2] In international collaborations, differences in organizational structures lead to complex management protocols. The study planning can get very complex when multiple countries are involved.

Selecting research sites usually depends upon the level of expertise available for the disease of interest in that center, estimated prevalence of the disease of interest in that region, the referral network, availability of research infrastructure including administrative and clinical staff, a track record of implementing similar clinical studies, and the willingness of the center to participate.[2]

27.3 Ethics Approval

Approaches to protecting human subjects participating in research differ among countries, requiring additional time and effort for compliance.[8] Each of the participating countries or even clinical sites usually have established mechanisms to assure the ethical conduct of research and the protection of human subjects, but the processes differ across different sites and countries. The study not only needs to be compliant with regulations of the funding agency and methods center, but it also needs to meet the expectations of each clinical site's own ethics review processes.

There is a demand for stronger links between research and local health care policy and practice. Local ethics boards often request justification showing the relevance of the proposed research study and impact of the study result to the local population. The study should be driven by each country's local and national agenda and be directly responsive to a country's demands.[9]

27.4 Consent Process

The standards of informed consent can be daunting for researchers when they face the pragmatic constraints of the field and cultural beliefs about consent in resource-limited countries.[10,11] Nevertheless, it is important to identify the key issues of the informed consent process and to promote the highest ethical standards of the research. Providing adequate and comprehensive information to potential participants and assessing the understanding of the entire research purposes prior to participants' consenting are fundamental. It is important to be aware that in developing countries, a number of potential factors often threaten voluntary informed consent, including poverty, illiteracy, disease burden, extreme need, marginalization, commercialization of medicine, and the social power of physicians.[12]

Culture in developing countries is dynamic and, although constantly changing, family-centered decision-making is more common than individual decision-making. In such societies, decision-making is the prerogative of a group that might be the extended family or even community leaders.[13] While facilitating the informed consent process, one needs to respect the local community customs and cultural expectations from where participants are drawn and at the same time respect individual autonomy.

It is important for non-Western research participants not to disengage from their cultures; Western procedures might have limitations and local cultures might dictate the norms.[11,13] There is also a need to reconstruct the standards of informed consent with reference to social and cultural conventions that might influence decision-making. Informed consent in non-Western countries should not be modeled only on Western standards; the choice of culturally acceptable strategies of decision-making in informed consent is central to people's definition of themselves in relation to their natural and social environment.[11,13] More flexibility in informed consent regulations and the need of Western ethics committees to be more familiar with the local context of the research can greatly improve informed consent procedures in clinical studies in LMICs.[10,13]

Both recruitment strategies and informed consent processes should be organized in consultation with the community's local authorities or advisory boards and should be in line with the local cultural norms. Careful planning, engagement of key actors, including peer counseling with local researchers and/or culture experts, is warranted prior to any clinical research study.

27.5 Motivating Coinvestigators

It is essential to keep investigators motivated through positive reinforcement throughout stages of the study. Increasing awareness, confidence, and motivation of investigators can be done by providing adequate salaries to offset lost revenue from practice, learning opportunities, and incentives of coauthorship and presenting papers at conferences. It is crucial to sustain strong personal relationships with coinvestigators via frequent communication at the outset of the study, throughout the clinical study and on study completion. Maintaining regular communication to boost morale and enthusiasm of the clinical sites is important.[2] Strong and trusting relationships among coinvestigators can create new understanding and overcome much adversity.[8] The relationship takes time to cultivate and can be done through teleconference calls, in-person investigator meetings, and social engagements. Note that both teleconferencing and in-person investigator meetings are challenging due to time differences and the need to travel internationally. Alternatively, an electronic newsletter approximately every few months to all participating sites can be a useful strategy for conveying information related to the study's status and other important issues.[2] It is significantly easier to collaborate with centers with passionate clinicians as well as experienced and enthusiastic research coordinators and assistants. Because most clinicians are extremely busy with their clinical work, the majority of the study organization often relies on the research coordinators and assistants. Committed research coordinators and assistants prevent delays in study start-up, and ensures good data quality and better communication. Selecting a suitable research coordinator is as important as having a suitable investigator.

27.6 Language Challenges

Differences in cultural backgrounds often result in differences in assumptions, expectations, roles, and work styles. This can lead to miscommunication among international researchers, especially when there is a language barrier. The expectations and responsibilities of all parties should be explicitly explained at the beginning of the study and documented in detail. Researchers should be aware that the coinvestigators might have different assumptions and expectations about how work and interactions should be conducted.[14] It is important to have basic knowledge about the coinvestigator's training and experience. It may be worthwhile to find out what they hope to gain professionally from the collaborative experience.

Due to language barriers with both research personnel and study participants, study documents need to be translated. It can often be challenging for site research personnel to have an in-depth understanding of the study due to language limitations. Translating the protocol, case report forms, and consent forms to other languages can be costly and pose a significant challenge.

Research coordinators should be alert and sensitive to cultural differences and the diverse needs of international clinical sites due to their cultural background.

27.7 Time Zone Difference

Research coordinators and investigators often need to deal with the practical challenges of working across different time zones. A certain amount of flexibility from all parties is necessary to accommodate the challenges of scheduling meetings and slower e-mail turnaround times.

27.8 Shortage of Research Staff

There is frequently a shortage of skilled research staff. The investigators from LMICs are often forced to cope with overly complicated institutional and government administration systems and procedures without a research assistant or administrative assistant. This can result in a disabling research environment and ultimately cause failure. It is important to identify potential supporting research staff, provide adequate salaries for protected research time, and provide training both at study initiation and throughout the study.

27.9 Data Collection Process

Expect variation in data collection processes and be prepared to work with numerous study protocol deviations. Data collection and data entry processes vary among countries, and what works in one country will not necessarily work in another country.[8] A pilot study should be considered, but at the same time, no amount of pilot testing can foresee all challenges in international research.[8]

27.10 Lower Data Quality

The loss to follow-up rate and percentage of missing data may be high due to large migrant populations in LMICs.[15] The international study population has higher heterogeneity by nature, which leads to relatively large random variation in clinical studies. The investigators need to be aware of this variability and that is the "noise in the system."

27.11 Timeline Delay

Everything takes longer in international research. International research almost always will take longer than expected and should include more generous time frames than would otherwise be required.[8]

27.12 Financial Challenges

Appropriate amount of monetary incentives to both physicians and patients should be established carefully.[16] In some instances, conducting clinical studies is seen more as a commercial activity. Level of funding is a critical issue as overfunding can be counterproductive in the long term. Overfunding of clinical studies will lead to "corruption of values" as the investigators would prefer to participate in overfunded studies for commercial gain, rather than in adequately funded studies of scientific and clinical value.[17] However, underfunding of clinical studies with a huge gap between the funding received by Western and developing nation researchers is also undesirable. Payments given to participants have always been a controversial issue. Although incentives increase participation and retention rates in a clinical study, they should not be undue, which might sway the informed consent process. However, adequate compensation should be provided for travel and loss of wages, which can be substantial for the poor in developing countries.[16]

The currency exchange rates can fluctuate widely, causing fluctuation in site payments. This can lead to both excessive and inadequate funding.[8] The administration of international funds is significantly more complex and often introduces delays in receiving financial payments.

There are direct costs associated with collaboration, and these expenses are essential, likely larger in international research, and should be included in grant budgets.[8]

27.13 Legal Considerations

Different countries have different laws and different legal systems—a fact often overlooked by researchers who are eager to collaborate internationally.[14] When working domestically, researchers may have little need to monitor legal requirements or consider the legal implications of their project decisions, largely because they can count on their institution's staff to handle the legal aspect. In international collaborations, the legal department of the researchers' home institution may be challenged by very different legal requirements and ways of reconciling legal mandates. Perhaps the most fundamental challenge in the case of mismatched laws is deciding whose laws apply in a given situation. Cross-national research may involve researchers from several nations with differing requirements. In some cases, contracts can be drawn up at the initiation of a collaboration, specifying whose laws will take precedence in the event of problems.[18] In the absence of such contracts, legal issues can be a project's greatest headache and the easiest way for researchers to get in trouble. This task requires expert management in every participating country.

There are often legal challenges around data sharing relevant to international collaborations.[18] For example, the European Union and the United States have different approaches to intellectual property. The former assumes that all parties of the collaboration will share intellectual property. The United States, through the Bayh–Dole Act, specifies that the parties of a collaboration have a right to intellectual property that they have created, but they are not expected to share that right with others who have not been involved in that creation.[18]

It is also important for researchers to recognize current sanctions against other countries and specific entities by their home country. It may not be possible to collaborate or have a partnership with researchers from a sanctioned country. Exemptions may be applied with the Minister of Foreign Affairs. This process can be both costly and time-consuming and a lawyer may need to be consulted.

27.14 Practical Application

The International Orthopaedic Multicenter Study in Fracture Care (INORMUS) is a large prospective cohort study of 40,000 men and women with musculoskeletal trauma in LMICs. INORMUS aims to determine what percentage of adult musculoskeletal trauma patients have major complications (mortality, reoperation, and infection) within 30 days post hospital admission and to determine factors associated with these major complications.[6] As of June 2018, 29,930 patients have been enrolled in the INORMUS study at 50 hospitals in 17 countries including China, Uganda, Kenya, Tanzania, South Africa, Nigeria, Botswana, Ghana, India, Pakistan, Nepal, Vietnam, Thailand, Philippines, Iran, Mexico, and Venezuela (▶Fig. 27.1). The INORMUS study is being managed and coordinated by the team at the Centre for Evidence-Based Orthopaedics (CEO) at McMaster University in Hamilton, ON, Canada.

27.14.1 Laying the Groundwork— The INORMUS Pilot Study

To assess the feasibility of the proposed INORMUS study, we conducted a pilot study at 14 hospitals with a wide geographic distribution in India.[7] Approximately 5,000 patients were enrolled in the

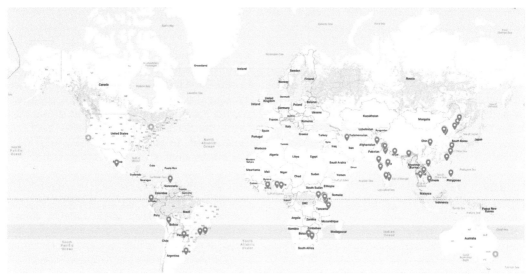

Fig. 27.1 INORMUS participating sites. Map data ©2019 Google.

pilot phase of the study between October 2011 and June 2012. This pilot study allowed us to develop our core study infrastructure and assess the feasibility of recruiting within our proposed study timelines. It also enabled us to refine our protocol and case report forms to ensure that our simplified study design and minimal dataset would facilitate data collection on a global scale. This pilot study also provided an opportunity for bidirectional learning in which all parties were able to share their respective expertise. Our successful completion of the pilot phase of INORMUS was made possible through our ability to leverage existing collaborative relationships with key researchers in India. Through these preexisting relationships, we were able to identify and engage a network of investigators and clinical sites, and to work collaboratively to resolve logistical challenges associated with the start-up and daily management of the study from the CEO methods center at McMaster University in Hamilton, ON, Canada.

Building International Partnerships and Collaborations

The success of the INORMUS pilot study in India demonstrated the feasibility of the INORMUS protocol and enabled our team to secure funding from the Canadian Institutes of Health Research (CIHR) in 2014 for the global phase of the study. However, we encountered a number of challenges during the initiation of the definitive study. These challenges included identifying and engaging local investigators in countries where our team had few or no existing relationships, evaluating potential sites' ability to participate in the study with respect to infrastructure and resources, and understanding local and/or national guidelines, policies, and practices for conducting research. These challenges highlighted the need to engage partners with local expertise in each global region. Consequently, we identified regional leads or "champions" for each geographic region. These individuals, who are all highly invested in improving the care of trauma patients, generated interest in the study through their personal contacts and through networking at local meetings and conferences. They also serve as liaisons between the local site investigators, the Principal Investigators, and the CEO methods center team. Their knowledge and expertise have been instrumental during all phases of the study including selection and evaluation of potential sites, site start-up and training, and ongoing conduct of the clinical study at sites within their regions.

Another need we identified early in the process of global expansion was the need to establish a larger central investigative team with established researchers to both develop study methodology and facilitate conduct of the study globally. This was particularly important for recruitment of patients from centers in geographically distant regions from Canada including Asia, Africa, and Latin America. In 2014, the George Institute for Global Health (TGI) in Sydney, Australia, joined the INORMUS team. TGI group has extensive experience in leading large-scale studies on injury prevention and management in India, China, and Southeast Asia. Their research offices in India and China are staffed with research personnel who are fluent in local languages and have a comprehensive understanding of both the local policies and the cultural sensitivities involved in conducting research in this geographic region. Additionally, TGI has a large and well-established network of surgeons and researchers who are highly invested in the care of trauma patients. TGI research teams serve as liaisons between the McMaster global methods center and our participating sites in China and India. They have played an integral role in all aspects of study management including site identification, initiation and training, monitoring data quality, and conducting on-site monitoring visits for all sites across India, China, Southeast Asia, and multiple sites in Africa. We were also successful in leveraging our initial CIHR funding to obtain significant funding from Australia's National Health and Medical Research Council (NHMRC) to support the INORMUS initiative in Asia and Africa.

Using the same collaborative model, we have partnered with the Institute for Global Orthopaedics and Traumatology (IGOT) at the University of California, San Francisco, to launch the INORMUS study in Latin America. The IGOT team is dedicated to the treatment of musculoskeletal injuries in LMICs through sustainable research and educational programs. A main focus of IGOT is to build research capacity of orthopaedic and trauma surgeons in resource-constrained environments through sustainable programs that address locally relevant research questions, quality and efficiency of care, and health care advocacy. Since its foundation in 2006, IGOT has established a network of over 28 partners and affiliates across 14 countries in Latin America, and has extensive experience in conducting research in this region. Our INORMUS study team is currently leveraging IGOT's expertise to expand the INORMUS study in Latin America and to pursue additional funding to support participating sites in this region.

INORMUS Study Organizational Structure and Study Management

This global study is being collaboratively led by a multinational team of Principal Investigators from CEO, TGI, and IGOT. The Principal Investigators are supported by established methods center infrastructure at all three institutions and a number of study committees consisting of key collaborators from around the world (▶Fig. 27.2).

The Operations Committee is comprised of a small number of key investigators from the three lead institutions. They provide guidance and direction to the overall study and will also be responsible for leading knowledge dissemination activities. The Global Steering Committee includes orthopaedic surgeons, research methodologists, and a statistician. This committee provides guidance and direction to the overall study, and is responsible for resolving any challenges that arise during the study. The Steering Committee's membership includes the members of the Operations Committee as well as region lead experts (▶Fig. 27.2). Each region's Lead and Co-Lead are also responsible for managing the clinical sites within each of their jurisdictions and reporting any issues to the Principal Investigators and Steering Committee members. At the completion of the study, the Steering Committee will oversee manuscript preparation on behalf of all study investigators and participating clinical sites.

The CEO global methods center at McMaster University is responsible for central coordination of the study. The CEO has established the necessary personnel and physical infrastructure to successfully lead global surgical studies and large observational studies. Research personnel include research methodologists, research project managers, research assistants, data managers, statisticians, and data analysts. Project Managers at the CEO methods center work closely with their counterparts at the GI and IGOT methods centers to manage the day-to-day activities of the study. Within their geographic regions, the GI and IGOT investigators and research personnel liaise between the clinical site investigators and the CEO methods center. They are actively engaged in identifying and selecting new site investigators, and assisting newly selected clinical sites with start-up activities including obtaining ethics approval, negotiating contracts, and developing local study processes.

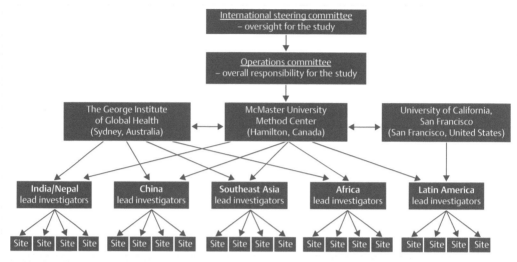

Fig. 27.2 The organizational structure of the INORMUS study.

The CEO methods center is responsible for overall data management for the clinical study. Project Managers at the CEO review and validate the clinical data, conduct remote data monitoring, address queries, prepare screening and enrolment reports, prepare study updates, and generate quality control reports. The INORMUS study teams at GI and IGOT communicate regularly with the clinical sites in their geographic regions, including following up on data quality issues, answering study-related questions, and conducting on-site monitoring visits as appropriate. In addition to this regular communication, all site investigators and research personnel receive regular updates on enrollment and study progress through electronic newsletters. Annual orthopaedic conferences and meetings of international research networks, including the Asociación de Cirujanos Traumatólogos de las Américas (ACTUAR), provide an opportunity for INORMUS collaborators to meet face to face. Ongoing concerns regarding participating clinical sites including contracting issues, data quality issues, and rates of recruitment or follow-up are escalated by the CEO, GI, and IGOT project management teams to the regional leads and Operations Committee. Any issues that cannot be unresolved by the regional leads are then escalated to Operations Committee and Steering Committee as appropriate.

INORMUS is among one of the largest cohort studies conducted to date in the field of orthopaedic surgery. We have succeeded in initiating 50 clinical sites and enrolling over 25,000 patients by engaging a collaborative global team of investigators and methods centers. Their expertise and dedication have been instrumental in understanding and working through the infrastructure limitations as well as the ethical, cultural, and operational challenges associated with conducting high-quality global research.

While the INORMUS study is poised to directly address a critical gap in our knowledge regarding the burden of trauma, the most important contribution of INORMUS is the establishment of global research infrastructure. The lessons learned from INORMUS in regard to building research capacity and the collaborative relationships that we have fostered will enable the global orthopaedic community to answer many important questions in injury care for years to come.

27.15 Conclusion

International collaboration brings opportunity—rapid completion of clinical studies, enhanced generalizability of the results of these studies, and a focus on questions that have evoked international curiosity. On the other hand, the requirements of conducting clinical research are much more complex and demanding in international collaborations and require additional effort, administrative skill, and patience.

The obstacles to conducting clinical studies in LMICs are numerous and fraught with ethical, political, and logistical considerations. It is important to initiate multinational cooperative groups to conducting large-scale cooperative studies. These studies will answer important clinical questions while simultaneously serving as models for future cooperative endeavors. It is also important for investigators working in LMIC setting to tailor clinical study designs and treatment paradigms to each region's unique resource profile. Impressive foundational work has been laid to initiate clinical studies in LMICs in many areas and we need to continue our efforts to increase comprehensive multinational and cooperative collaboration in the future.

Overall, international clinical research can be productive and extremely gratifying, but it is not for the faint-hearted.

Definitions

- **Case report form CRF:** A paper or electronic questionnaire specifically used in clinical study research to collect the specific data in order to answer the research questions.
- **Informed consent:** A process for getting permission before conducting a health care intervention on a person, or for disclosing personal information. It is the process where a participant is informed about all aspects of the study, which are important for the participant to make a decision and after studying all aspects of the study the participant voluntarily confirm their willingness to participate in a particular clinical study and significance of the research for advancement of medical knowledge and social welfare. Informed consent is an ethical and legal requirement for research involving human participants.

References

[1] Katsouyanni K. Collaborative Research: Accomplishments & Potential. Environ Health 2008;7:3
[2] Minisman G, Bhanushali M, Conwit R, et al. Implementing Clinical Trials on an International Platform: Challenges and Perspectives. J Neurol Sci 2012;313(1–2):1–6
[3] Butrous G. International Cooperation to Promote Advances in Medicine. Ann Thorac Med. 2008;3(3):79–81
[4] Franzen SRP, Chandler C, Siribaddana S, Atashili J, Angus B, Lang T. Strategies for Developing Sustainable Health Research Capacity in Low and Middle-Income Countries: A Prospective, Qualitative Study Investigating the Barriers and Enablers to Locally Led Clinical Trial Conduct in Ethiopia, Cameroon and Sri Lanka. BMJ Open 2017;7(10):e017246
[5] Grover S, Xu M, Jhingran A, et al. Clinical Trials in Low and Middle-Income Countries: Successes and Challenges. Gynecol Oncol Rep 2016;19:5–9
[6] Investigators I; INORMUS Investigators. INternational ORthopaedic MUlticentre Study (INORMUS) in Fracture Care: Protocol for a Large Prospective Observational Study. J Orthop Trauma 2015;29(Suppl 10):S2–S6
[7] Foote CJ, Mundi R, Sancheti P, et al. INORMUS Investigators. Musculoskeletal Trauma and All-Cause Mortality in India: A Multicentre Prospective Cohort Study. Lancet 2015;385(Suppl 2):S30
[8] Green LA, Fryer GE Jr, Froom P, Culpepper L, Froom J. Opportunities, Challenges, and Lessons of International Research in Practice-Based Research Networks: The Case of an International Study of Acute Otitis Media. Ann Fam Med 2004;2(5):429–433
[9] Alemayehu C, Mitchell G, Nikles J. Barriers for Conducting Clinical Trials in Developing Countries - A Systematic Review. Int J Equity Health 2018;17(1):37
[10] Mystakidou K, Panagiotou I, Katsaragakis S, Tsilika E, Parpa E. Ethical and Practical Challenges in Implementing Informed Consent in HIV/AIDS Clinical Trials in Developing or Resource-Limited Countries. SAHARA J 2009;6(2):46–57
[11] Crigger NJ, Holcomb L, Weiss J. Fundamentalism, Multiculturalism and Problems of Conducting Research with Populations in Developing Nations. Nurs Ethics 2001;8(5):459–468
[12] Castillo FA. Limiting Factors Impacting on Voluntary First Person Informed Consent in the Philippines. Developing World Bioeth 2002;2(1):11–20
[13] Shaibu S. Ethical and Cultural Considerations in Informed Consent in Botswana. Nurs Ethics 2007;14(4):503–509
[14] Anderson MS. International Research Collaborations: Anticipating Challenges Instead of Being Surprised. In: Europa World of Learning. 61st ed. Vol. 1. London: Routledge; 2010:14–18
[15] Bao J, Hafner R. Conducting High-Quality Tuberculosis Clinical Trials in China: Opportunities and Challenges. Int J Tuberc Lung Dis 2017;21(11):1094–1100
[16] Devasenapathy N, Singh K, Prabhakaran D. Conduct of Clinical Trials in Developing Countries: A Perspective. Curr Opin Cardiol 2009;24(4):295–300
[17] Yusuf S. Clinical Research and Trials in Developing Countries. Stat Med 2002;21(19):2859–2867
[18] Anderson MS, Steneck NH, eds. International Research Collaborations: Much to Be Gained, Many Ways to get in trouble. New York, NY: Routledge; 2011:xiii, 296

Further Readings

Anderson MS, Steneck NH, ed. International Research Collaborations: Much to Be Gained, Many Ways to get in trouble. New York, NY: Routledge; 2011:18
Global Health Trials: an online community for researchers in global health to share their knowledge, tools and methods for conducting health research. https://globalhealthtrials.tghn.org/

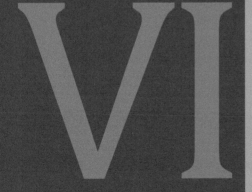

Part VI

A Coordinator's Toolbox

VI

Toolbox A	*286*
Toolbox B	*288*
Toolbox C	*290*
Toolbox D	*292*
Toolbox E	*293*
Toolbox F1	*299*
Toolbox F2	*300*
Toolbox F3	*301*
Toolbox F4	*302*
Toolbox F5	*303*
Toolbox F6	*304*
Toolbox F7	*305*
Toolbox F8	*306*
Toolbox F9	*308*
Toolbox F10	*309*
Toolbox F11	*310*
Toolbox G	*312*

Toolbox A

Anticipated Research Study Expenses and Justification

Expense	Description of tasks	Justification of expense	Year 1	Year 2	Total for years 1 and 2
Clinical research project manager	Submit application to ethics, ensure protocol compliance for each study participant, perform interim and final statistical analyses for functional data, and write manuscript	Institutional base salary rate of $40.00/h with 4% in lieu of pension and benefits: $81,120.00 × 0.80 FTE = $64,896.00	$64,896.00	$64,896.00	$129,792

Clinical research coordinators A and B	Recruit study participants and conduct all visits and paperwork for study follow-ups at Campus A or B. Ensure compliance of each study event/data point per participant:
	• Informed consent
	• Inclusion/exclusion
	• Basic demographics
	• Waist circumference
	• Operative information
	• Device information
	• PROMs
	  ◦ WOMAC
	  ◦ HOOS
	  ◦ EQ-5D
	  ◦ VAS pain score
	• Pre-post Hgb
	• Complications
	• Readmissions
	• TUG
	• TSC
	• IR and ER ROM at flexion and extension
		Institutional base salary rate of $35.00/h with 4% in lieu of pension and benefits: $70,980.00 × 0.4 FTE = $28,392.00	$28,392.00 + $28,392.00	$28,392.00 + $28,392.00	$113,568

Laboratory technician	Install and calibrate motion capture apparatus for patients undergoing gait analyses at biomechanics laboratory, and follow gait analyses protocol for all study participants. Ensure compliance to the collection of motion capture for gait analysis data	Collaborating center base salary rate of $28.00/h with 4% in lieu of pension: $56,784 × 0.4 FTE = $22,713.60	$22,713.60	$22,713.60	$45,427
Motion capture and data processing analyst	Organization and processing of kinematic, kinetic, and EMG data of all subjects. Approximately 150 h total over the course of the study	Collaborating center base salary rate of $39.91/h with 4% in lieu of pension: $41.506/h × 150 h = $6225.90		$6225.90	$6226

(Continued)

Expense	Description of tasks	Justification of expense	Year 1	Year 2	Total for years 1 and 2
Ethics fees	Initial fee and annual renewal fees for industry-sponsored study	Initial fee of $5,000 and annual renewal fee of $1,000 for year 2	$5,000.00	$1000.00	$6,000
Patient stipend for substudy participation	Study participants participating in gait substudy will receive a $50 gift card at the beginning, middle, and at the end of study participation	30 study participants in total × ($50 per gift card) × 3 timepoints, assuming no attrition = $4,500.00		$4,500.00	$4,500
Dissemination of results	Open access fee for one orthopaedic journal	Average cost of $3,000		$3,000.00	$3,000
Indirect costs	Institutional overhead fee that covers basic administrative support, contracts, and office supplies	Institutional overhead fee of 30%	$44,818.08	$47,735.85	$92,554
				Total costs	$401,067

Abbreviations: EMG, electromyography; EQ-5D, EuroQol-5D; ER, external rotation; Hgb, hemoglobin; HOOS, hip disability and osteoarthritis outcome score; IR, internal rotation; PROMs, patient-reported outcome measures; ROM, range of motion; TSC, timed stair climb; TUG, timed up and go; VAS, Visual Analog Scale; WOMAC, Western Ontario and McMaster Universities Osteoarthritis Index.

Toolbox B

Sample Site Trial Master File/Investigator Site File Table of Contents

1.	Delegation log
2.	Site personnel CVs
3.	Site personnel training documents
4.	Initial Ethics Committee correspondence and approval
5.	Approved informed consent form
6.	Ethics amendments and correspondence
7.	Continuing Ethics Review correspondence and approvals
8.	Serious adverse events reported to Ethics Committee
9.	Serious adverse events correspondence
10.	Protocol deviations reported to Ethics Committee
11.	Protocol deviation correspondence
12.	Study protocol
13.	Investigator's Brochure
14.	FDA Form 1572
15.	Investigational product accountability log
16.	Case report forms
17.	Clinical site manual
18.	DSMB/DSMC reports
19.	Monitoring visit log
20.	Monitoring reports
21.	Notes to file
22.	Clinical trial agreements/contracts
23.	Significant correspondence

Abbreviations: CV, curriculum vitae; DSMB/DSMC, Data Safety and Monitoring Board/Data Safety and Monitoring Committee; FDA, Food and Drug Administration.

Sample Methods Center Trial Master File Table of Contents

1.	Delegation log
2.	Ethics Committee approval letter(s)
3.	Feasibility questionnaire
4.	Clinical site initiation checklist
5.	Data management plan
6.	Site monitoring plan
7.	Data Safety and Monitoring Committee (DSMC) charter
8.	Adjudication Committee charter
9.	Executive Committee charter
10.	Steering Committee charter
11.	Study protocol
12.	Investigator's Brochure
13.	Investigational product accountability log
14.	Case report forms
15.	Clinical site manual
16.	Randomization plan
17.	Statistical analysis plan
18.	Adjudication study-specific procedure
19.	DSMB/DSMC study-specific procedure
20.	Notes to file
21.	Significant correspondence
Abbreviation: DSMB, Data Safety and Monitoring Board.	

Toolbox C

General Checklist for a Successful Ethics Submission

Please check with your specific ethics committee for local requirements. This is meant to be a sample of what is typically required.

Section	Information required
Administrative information	☐ Principal investigator's name and affiliation
	☐ Research team members' names and affiliations
Project summary	☐ Lay person statement written using grade 8 level English (or the language used by the review committee)
	☐ Avoid using technical terminology
Background information	☐ Brief description of the context and reasons why the research is needed
	☐ Study objectives and/or hypothesis
	☐ Include references
Methodology	☐ Brief description of methodology so the committee can judge the scientific validity
	☐ Sample size target
	☐ Brief statistical analysis plan
Benefits and harms/safety	☐ Description of possible harms and how they will be mitigated
	☐ Brief description of possible benefits to participants
	☐ If your research involves using an experimental medical product, all available safety data should be provided
Recruitment process	☐ A detailed description of the recruitment process including who, when, where, and how participants will be approached
Informed consent	☐ Details of exactly how the consent process will be undertaken
	☐ An informed consent form written in the primary language of the participants (or multiple languages if required)
	☐ The language used should be written in a way that is appropriate for the participants (generally grade 8 level language)
Data collection and management	☐ Description of what information will be collected from participants and how this will be done
	☐ Details of how the data will be protected and stored
	☐ Plan to protect confidentiality/privacy of participants
Statement of remuneration	☐ Detail whether participants will receive remuneration (e.g., cash, gift cards, parking passes, nonmonetary gifts)
	☐ If applicable, insurance coverage for participants should be detailed
Disclosures	☐ All potential and actual conflicts of interest should be detailed
	☐ If there are conflicts, outline a plan to minimize them
	☐ You may be required to disclose whether a previous decision was made regarding this clinical study (e.g., another site's ethics committee)

(Continued)

Section	Information required
Budget	☐ If funded, provide a statement outlining the budget used to conduct this research and exact details of how the money will be spent
Signatures	☐ Principal investigator and/or local principal investigator
	☐ Sometimes further signatures are needed such as those of clinic managers, specific hospital departments, and/or university department chairs
Attachments	☐ A full protocol is typically required to be submitted
	☐ Full informed consent form, if applicable
	☐ Investigator's brochure, for regulated studies
	☐ Data collection forms, case report forms, or questionnaires
	☐ Recruitment materials/advertisements, if applicable

Toolbox D

Checklist of Actions during Study Start-Up

Study start-up checklist		
Identify and contact sites	Identify suitable sites/local investigators	☐
	Contact suitable sites	☐
	Confidentiality agreement required?	☐
Feasibility assessment	Feasibility questionnaire	☐
	Site visit/contact	☐
Clinical trial agreement negotiation	Setting legal terms and conditions	☐
	Negotiating budget and intellectual property	☐
Regulatory approval	Provide necessary documents from central approval	☐
	Collect documents for local approval	☐
Site initiation visit	Training site staff	☐
	Review protocol and study procedures	☐
	Check required documents	☐
	Pharmacy initiation visit	☐
Site activation	Initiate patient recruitment	☐
	Continue monitoring of patient enrolment	☐

Toolbox E

Sample Information Sheet/Consent Form for Medical Research

A Consent Form should contain the elements identified on the following pages to ensure that research participants have sufficient information to make a fully informed and free decision about whether to participate in the research study.

This form should be used as a guideline and may not be applicable to all types of studies.

- Use of 12-point font is recommended. Larger type may be necessary for elderly or visually compromised participants. Avoid italics or ornate type.
- Use of questions or headings to highlight the various elements is strongly recommended.
- Use of bullets, tables, and charts is also recommended.
- Use of "white space" makes the document easier to read.
- Include a page header or footer, numbering on each page with the protocol reference, version number and/or date, the version number and/or date of the Consent Form; and include a space for subject initials on each page of the consent.
- If the investigators propose to include their own patients in a study, the invitation to participate should be made and the informed consent should be obtained by persons on whom the participants have no dependency.

If the clinical trial is _not_ registered, please include this statement in the information sheet/consent form:

"This clinical trial will not be registered with a recognized, publicly-accessible clinical trial registry and therefore it is unlikely the study results will be published by established medical journals."

Use Appropriate Letterhead

Participant Information Sheet

Title of Study:
Locally Responsible Investigator and Principal Investigator, Department/Hospital/Institution:
Coinvestigator(s), Department/Hospital/Institution:
Sponsor: for example, pharmaceutical company, granting agency, university, or hospital.

You are being invited to participate in a research study conducted by Dr. ... because you have ... *[insert the participant's condition or circumstance that makes them eligible for the study. If the study is recruiting healthy volunteers, indicate: ... because you are a healthy individual. If this is a student project, indicate:* "This is a student research project conducted under the supervision of Dr. ... *[insert name].* The study will help the student learn more about the topic area and develop skills in research design, collection and analysis of data, and writing a research paper.

In order to decide whether or not you want to be a part of this research study, you should understand what is involved and the potential risks and benefits. This form gives detailed information about the research study, which will be discussed with you. Once you understand the study, you will be asked to sign this form if you wish to participate. Please take your time to make your decision. Feel free to discuss it with your friends and family, or your family physician.

.... *[insert name of Hospital or Institution]* and the Investigator Dr. ... *[insert Locally Responsible Investigator's name]* are under contract with the Sponsor of this study and are receiving compensation to cover the costs of conducting the study.

Describe any conflict of interest that exists or may appear to exist as it relates to any of the investigators and this study. A conflict of interest exists if there is potential benefit to the investigator(s) beyond the professional benefit from academic achievement or presentation of the results.

(Continued)

Why is this research being done?
Explain in layman's terms the background for the study.

What is the purpose of this study?
Explain in layman's terms the purpose of the study.

What will my responsibilities be if i take part in the study?
If you volunteer to participate in this study, we will ask you to do the following things:

Describe the procedures chronologically using simple language, short sentences, and short paragraphs. The use of subheadings helps organize this section and increases readability. Medical and scientific terms should be defined and explained. The more invasive the procedures, the more detail should be provided.

Identify all procedures that are experimental.

Explain the following to the participant:
- *What will happen at each visit including the specifics of any procedures, tests, questionnaires, interviews.*
- *Include screening visits.*
- *What is being done as part of the research versus what is being done as part of standard care.*
- *The frequency of procedures, tests, etc.*
- *The location of procedures, tests, etc.*
- *How the participant will be assigned to study groups, with a lay description of the randomization process, if applicable, and explanation of the chances of being assigned to any group.*

For example: The participants in the study will be assigned at random, that is, by a method of chance (like a flip of a coin), to one of two groups. You will have a [specify one in two, three in four, etc.] chance of being in the group that receives Drug A and [specify one in two, three in four, etc.] chance of being in the group that receives Drug B. Neither you nor your study doctor will know which group you are in. However, in the case of an emergency, the code can be broken.

- *The length of time for each visit.*
- *The total time commitment for participation, i.e., number of weeks/months.*
- *The drugs that will be administered and their therapeutic action in lay terms [e.g., "hydrochlorothiazide," which is a "water pill" designed to help get rid of excess fluid in your body].*
- *The need for "washout" of any drugs the patient is currently taking and the potential risks/discomforts of this.*
- *Any follow-up contacts by phone or mail and what is involved, how long each will take.*

If the trial involves a placebo rather than an active comparator, describe what a placebo is and indicate what the chance is of receiving the placebo versus the active drug(s). Indicate whether the patient's condition may fail to improve or worsen on placebo.

For example: This is a placebo-controlled study. That means you will be assigned by chance (like a flip of a coin) to a group of people who receive either (Drug A) or a placebo. A placebo is an inactive sub-stance, like a sugar pill. In this study, you have a 50% chance of receiving the placebo and a 50% chance of receiving Drug A. If you receive placebo, it is possible that your ... [specify condition] may not improve or may worsen. Your condition will be carefully monitored. If it does worsen, the study doctor will ... [specify action to be taken].

Provide details about the collection of specimens or human tissues. Indicate the following:

- *What the sample(s) are to be used for, for example, for the current study only, or for future unknown research (banking).*
- *Where and how the samples will be stored.*
- *Whether the participant will receive the results of the testing.*
- *Whether the sample(s) will be linked to the participant.*
- *How long they will be stored.*
- *How they will be disposed of.*
- *Describe the possibility for commercialization of research findings and what the subject may expect in way of compensation.*

(Continued)

For example: The sample(s) will be discarded or destroyed once they have been used for the purposes described above. The samples will be used for research and such use may result in inventions or discoveries that create new products or diagnostic or therapeutic agents. In some instances, these inventions and discoveries may be of potential commercial value and may be patented and licensed by the researchers/ sponsor. You will not receive any money or other benefits derived from any commercial or other products that may be developed from use of the specimens.

what are the possible risks and discomforts?

Describe any reasonably foreseeable risks, harms, discomforts, inconveniences (including, e.g., physical, psychological, emotional, financial, and social) to the participant (and, when applicable, to an embryo, fetus, or nursing infant) and how these will be managed.

- *If there are risks to participation, describe them for each procedure and drug.*
- *Group the risks into those that are frequent, occasional, or rare and give the frequencies for each of these groups (e.g., "rare": <1 in 1,000 patients).*
- *List all side effects, no matter how rare, that are life-threatening or potentially life altering (e.g., visual loss, anaphylaxis, paralysis, aplastic anemia).*
- *Explain the ramifications of some risks (e.g., what is the importance to the participant if liver enzyme tests indicate an abnormality?).*
- *Studies that present real and potential risks of fetal or reproductive harm should have a description of this risk. If reproductive risk exists, participants should be advised not to become pregnant (or father a baby) while in this study.*

For studies affiliated with [Catholic Hospital], insert either of the following pregnancy clauses:

Pregnancy and this study are not compatible. Due to the risk of potential risk to the fetus, women who are pregnant, or planning to become pregnant, are therefore excluded from this study. Women of child-bearing potential are advised to discuss appropriate family planning with their doctor if they are interested in enrolling in this study. Unless you have had a hysterectomy, a tubal ligation, are postmenopausal, or not at risk of pregnancy, you are advised to practice an appropriate method of family planning.

Or

It is not known whether xxx (name of drug) may cause side effects to pregnant women, to an unborn child (an embryo or a fetus), or to children of breastfeeding women. Because of these unknown risks, if you are pregnant or trying to become pregnant, you cannot enter the study. If you are breastfeeding a child, you cannot enter the study.

If you can have children, you are required to have a negative pregnancy test result before enrolling in the study. You are a woman who can have children if:

- You have not completed menopause.
- You have not had a hysterectomy.
- You have not had surgery to become sterile (i.e., a tubal ligation).
- Your sexual partner has not had surgery to become sterile (i.e., a vasectomy).

If you are sexually active and can have children, you must not become pregnant during the time you are participating in the study, and for a period of xx months after the study.

If you miss a menstrual period or think you might be pregnant during the study, you must tell the study doctor immediately.

If you become pregnant during the study or within xx days from your last dose of the study drug, the study doctor will ask to follow the outcome of your pregnancy and the condition of your newborn.

Men who are participating in this study also need to understand the danger of taking the study drug whose effects on a fetus are unknown. Female partners of male participants cannot be pregnant during the time their male partner is participating in the study, and for xx days after the last dose of the study drug. Please speak to a doctor to discuss which family planning method is best suited for you.

- *If the risk of fetal harm is not known, then indicate it is not known.*
- *If there are no risks associated with the research, then indicate no known risks.*
- *Wherever possible, present risks in a table format to enhance participant comprehension.*

(Continued)

In addition to the risks listed above, you may experience a previously unknown risk or side effect *[not necessary for no-risk or minimal-risk studies]*.

If you choose to take part in this study, you will be told about any new information that might affect your willingness to continue to participate in this research.

How many people will be in this study?
Indicate the numbers locally and the total number for a multisite study.

What are the possible benefits for me and/or for society?
Describe benefits to participants expected from the research. If the participant will not benefit personally from participation, clearly state this fact.

For example: We cannot promise any personal benefits to you from your participation in this study. However, possible benefits include ... [specify benefits]. Your participation may help other people with ... [specify, e.g., cancer] in the future. If there is likely to be no medical benefit to participation, then state: There are no medical benefits to you from your taking part in this study.

If I do not want to take part in the study, are there other choices?
It is important for you to know that you can choose not to take part in the study. There are other choices such as ... [specify choices]. Your study doctor will discuss these with you.
Or
An alternative to the procedures described above is not to participate in the study and continue on just as you do now. Your study doctor will discuss this alternative with you.

Describe how you would care for a participant who is not part of this research study or describe the options that you would normally offer a person who did not participate in the study. If applicable, include supportive care as an option.

If the study involves patients, the following statement must be added at the end of this section: Choosing not to participate in this study will in no way affect your care or treatment.

What information will be kept private?
Your data will not be shared with anyone except with your consent or as required by law. All personal information such as your name, address, phone number, OHIP number, and family physician's name will be removed from the data and will be replaced with a number. A list linking the number with your name will be kept in a secure place, separate from your file. The data, with identifying information removed, will be securely stored in a locked office in the research laboratory.

For the purposes of ensuring the proper monitoring of the research study, it is possible that a member of the Hamilton Integrated Research Ethics Board, a Health Canada representative *[include Health Canada if this is a clinical trial involving a drug, device, or natural health product regulated by Health Canada]* or ... *[list the designated institutions where relevant, such as the U.S. Food and Drug Administration]*, and representatives of ... *[name of the sponsoring company if relevant]* may consult your research data and medical records. However, no records that identify you by name or initials will be allowed to leave the hospital. By signing this consent form, you or your legally acceptable representative authorizes such access.

If information will be released to any other party for any reason, state the person/agency to whom the information will be furnished, the nature of the information, and the purpose of the disclosure.

In order to permit access to a participant's health records if they are admitted to another hospital during the study, or if they die during their participation, it is recommended that you include the following wording:

If you are admitted to another hospital for any reason or die from natural or other causes while participating in this study, your medical records will be requested in order to collect information relevant to your study participation. By signing this Consent Form, you are allowing such access.

If the results of the study are published, your name will not be used and no information that discloses your identity will be released or published without your specific consent to the disclosure. However, it is important to note that this original signed consent form and the data that follow may be included in your health record.

(Continued)

If activities are to be audio- or videotaped or digitally recorded, describe the participant's right to review/edit the tapes, who will have access, if they will be used for educational purposes, and when they will be erased. For example: video tapes will be viewed only by members of the research team and they will be destroyed after .... *[specify number of]* years.

Can participation in the study end early?

If you volunteer to be in this study, you may withdraw at any time and this will in no way affect the quality of care you receive at this institution. *Indicate whether the participant has the option of removing data and/or tissue already collected. For example:* You have the option of removing your data from the study. You may also refuse to answer any questions you do not want to answer and still remain in the study. The investigator may withdraw you from this research if circumstances arise that warrant doing so.

Will I be paid to participate in this study?

If you agree to take part, we will reimburse you $_____ (indicate amount) for study-related expenses. In the event that you cannot complete the requirements of the study, you will receive a prorated amount at the rate of $X/h/session. *Indicate if the amount is prorated for study visit completion.*

will there be any costs?

Tell participants what charges they or their insurance will have to pay. Your participation in this research project may involve additional costs to you for *[indicate source of cost, e.g., drugs, device, diagnostic procedure, therapeutic procedure].* Your health care insurance probably will not pay for all of these additional costs. *Also, tell participants what they may expect to receive for free.* For example: Your participation in this research project will not involve any additional costs to you or your health care insurer.

What happens if I have a research-related injury?

If you are injured as a direct result of taking part in this study, all necessary medical treatment will be made available to you at no cost. Financial compensation for such things as lost wages, disability, or discomfort due to this type of injury is not routinely available. However, if you sign this consent form, it does not mean that you waive any legal rights you may have under the law, nor does it mean that you are releasing the investigator(s), institution(s), and/or sponsor(s) from their legal and professional responsibilities. *There should be no exculpatory language whereby the participant waives, or appears to waive, any of their legal rights, including any release of the sponsor, institution, or its agents from liability for negligence.*

If I have any questions or problems, whom can I call?

If you have any questions about the research now or later, or if you think you have a research-related injury, please contact... *For greater than minimal risk, include night/emergency phone numbers.*

Consent Statement

- *Not all of the following signature lines are required.*
- *Please select the signature lines that are appropriate for your study.*

Participant: *(required for participants capable of consent)*

I have read the preceding information thoroughly. I have had an opportunity to ask questions and all of my questions have been answered to my satisfaction. I agree to participate in this study. I understand that I will receive a signed copy of this form.

Name	Signature	Date

Person obtaining consent: *(required for all studies)*

(Continued)

I have discussed this study in detail with the participant. I believe the participant understands what is involved in this study.

Name, role in study	Signature	Date

Investigator: *(required for studies that include a medical act)*
In my judgment, this participant has the capacity to give consent, and has done so voluntarily.

Name, MD	Signature	Date

Legally authorized representative: *(required if child is under age 16 or participant is incapable of consent)*
I have read the preceding information thoroughly. I have had an opportunity to ask questions and all of my questions have been answered to my satisfaction. I understand that I will receive a signed copy of this form.
I give my permission for _____to participate in this study.

Name, relationship to participant	Signature	Date

Witness: *(required if participants are unable to read, or if translation is necessary)*
I was present when the information in this form was explained and discussed with the participant. I believe the participant understands what is involved in this study.

Name, MD	Signature	Date

• *Include the following statement at the end of the signature page*

This study has been reviewed by the *ethics committee*. The *ethics committee* is responsible for ensuring that participants are informed of the risks associated with the research and that participants are free to decide if participation is right for them. If you have any questions about your rights as a research participant, please call *contact information*.

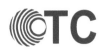

Toolbox F1

Patient Contact Form

(Please do not send this form to sponsor; it must remain at the site.)

A.　Primary contact information for patient

1. Name _____
2. Address _____
3. Postal/zip code + city _____
4. Phone number _____
5. Mobile phone number _____
6. E-mail _____

B.　Alternate contact information for patient (optional)

1. Name _____
2. Relation to patient _____
3. Address _____
4. Postal/zip code + city _____
5. Phone number _____
6. Mobile phone number _____
7. E-mail _____

C.　General practitioner contact information

1. Name _____
2. Address _____
3. Postal/zip code + city _____
4. Phone number _____
5. E-mail _____

Toolbox F2

Patient Screening Form

A. Inclusion criteria

		Yes	No
1.	Age 50 y or older	☐	☐
2.	Fracture of the femoral neck, confirmed with anteroposterior and lateral hip radiographs, CT, or MRI	☐	☐
3.	... (list all other inclusion criteria)	☐	☐

		N.A.		
4.	Signed informed consent by patient (or proxy)	☐	☐	☐

B. Exclusion criteria

		Yes	No
1.	Patient is not eligible for treatment A or B	☐	☐
2.	... (list all other exclusion criteria)	☐	☐
3.	Likely problems, in the judgment of the investigators, with maintaining follow-up (e.g., patients have no fixed address)	☐	☐
4.	Patient is enrolled in another ongoing drug or surgical intervention study	☐	☐

C. Patient status

☐ Included: Date of randomization: ☐☐ - ☐☐☐ - ☐☐☐☐ (dd-mmm-yyyy)

        Allocated to: ☐ Treatment A

                          ☐ Treatment B

☐ Excluded

☐ Missed (i.e., patient was eligible, but was not enrolled due to error)

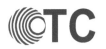

Toolbox F3

Baseline Data and Patient Characteristics
Complete the following questions for all included patients after randomization.

1. **Date of birth** ☐☐ - ☐☐☐ - ☐☐☐☐
   dd - mmm - yyyy

2. **Gender at birth**
   ☐ Male
   ☐ Female

3. **Height** ☐☐☐.☐ ☐ inch
   ☐ cm

4. **Weight** ☐☐☐.☐ ☐ lb
   ☐ kg

5. **ASA class**
   ☐ ASA 1
   ☐ ASA 2
   ☐ ASA 3
   ☐ ASA 4
   ☐ ASA 5

6. **Smoking history**
   ☐ Smokes currently   Since age: ☐☐ (y)
   ☐ Quit smoking   Age began: ☐☐ (y)
   ☐ Never smoked   Age stopped: ☐☐ (y)

7. **Medication use before trauma**
   (check all that apply)
   ☐ No, patient is not taking any of the following:
   ☐ NSAIDs
   ☐ Analgesic opioid
   ☐ Anti-hypertension medications
   ☐ General cardiac medications
   ☐ Pulmonary (respiratory system) medications
   ☐ Osteoporosis medications

8. **Independence in activities of daily living before trauma**
   ☐ Yes
   ☐ No: ☐ Patient needed help with bathing or showering
   ☐ Patient needed help with getting (un)dressed
   ☐ Patient needed help with toileting
   ☐ Patient needed help with transfer from bed to chair
   ☐ Patient needed help with eating
   ☐ Patient used incontinence materials

9. **Comments** (optional) _____
   _____
   _____

Abbreviations: ASA, American Society of Anesthesiologists; NSAIDs, nonsteroidal anti-inflammatory drugs.

Toolbox F4

Medication Record

1. **Medication use** ☐ None

2. **Drug name** **Date started** **Date stopped** **Continues**

(Generic preferred, but use brand name for combination)

	dd	mmm	yyyy	dd	mmm	yyyy	
_____	☐☐ -	☐☐☐ -	☐☐☐☐	☐☐ -	☐☐☐ -	☐☐☐☐	☐
_____	☐☐ -	☐☐☐ -	☐☐☐☐	☐☐ -	☐☐☐ -	☐☐☐☐	☐
_____	☐☐ -	☐☐☐ -	☐☐☐☐	☐☐ -	☐☐☐ -	☐☐☐☐	☐
_____	☐☐ -	☐☐☐ -	☐☐☐☐	☐☐ -	☐☐☐ -	☐☐☐☐	☐
_____	☐☐ -	☐☐☐ -	☐☐☐☐	☐☐ -	☐☐☐ -	☐☐☐☐	☐
_____	☐☐ -	☐☐☐ -	☐☐☐☐	☐☐ -	☐☐☐ -	☐☐☐☐	☐
_____	☐☐ -	☐☐☐ -	☐☐☐☐	☐☐ -	☐☐☐ -	☐☐☐☐	☐
_____	☐☐ -	☐☐☐ -	☐☐☐☐	☐☐ -	☐☐☐ -	☐☐☐☐	☐
_____	☐☐ -	☐☐☐ -	☐☐☐☐	☐☐ -	☐☐☐ -	☐☐☐☐	☐
_____	☐☐ -	☐☐☐ -	☐☐☐☐	☐☐ -	☐☐☐ -	☐☐☐☐	☐
_____	☐☐ -	☐☐☐ -	☐☐☐☐	☐☐ -	☐☐☐ -	☐☐☐☐	☐

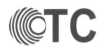
Toolbox F5

Trauma, Injury, and Fracture Details

1. **Date and time of trauma**

   ☐☐ - ☐☐☐ - ☐☐☐☐ ☐☐:☐☐
   dd   mmm   yyyy   hh   mm

2. **Date and time of emergency department presentation**

   ☐☐ - ☐☐☐ - ☐☐☐☐ ☐☐:☐☐
   dd   mmm   yyyy   hh   mm

3. **Date and time of hospital admission**

   ☐☐ - ☐☐☐ - ☐☐☐☐ ☐☐:☐☐
   dd   mmm   yyyy   hh   mm

4. **Mechanism of injury**

   ☐ Fall
   ☐ Spontaneous (stress) fracture
   ☐ Other, specify: _____

5. **Fractured side**

   ☐ Left
   ☐ Right

6. **Previous surgeries to the affected hip**

   ☐ Yes, (specify) _____
   ☐ No

7. **Additional injuries**

   ☐ No (you may skip question 8)
   ☐ Yes

8. **If yes, specify additional injuries** (check all that apply, and specify injures as applicable)

   ☐ Lower extremity (ipsilateral):
   ☐ Lower extremity (contralateral): _____
   ☐ Upper extremity: _____
   ☐ Head: _____
   ☐ Face: _____
   ☐ Neck: _____
   ☐ Thorax: _____
   ☐ Abdomen: _____
   ☐ Pelvis: _____
   ☐ Spine: _____

9. **Garden classification**

   ☐ Undisplaced   ☐ Garden I
                       ☐ Garden II
   ☐ Displaced   ☐ Garden III
                       ☐ Garden IV

10. **Pauwels classification**

    ☐ Pauwels I
    ☐ Pauwels II
    ☐ Pauwels III

Toolbox F6

Vital Signs at Hospital Presentation
(List the first recording upon presentation to the emergency department.)

1. **Was the examination performed?** ☐ Yes (complete below)
☐ No, specify why: _____

2. **Date and time of measurement** ☐☐ - ☐☐☐ - ☐☐☐☐ ☐☐:☐☐
dd   mmm   yyyy   hh   mm

3. **Heart rate** ☐☐☐ (beats per min)

4. **Respiratory rate** ☐☐☐ (resp. per min)

5. **Temperature** ☐☐☐.☐   °C
°F

6. **Blood pressure (mean of 3 readings;** Systolic: ☐☐☐ (mm Hg)
patient in sitting position for 5 min) Diastolic: ☐☐☐ (mm Hg)

7. **Comments (optional)** _____
_____
_____

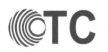

Toolbox F7

Hospital Discharge Form

1. **Date of hospital discharge**
   □□ - □□□ - □□□□
   dd   mmm   yyyy

2. **Discharge destination**
   ☐ Home
   ☐ Elderly care facility
   ☐ Skilled nursing facility
   ☐ Rehabilitation facility
   ☐ Transferred to other hospital
   ☐ Other, specify: _____

3. **Weight-bearing status at discharge**
   ☐ Non–weight bearing
   ☐ Partial weight bearing
   ☐ Full weight bearing

4. **Aid(s) use at discharge (check all that apply)**
   ☐ Patient is bedridden
   ☐ Wheelchair
   ☐ Two crutches
   ☐ One crutch
   ☐ Cane
   ☐ Other, specify: _____
   ☐ None; patient is ambulatory

5. **Comments (optional)**
   _____
   _____
   _____

Toolbox F8

Follow-Up Form

(This form should be completed at each follow-up visit.)

1.	**Follow-up number**	☐ 1 wk	☐ 3 mo
		☐ 2 wk	☐ 6 mo
		☐ 6 wk	☐ 12 mo

2. **Date of follow-up** ☐☐ - ☐☐☐ - ☐☐☐☐
 dd   mmm   yyyy

3. **For EACH of the following, indicate if** *the investigator* **has completed the forms**
☐ Follow-up form (this form)
☐ Katz index
☐ Adverse event form (if applicable)
☐ Revision surgery form (if applicable)
☐ Early withdrawal form (if applicable)

4. **For EACH questionnaire, indicate if patient has completed**
☐ Pain questionnaire (Visual Analog Scale)
☐ EQ-5D-5L
☐ SF-12
☐ Health consumption questionnaire

5. **Visit status**
☐ Complete: all required forms are completed
☐ Partially complete; specify why:
_____

6. **Patient's living status at follow-up**
☐ Home
☐ Elderly care facility
☐ Skilled nursing facility
☐ Rehabilitation facility
☐ Hospitalized
☐ Other, specify: _____

7. **Weight bearing status at follow-up**
☐ Non–weight bearing
☐ Partial weight bearing
☐ Full weight bearing

8. **Aid(s) use at follow-up (check all that apply)**
☐ Patient is bedridden
☐ Wheelchair
☐ Two crutches
☐ One crutch
☐ Cane
☐ Walker
☐ Other, specify: _____
☐ None; patient is ambulatory

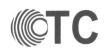

Follow-Up Form
(This form should be completed at each follow-up visit)

9. **Were X-rays taken at this follow-up?**
   - ☐ Yes
   - ☐ No

   (Please complete X-ray evaluation form)
   Specify why: _____

10. **Has patient visited the ED for their hip fracture since last follow-up?**
    - ☐ No
    - ☐ Yes

    Patient visited the ED ☐☐ times
    Specify why: _____

11. **Has patient had any adverse events (AEs) or complications since last follow-up?**
    - ☐ No
    - ☐ Yes,

    Patient had ☐☐ (number) of AEs
    (please complete an adverse event form for each event)

12. **Has patient had any revision surgeries since last follow-up?**
    - ☐ No
    - ☐ Yes

    Patient had ☐☐ (number) of surgeries
    (please complete a revision surgery form for each intervention)

13. **Comments (optional)**
    _____
    _____
    _____

Toolbox F9

Revision Surgery Form

1. **Date of revision surgery**
☐☐ - ☐☐☐ - ☐☐☐☐
dd   mmm   yyyy

2. **Specify procedure
(NB: complete a new form for
EACH revision surgery)**
☐ Soft-tissue procedure, please specify:
_____
☐ Supplemental osteosynthesis material, please
     specify: _____
☐ Implant removal
☐ Implant exchange, please specify:

_____

☐ Other, please specify:

_____

3. **Indication for surgery**
☐ Hip dislocation
☐ Wound closure
☐ Superficial infection
☐ Deep infection
☐ Malpositioned osteosynthesis material
☐ Implant failure:
     ☐ Loosening
     ☐ Breakage
     ☐ Other, please specify:

     _____

☐ Periprosthetic femur fracture
☐ Avascular necrosis
☐ Painful hardware
☐ Nonunion
☐ Other, please specify:

_____

4. **Was patient (re)admitted to
hospital for this procedure?**
☐ Yes (complete questions 5 and 6)
☐ No
☐ Not applicable; procedure occurred during initial
     hospitalization
☐ Not applicable; procedure occurred during hospi-
     talization for another problem

5. **Hospital admission date**
☐☐ - ☐☐☐ - ☐☐☐☐
6. **Hospital discharge date**
☐☐ - ☐☐☐ - ☐☐☐☐
dd   mmm   yyyy

7. **Comments (optional)**
_____
_____
_____

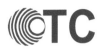

Toolbox F10

Adverse Event Form

1. **Date of diagnosis**

☐☐ - ☐☐☐ - ☐☐☐☐
dd   mmm   yyyy

2. **Specify adverse event (NB: complete a new form for EACH adverse event)**

☐ Superficial infection
☐ Deep infection
☐ Sepsis
☐ Acute respiratory distress syndrome
☐ Multiorgan failure
☐ Deep vein thrombosis
☐ Avascular necrosis
☐ Pulmonary embolism
☐ Pneumonia
☐ Hardware failure
☐ Delayed union
☐ Nonunion
☐ Death (please complete early withdrawal form)
☐ Other, please specify:

_____

3. **Was patient (re)admitted to hospital for this adverse event?**

☐ Yes (complete questions 4 and 5)
☐ No
☐ Not applicable; procedure occurred during initial hospitalization
☐ Not applicable, procedure occurred during hospitalization for another problem

4. **Hospital admission date**

☐☐ - ☐☐☐ - ☐☐☐☐
dd   mmm   yyyy

5. **Hospital discharge date**

☐☐ - ☐☐☐ - ☐☐☐☐
dd   mmm   yyyy

6. **Relation to treatment arm, according to the attending physician**

☐ Related
☐ Probably related
☐ Possibly related
☐ Not related

7. **Outcome of adverse event**

☐ Resolved without subsequent impairment
☐ Resoled with subsequent impairment
☐ Ongoing (please update form when resolved)
☐ Fatal (please complete early withdrawal form)

8. **Date resolved**

☐☐ - ☐☐☐ - ☐☐☐☐   ☐ Not resolved
dd   mmm   yyyy

9. **Comments (optional)**

_____

Toolbox F11

Early Withdrawal Form

1. **Date of early withdrawal from this study**

☐☐ - ☐☐☐ - ☐☐☐☐
dd   mmm   yyyy

2. **Reason for withdrawal**

☐ Death (please complete Adverse Event form)
☐ Unable to locate patient or proxy
☐ Patient withdrew consent
☐ Other, please specify:

_____

3. **Date of last hospital visit**

☐☐ - ☐☐☐ - ☐☐☐☐
dd   mmm   yyyy

4. **Has patient visited the hospital since last follow-up?**

☐ No (form is complete)
☐ Yes (please complete questions below)

5. **Patient's living status at last hospital visit**

☐ Home
☐ Elderly care facility
☐ Skilled nursing facility
☐ Rehabilitation facility
☐ Hospitalized
☐ Other, specify: _____
☐ Not documented

6. **Weight-bearing status at last hospital visit**

☐ Non–weight bearing
☐ Partial weight bearing
☐ Full weight bearing
☐ Not documented

7. **Aid(s) use at last hospital visit (check all that apply)**

☐ Patient is bedridden
☐ Wheelchair
☐ Two crutches
☐ One crutch
☐ Cane
☐ Walker
☐ Other, specify: _____
☐ None; patient is ambulatory
☐ Not documented

8. **Were X-rays taken at the last hospital visit?**

☐ Yes   (Please complete X-ray evaluation form)
☐ No

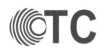

Early Withdrawal Form

9. **Has patient visited the emergency department (ED) for their hip fracture since last follow-up?**
    ☐ No Patient visited the ED ☐☐ times
    ☐ Yes Specify why: _____

10. **Has patient had any adverse events or complications since last follow-up?**
    ☐ No Patient had ☐☐ (number) of AEs
    ☐ Yes (Please complete an adverse event form for each event)

11. **Has patient had any revision surgeries since last follow-up?**
    ☐ No Patient had ☐☐ (number) of surgeries
    ☐ Yes (Please complete a revision surgery form for each intervention)

12. **Comments (optional)**
    _____
    _____
    _____

Toolbox G

Study Closeout Checklist

Study Name: _____

Investigator: _____ Sponsor: _____ Date of Closure: _____

Participants:
- All assessments, visits, and source documents complete
- Ongoing adverse events resolved or updated
- Have returned all study materials (study drug/device, equipment, diaries, etc.)
- Compensation paid
- Contact information updated
- Follow-up care arranged (if applicable)
- Notified of early termination (if applicable)

Data:
- All Case Report Forms (CRFs) complete
- Source data verification complete
- Queries resolved
- Investigator reviewed/signed CRFs
- CRFs submitted to sponsor or entered into database as applicable

Investigational Product:
- Inventory
- Disposition and accountability records complete and accurate
- Final disposition complete (e.g., returned or destroyed) and documented

Study Supplies:
- Advertising removed
- Study supplies returned, released, or destroyed (e.g., collection tubes, shipping boxes)
- Study equipment returned
- Unused CRFs, binders, labels, forms, etc., returned or destroyed

Study Samples:
- All biological samples processed
- All biological samples shipped to sponsor or study lab
- Unused samples destroyed or appropriately stored/labeled for future use

Investigator Site File:
- All logs completed (e.g., screening/enrollment log, site visit log, delegation of authority log)
- All signed informed consents filed
- All essential documents filed
- All correspondence filed

(Continued)

Ethics:
- All documents submitted (e.g., safety reports, protocol deviations)
- Ethics committee notified of study closure (final report)

Sponsor:
- Closeout meeting scheduled (key personnel available, room booked, medical records available)
- All previous issues resolved
- All documents submitted
- Questions to be addressed:
  - Participant follow-up
  - Length of record retention
  - Process for audit/inspection
- Sponsor final closeout letter received and filed

Site:
- All bills paid; payments received
- Account closed
- Staff and service providers notified of study closure
- Study files boxed and securely stored for retention period

Index

Note: Page numbers set in **bold** indicate headings.

A

additional study oversight committees **271**, **273**
– adjudication committee 273
– data safety monitoring committee/data safety monitoring boards 271
– steering committee 271
adjudication 275
adjudication committee **273**
adverse event 22, 67
adverse event form 309
Africa **159**
agreements, research contracts **161**, **162**, **163**
– parts of 162, 163
–– parties 162
–– preamble 163
– types of 161, 162
–– collaboration 161
–– grant funding 161
–– industry-initiated study agreement 162
–– industry involved in investigator initiated study 162
–– sites 162
analysis of survey data **90**
analytic approach 105
angel investor 129
anticipated research study expenses and justification 286
assessing and reporting adverse events **65**
– monitoring randomized controlled trial 65
attrition 212
audit committe **274**
autocratic leaders **2**

B

baseline data and patient characteristics 301

C

case report forms (CRF) **197**
– design guidelines 197
case report forms (CRF) **194**
center/sponsor study management **207**
– continual monitoring of study data and outcomes 207
center study design **71**
centralized monitoring **262**
centralized versus decentralized budgetary management **131**
CFR 313
chain-referral (snowball) sampling **96**
clauses **163**
– clause content determined by the study 163
– standard clauses 163
clinical trial agreement 175
clinical trial agreement negotiation **171**
closeout visit (COV) **261**
cluster sampling **86**
Code of Federal Regulations (CFR) 33
coercion 192
collaboration **161**
collaborative research focus group discussion guide **107**
communicating with staff **6**, **7**
– relationship/team building 7

– strategies 6
– with external staff 7
communication 13, **19**
– clinical study 13
– with ethics committee 19
– with sponsor 19
communication **39**
complexity of questions **84**
confidentiality agreement 175
contemporaneous 17
content of study **85**
– knowledge about question 85
– need to consult records 85
contingency budget **134**
COV 313
critical appraisal 56
cross-sectional survey **81**

D

data analysis **76**, **77**
– dealing with confounding 76
– handling missing outcome data 77
data collection, in clinical study **193**
data dissemination committe **274**
data management **17**
data management software **101**
data safety monitoring committee/data safety monitoring boards **271**
decision-making capacity 192
Declaration of Helsinki (1964) 110
delaying factors **174**
delegation of duties **14**
democratic leaders **3**
descriptive approach **100**
descriptive field notes 105

designing recruitment plan **45**
desirable characteristics, highly qualified research coordinator **29**, **30**, **31**, **32**, **33**, **34**
– clinical experience 34
– communication skills 29
– computer skills and project management 33
– financial or grant management 34
– interpersonal skills 30
– positive attitude 31
– professional skills 31
– regulatory and ethics guidelines 32
– team building skills 30
– writing skills 34
digital storytelling **229**
direct costs **132**
direct observation 97, 105
discussion guide 105
dissemination 106
– format 106
dissemination 275, 105
double-blind studies 117
duties **16**, **17**, **18**, **19**
– data management 17
– participant care 16, 17
–– conducting study visits 17
–– human participants, protection of 16
–– informed consent 16
–– participant advocate 16
– study planning, coordination, and administration 18, 19
–– communication with ethics committee 19
–– communication with sponsor 19
–– essential documents management 19
–– standard operating procedures 18
–– training 18

E

early withdrawal form
310
electronic case report
forms, datasheets
on **195**
electronic data capture
194
electronic data capture
system 201
emergency unblinding 67
emotional intelligence **3**
enthusiasm **40**
essential documents 22
essential documents
management **19**
ethics committee 22
ethics submissions 290,
**155, 156, 157, 158,
159**
– checklist for 290
– research ethics com-
mittee 155, 156, 157,
158, 159
– – Africa 156
– – Asia 156
– – Europe 156
– – multicenter human
studies and interna-
tional studies 159
– – North America 155
– – review process 157,
158, 159
– – – Asia 159
– – – Australia 158
– – – Europe 158
– – – financial benefits, cost,
and any conflicts of
interest 158
– – – informed consent
process 158
– – – North America 158
– – – risk and benefits 157
– – – safety and privacy of
participants/personal
health information
158
– – – scientific design 157
– – – study population
selection and
recruitment 158
ethnography **95**
evidence-based medicine
50, 51, 52, 53, 54, 55
– clinical research 55
– criticism of 54
– history of 50

– practical application
55
– – clinical example 55
– principles of 51, 52,
53
– – best available evi-
dence 51
– – – hierarchy of evidence
51
– – evaluate available
evidence 52, 53
– – – critical appraisal 52
– – – judicious and
reasonable 53
– – evidence in care for
individual patients 53
– – – shared decision-
making 53
evidence-based medicine
56
explanatory approach
100
external validity 212
extreme case sampling
106

F

face-to-face interviews **83**
facilitator 106
facilitator bias 103
feasibility **171**
feasibility questionnaire
175
financial lifecycle **131**
follow-up **203, 204, 205,
206, 207, 209, 210,
211, 212**
– important 203
– participants lost to
204
– practical application
212
– strategies to minimize
loss to 205, 206, 207,
209, 210, 211
– – center/sponsor study
management 207
– – – continual monitoring
of study data and
outcomes 207
– – local site study man-
agement to maintain
207, 209, 210
– – – communication
strategies between
participants and
research staff 210

– – – data monitoring and
quality control 209
– – – finding missing
participants 210
– – – reducing study
burden 209
– – – relationships 210
– – – subject selection and
informed consent
207
– – retention strategies
211
– – – participant incentives
211
– – study design strate-
gies 205, 206, 207
– – – conduct pilot study
206
– – – identifying primary
outcome early 205
– – – inclusion/exclusion
criteria 205
– – – reduction of study
burden 206
– – – sample size 206
– – – stakeholder engage-
ment 207
follow-up form 306
follow-up question 106
formative approach **100**
free open access medical
information **228**
funding phase **130**

G

good clinical practice
(GCP) and research
conduct **109, 110,
115, 117**
– checklist for clinical
research coordinators
117
– clinical studies 109
– globalization and
universal adoption
of 115
– guidelines 110
good manufacturing
practice 117
grant funding **161**
grant writing **120, 122,
123, 124, 125, 127,
128, 129**
– getting started 120,
122, 123, 124, 125,
127, 128

– – start early 120, 122,
123, 124, 125, 127,
128
– – – background 125
– – – budget 127
– – – compelling research
proposal 124
– – – follow instructions
123
– – – identify funding agencies and
resources 120
– – – investigators/research
team/environment
127
– – – methodology 125
– – – obtain ethics approval
124
– – – resubmissions 128
– – – review funding agency
specifications 122
– – – significance 125
– – – study summary 124
– – – supporting
documentation 128
– – – understand how grant
applications reviewed
122
– rejection 129
grounded theory **95**

H

Health Canada Division
5 33
Health Canada Guidance
Document 154
highly qualified research
coordinator **24, 25,
28, 29, 30, 31, 32, 33,
34, 35**
– decision to hire 24
– desirable character-
istics 29, 30, 31, 32,
33, 34
– – clinical experience 34
– – communication skills
29
– – computer skills and
project management
33
– – financial or grant
management 34
– – interpersonal skills 30
– – positive attitude 31
– – professional skills 31
– – regulatory and ethics
guidelines 32

-- team building skills 30
-- writing skills 34
- hiring process 25
- interview 28
- making decision 29
- newly hired research coordinator 35
- role of 24
homogenous sampling 106
hospital discharge form 305
hospital presentation, vital signs at 304
household drop-off survey 93
human participants, protection of **16**

I

identifying eligible patients **43**
indirect costs **132**
industry-initiated study agreement **162**
informed consent **39**
- form 39
informed consent 192, **16**, 47
intellectual property **166**
intention-to-treat analysis 67
internal audits **153**
internal validity 212
International Ethical Guidelines for Biomedical Research Involving Human Subjects (1982) 110
international research **276**, **277**, **278**, **279**
- consent process 277
- data collection process 278
- financial challenges 278
- language challenges 278
- legal considerations 279
- lower data quality 278
- motivating coinvestigators 277
- practical application 279
- shortage of research staff 278

- study planning phase 276
- timeline delay 278
- time zone difference 278
investigator 22
investigator site file 175, 22

K

key expenses **131**
knowledge dissemination **223**, **224**, **225**, **226**, **227**, **228**, **229**, **230**
- barriers to implementation 229, 230
-- audience 229
-- institutions 229
-- knowledge users 229
-- predatory journals 230
-- researchers 229
- developing effective dissemination plan 224
- maximizing uptake of 223
- nontraditional 227, 228, 229
-- academic social networks 227
-- blogs and podcasts 228
-- digital storytelling 229
-- free open access medical information 228
-- preprints 228
-- twitter 227
- practical application 230
-- traditional 225, 226, 227
-- conference presentation 225
-- departmental research day 226
-- institute website and newsletter 226
-- journal publication 225
-- policy brief 226
-- press release 226
-- research report 227

L

laissez-faire leadership **3**
leadership/management **2**, **3**, **4**, **5**, **6**, **7**, **8**, **10**
- communicating with staff 6, 7
-- relationship/team building 7
-- strategies 6
-- with external staff 7
- management competence 10
-- managing up and managing down 10
-- professional development 10
- mentoring new staff 4, 5, 6
-- mentoring 5
-- orientation 4
-- performance reviews 6
- motivational workplace 3, 4
-- emotional intelligence 3
-- mandates and vision 4
-- physical environment 4
- organization 8
-- documentation 8
-- time management 8
- styles 2, 3
-- autocratic leaders 2
-- democratic leaders 3
-- laissez-faire leadership 3
legally authorized representative **190**
legible 17
lengthy questions **85**
local site study management **207**, **209**, **210**
- communication strategies between participants and research staff 210
- data monitoring and quality control 209
- finding missing participants 210
- reducing study burden 209
- relationships 210
- subject selection and informed consent 207
longitudinal survey **82**

M

main question 106
management committee **267**, **268**, **269**, **270**
- additional team members 270
- co-investigators 268
- database managers 269
- financial analysts/business analysts 269
- research assistants 270
- study manager 269
- study monitors 270
- study principal investigator 267
- study statistician 270
management competence **10**
- managing up and managing down 10
- professional development 10
maximal variation sampling 106
medication record 302
mentoring new staff **4**, **5**, **6**
- mentoring 5
- orientation 4
- performance reviews 6
methods center 154
monitoring committe **274**
monitoring, in clinical study **258**, **259**, **260**, **261**, **262**, **264**, **265**, **266**
- after visit 266
- centralized 262
- closeout visit 261
- data and safety monitoring committee 265
- managing expectations 266
- qualifications 258
- reports 262
- responsibilities, extent, and nature of 258
- risk-based 264
- routine monitoring visits 260
- site initiation visit 260

- site selection visit 259
- visits 259
motivational workplace **3, 4**
- emotional intelligence 3
- mandates and vision 4
- physical environment 4
multicenter study design **71**

N

narrative approach 106
negotiating study budget **132**
nontraditional knowledge dissemination **227, 228, 229**
- academic social networks 227
- blogs and podcasts 228
- digital storytelling 229
- free open access medical information 228
- preprints 228
- twitter 227
Nuremberg Code (1947) 110

O

observational studies **68, 69, 70, 71, 72, 73, 74, 75, 76, 77, 79, 80**
- bias associated with 69
- data analysis 76, 77
-- dealing with confounding 76
-- handling missing outcome data 77
- data collection 75
- designing 70
- ethical considerations/ data handling 74
- keep staff informed and committed during study 76
- outcomes and other study parameters 73
- patient inclusion in prospective studies 76

- performing study 75
-- initiation phase 75
- practical application 79, 80
-- background 79
-- ethical considerations 80
-- patients 79
-- sample size 79
-- statistical analysis 80
-- study design 79
-- study objective 79
-- study outcomes and other parameters 79
-- treatment 79
- pros and cons of 69
- reporting 77
- retrospective or prospective study design 71
- single-center or multicenter study design 71
- statistical analysis plan 74
- study parameters 73
- study population 72
-- inclusion and exclusion criteria 72
-- sample size 72
- study procedure 74
- treatment and procedures 72
- types of 68, 69
-- case-control studies 68
-- case series 69
-- cohort studies 68
observer bias 103
obtaining informed consent **187, 188**
- elements of 188
- process 187
- voluntary consent 188
open-label study 67
opportunistic sampling 106

P

paper case report forms, datasheets on **195**
participant adherence **64**
participant advocate **16**
participant care **16, 17**
- conducting study visits 17

- human participants, protection of 16
- informed consent 16
- participant advocate 16
participant observation 106
patient contact form 299
patient-reported outcome measure 201
patient screening form 300
phenomenology **95**
phishing scams 36
pilot testing **89**
placebo 117
planning budget **131**
policy approach 106
population **84**
- access to potential participants/respondents 84
- geographic restrictions 84
- literacy level of respondents 84
pragmatic trials 117
premature study termination **136**
preplanning phase **130**
prescreening **178**
- phase 178
prescreening **178**
probes 106
problem-solving approach 106
prospective study design **71**
protocol adherence **173**
protocol development **37**
protocol deviation 22
publication clause **167**
purposive sampling **96**

Q

qualitative research **94, 95, 96, 97, 98, 99, 100, 101, 102, 103**
- advantages of 94
- ambiguities 102
- data analysis and interpretation 100, 101
-- data management software 101
-- qualitative data analysis approaches 100
--- descriptive approach 100

--- explanatory approach 100
--- formative approach 100
--- transformative approach 100
-- qualitative data coding 100
- data collection 97, 98, 99, 100
-- collecting initial demographic details 99
-- focus group 97
-- guide/interview script development 98
-- interview 97
-- interview/focus group question development 99
-- observation 97
-- obtaining adequate responses 99
-- transcription of interviews and focus groups 100
- designing and conducting the study 95
-- general study details 95
-- research objectives 95
-- research question 95
- frequency 103
- generalizability 102
- informed consent 102
- practical application 103
- protecting confidentiality 102
- reporting and disseminating study 102
-- authorship 102
-- publish 102
- sample size 96
- sampling 96
-- chain-referral (snowball) sampling 96
-- purposive sampling 96
-- quota sampling 96
- study methods 95
-- ethnography 95
-- grounded theory 95
-- phenomenology 95
- types of bias associated with 103

-- strategies for managing bias 103
- verses quantitative research 94
qualitative research **94**
query 22
question **84, 88**
- order 88
- screening 84
- wording 88
question bias 103
questionnaire 93
questionnaire layout **87**
questionnaires **82**
questions **86**
- types of 86
quota sampling **96**

R

random assignment (randomization) **60**
randomization 47, 67
randomized controlled trials **59, 60, 61, 62, 63, 64, 65**
- assessing and reporting adverse events 65
-- monitoring randomized controlled trial 65
- blinding 61
- outcome measurement 62
-- reliability and validity of 62
- participant adherence 64
- quality control and data collection 62
- random assignment (randomization) 60
- recruitment of study participants 63
-- tips for coordinators 63
- study design 59
- study population 59
random sampling **86**
- cluster sampling 86
- simple random sampling 86
- stratified sampling 86
recruitment **180, 186**
- checklist 186
- improve 180
- plan and contact methods 180

recruitment **178, 42**
recruitment plan 47
reflective field notes 106
regulatory approval 175
regulatory trials **237, 238, 239, 240, 241, 242, 243, 244**
- expedited reporting 243
- practical application 244
- regulation and international harmonization 237, 238, 239, 240, 241, 242
-- follow detailed protocol 240
-- good clinical practice 239
-- reporting and public disclosure of interventional clinical trial results 241
-- role of regulatory agency 237
-- safety reporting 242
-- standard clinical trials and regulatory trials 238
-- structure of regulatory trials 238
-- trial registration 240
- research coordinator's responsibilities 242
reliability, survey **90**
remote data entry **194**
remote data entry system 201
reporting bias 103
research budget **130, 131, 132, 134, 135, 136**
- ongoing monitoring of 135, 136
-- amending study budget 136
-- invoicing and payments 135
- planning and creating 130, 131, 132, 134, 135
-- associated with budgetary planning 135
-- centralized versus decentralized budgetary management 131
-- contingency budget 134
-- direct and indirect costs 132

-- financial lifecycle 131
-- funding phase 130
-- key expenses 131
-- negotiating study budget 132
-- planning budget 131
-- preplanning phase 130
research contracts **161, 162, 163, 165, 166, 167**
- agreements 161, 162, 163
-- parts of 162, 163
--- parties 162
--- preamble 163
-- types of 161, 162
--- collaboration 161
--- grant funding 161
--- industry-initiated study agreement 162
--- industry involved in investigator initiated study 162
--- sites 162
- clauses 163
-- clause content determined by the study 163
-- standard clauses 163
- intellectual property 166
- practical application 165
- publication clause 167
- signatories 165
- study budget 165
research coordinator **12, 13, 14, 16, 17, 18, 19, 20**
- delegation of duties 14
- duties 16, 17, 18, 19
-- data management 17
-- participant care 16, 17
--- conducting study visits 17
--- human participants, protection of 16
--- informed consent 16
--- participant advocate 16
-- study planning, coordination, and administration 18, 19
--- communication with ethics committee 19

--- communication with sponsor 19
--- essential documents management 19
--- standard operating procedures 18
--- training 18
- education and certification 13
- necessary 12
- practical application 20
research ethics committee **155, 156, 157, 158, 159**
- Africa 156
- Asia 156
- Europe 156
- multicenter human studies and international studies 159
- North America 155
- review process 157, 158, 159
-- Africa 159
-- Asia 159
-- Australia 158
-- Europe 158
-- financial benefits, cost, and any conflicts of interest 158
-- informed consent process 158
-- North America 158
-- risk and benefits 157
-- safety and privacy of participants/personal health information 158
-- scientific design 157
-- study population selection and recruitment 158
research finances **130, 131, 132, 134, 135, 136**
- ongoing monitoring of research budget 135, 136
-- amending study budget 136
-- invoicing and payments 135
- planning and creating research budget 130, 131, 132, 134, 135
-- associated with budgetary planning 135

-- centralized versus decentralized budgetary management 131
-- contingency budget 134
-- direct and indirect costs 132
-- financial lifecycle 131
-- funding phase 130
-- key expenses 131
-- negotiating study budget 132
-- planning budget 131
-- preplanning phase 130
- practical application 136
- study termination 136
-- premature study termination 136
research methods **82**, **83**
- face-to-face interviews 83
- questionnaires 82
- telephone interviews 83
research question **84**, **85**
- complexity of questions 84
- lengthy questions 85
- screening questions 84
- subject matter 84
research tool design **86**, **87**, **88**
- questionnaire layout 87
- question order 88
- question wording 88
- training interviewers 88
- types of questions 86
resources, survey **85**
- cost 85
- facilities 85
- personnel 85
retention 212
retention strategies **211**
- participant incentives 211
retrospective study design **71**
revision surgery form 308
risk-based monitoring **264**

S

sample site trial master file/investigator site file table of contents 288
sampling **86**, **96**, 103
- bias 103
- chain-referral (snowball) sampling 96
- nonrandom sampling 86
- purposive sampling 96
- quota sampling 96
- random sampling 86
-- cluster sampling 86
-- simple random sampling 86
-- stratified sampling 86
saturation 106
schedule of events 138
screening **182**, **185**, **186**, **84**
- checklist 186
- mechanism 182
- phase 185
- questions 84
severe adverse event 67
shared decision-making 56
signatories **165**
simple random sampling **86**
single study design **71**
site activation **173**
site audit **251**, **252**, **253**, **254**, **255**, **256**, **257**
- big picture 253
- documentation 253
- final audit meeting 255
- informal conversations in between audit events 255
- meetings and interviews with auditors 254, 255
-- audit interviews 254
-- daily briefings 255
-- start-up meeting 254
- monitoring and auditing, difference 251, 252
-- first line of defense: procedures 251
-- second line of defense: monitoring 252

-- third line of defense: auditing 252
- practical application 257
- report and corrective action/preventive action plan 256
site initiation visit **172**
soft skills 36
source documents 22
sponsor 154, 22
stakeholder engagement **207**
standard operating procedure 22
standard operating procedures **18**
statistical analysis plan **74**
steering committee **271**
stratified sampling **86**
study closeout checklist 312
study closure **214**, **215**, **216**, **217**, **219**
- closeout visit 216
- practical application 219
- process of 215, 216
-- closeout visit 215, 216
--- biological samples 215
--- data 215
--- investigational product 215
--- other parties 216
--- participants 215
--- reporting 215
--- trial master file/investigator site file 215
- reasons for 214
- record retention 217
- with ethics committee 217
-- administrative issues 217
-- final report to sponsor 217
study design strategies **205**, **206**, **207**
- conduct pilot study 206
- identifying primary outcome early 205
- inclusion/exclusion criteria 205
- reduction of study burden 206
- sample size 206

- stakeholder engagement 207
study planning, coordination, and administration **18**, **19**
- communication with ethics committee 19
- communication with sponsor 19
- essential documents management 19
- standard operating procedures 18
- training 18
study screening **178**
study start up 292, **170**, **171**, **172**, **173**, **174**
- checklist of actions 292
- delaying factors 174
- drug, device, or procedure 174
- guidelines for good clinical practice 174
- meeting recruitment goals 173
- phase 170, 171, 172, 173
-- clinical trial agreement negotiation 171
-- feasibility 171
-- identify and contact sites 170
-- regulatory and ethics approval 172
-- site activation 173
-- site initiation visit 172
- practical application 174
- protocol adherence 173
study termination **136**
- premature study termination 136
subject matter **84**
substitute decision maker 47
surveys 81, **82**, **83**, **84**, **85**, **86**, **87**, **88**, **89**, **90**, **91**
- analysis of survey data 90
- method 84, 85
-- bias issues 85
--- interviewer bias 85
---- respondent identity 85
--- social desirability 85
-- content of study 85

––– knowledge about question 85
––– need to consult records 85
–– population 84
––– access to potential participants/respondents 84
––– geographic restrictions 84
––– literacy level of respondents 84
–– research question 84, 85
––– complexity of questions 84
––– lengthy questions 85
––– screening questions 84
––– subject matter 84
–– resources 85
––– cost 85
––– facilities 85
––– personnel 85
– pilot testing 89
– practical application 91
– reliability and validity 90
– research, ethics of 90
– research methods 82, 83

–– face-to-face interviews 83
–– questionnaires 82
–– telephone interviews 83
– research tool design 86, 87, 88
–– questionnaire layout 87
–– question order 88
–– question wording 88
–– training interviewers 88
–– types of questions 86
– sample and sampling 86
–– nonrandom sampling 86
–– random sampling 86
––– cluster sampling 86
––– simple random sampling 86
––– stratified sampling 86
– study 81, 82
–– cross-sectional survey 81
–– longitudinal survey 82
– translation 89

T
target population **180**
TCPS2 313
telephone interviews **83**
TMF 313
traditional knowledge dissemination **225**, **226**, **227**
– conference presentation 225
– departmental research day 226
– institute website and newsletter 226
– journal publication 225
– policy brief 226
– press release 226
– research report 227
training **41**
training interviewers **88**
transformative approach **100**
translation **89**
trauma, injury, and fracture details 303
trial master file (TMF) **149**, **151**, **152**, **153**
– at methods center 151
– at participating clinical site 149

– clinical site manual 152
– documentation 149
– document control and 152
– internal audits 153
– practical application 153
Tri-Council Policy Statement 2 (TCPS2) 33
typical sampling 106

U
undue influence 192

V
validity, survey **90**
voluntary consent **188**

W
World Medical Association (WMA) 110
writing committee **274**